Orthodontically
Driven Corticotomy

Orthodontically Driven Corticotomy

Tissue Engineering to Enhance Orthodontic and Multidisciplinary Treatment

Edited by

Dr Federico Brugnami
Diplomate of The American Board of Periodontology
Private Practice Limited to Periodontics, Oral Implants and Adult Orthodontics,
Rome, Italy

Dr Alfonso Caiazzo
Visiting Clinical Assistant Professor
Department of Oral and Maxillofacial Surgery,
MGSDM Boston University
Private Practice, Centro Odontoiatrico Salernitano
Salerno, Italy

WILEY Blackwell

Library of Congress Cataloging-in-Publication Data

Orthodontically driven corticotomy : tissue engineering to enhance orthodontic and multidisciplinary treatment / edited by Dr. Federico Brugnami, Dr. Alfonso Caiazzo.
    p. ; cm.
  Includes bibliographical references and index.
  ISBN 978-1-118-48687-0 (cloth)
I. Brugnami, Federico, 1967– editor.   II. Caiazzo, Alfonso, 1968– editor.
[DNLM: 1. Orthodontics–methods.   2. Oral Surgical Procedures–methods.   3. Tissue Engineering.
4. Tooth Movement–methods. WU 400]
  RK521
  617.6′43–dc23

                                     2014016567

A catalogue record for this book is available from the British Library.

1   2015

Federico Brugnami

To Stefania and Giulia, my family and center of gravity, for all the time that writing this book has been taking away from them.

Alfonso Caiazzo

To Antonia, my love.

Contents

Dr Federico Brugnami
Diplomate of The American Board of
Periodontology
Private Practice Limited to Periodontics,
Oral Implants and Adult Orthodontics,
Rome, Italy
fbrugnami@gmail.com

Dr Alfonso Caiazzo
Visiting Clinical Assistant Professor
Department of Oral and Maxillofacial Surgery,
MGSDM Boston University
Private Practice, Centro Odontoiatrico
Salernitano
Salerno, Italy

Neal C. Murphy, DDS, MS
Department of Orthodontics, Case Western
Reserve University School of Dental Medicine,
Cleveland, OH, USA
Department of Periodontics, Case Western
Reserve University School of Dental Medicine,
Cleveland, OH, USA

M. Thomas Wilcko, DDS, MS
Department of Periodontics, Case Western
Reserve University School of Dental Medicine,
Cleveland, OH, USA

Nabil F. Bissada, DDS, MSD
Department of Periodontics, Case Western
Reserve University School of Dental Medicine,
Cleveland, OH, USA

Ze'ev Davidovitch, DMD, Cert Ortho
Department of Orthodontics, Case Western
Reserve University School of Dental Medicine,
Cleveland, OH, USA
Chairman Emeritus, Department of
Orthodontics, Harvard University
School of Dental Medicine, Cambridge,
MA, USA

Donald H. Enlow, PhD
Department of Orthodontics, Case Western
Reserve University School of Dental Medicine,
Cleveland, OH, USA

Jesse Dashe, MD
Department of Orthopedic Surgery,
Boston University Medical Center,
Boston, MA, USA

Donald J. Ferguson, DMD, MSD
European University College (Formerly
Nicolas & Asp University College), Dubai
Healthcare City, UAE

Pushkar Mehra, BDS, DMD
Department of Oral and Maxillofacial Surgery,
Boston University Henry M. Goldman School
of Dental Medicine, Boston, MA, USA

Hasnain Shinwari, BDS, DMD
Department of Oral and Maxillofacial Surgery,
Boston University Henry M. Goldman School
of Dental Medicine, Boston, MA, USA

Serge Dibart, DMD
Department of Periodontology and
Oral Biology, Boston University
Henry M. Goldman School of Dental
Medicine, Boston, MA, USA
Private Practice Limited to Periodontics and
Implant Dentistry, Boston, MA, USA

Elif I. Keser, DDS, PhD
Department of Orthodontics, Boston
University Henry M. Goldman of Dental
Medicine, Boston, MA, USA
Private Practice, Istanbul, Turkey

Birte Melsen
Department of Orthodontics, School of
Dentistry, Aarhus University, Aarhus,
Denmark

Cesare Luzi, DDS, MSc
Department of Orthodontics, School of
Dentistry, Aarhus University, Aarhus,
Denmark
University of Ferrara, Ferrara, Italy
Private Practice Limited to Orthodontics,
Rome, Italy

**Nagwa Helmy El-Mangoury, DDS,
FDSRCSEd, MS, PhD**
Department of Orthodontics & Dentofacial
Orthopedics, Cairo University Faculty of
Dentistry, Cairo, Egypt

Helmy Y. Mostafa, DDS, CAGS, DScD
Mangoury & Mostafa Research Group
Private Practice of Orthodontics, Binghamton &
Endicott, New York, NY, USA

Raweya Y. Mostafa, DDS
Mangoury & Mostafa Research Group
Private Practice of Orthodontics,
Cairo, Egypt

"How long will my orthodontic treatment last, doctor?"

Very often the answer to this uncomfortable question disappoints the patient and frustrates the orthodontist. In the mid-20th century many orthodontists quoted "open-ended" fees, adjusting to variance in tissue response and leaving the patient to decide when they were "finished." But evolving practice customs and third-party fee limits have painted many 21st-century doctors into a corner, demanding standards of excellence that are often difficult to achieve on the predictable basis which one fee demands.

This is because our patients, like all biological systems, are characterized by great heterogeneity and unpredictable confounding variables. So the inflexible strictures of fixed fees often impose unrealistic expectations, and early successes must subsidize laggards and inefficient biomechanics. Fortunately, many innovative techniques have evolved to soften these blows to efficient clinical management. Some propose surgically facilitated orthodontic therapies (SFOTs), which encompass major surgery and hospitalization. More refined outpatient methods, herein referred to as Orthodontically Driven Corticotomy (ODC), have promised even greater innovations for forward-thinking professionals.

All modern incarnations of the 19th-century corticotomy share the common attribute of accelerated tooth movement if adjustments are made biweekly. But the benefits of ODC are far more important than speed alone. The benefits of Periodontally Accelerated Osteogenic Orthodontics® (PAOO®), for example, define a new era of practical tissue management by literally engineering novel epigenetic expression. The full expression of ODC also carries salutary benefits to supporting tissue, including better protection for the periodontium. This is true regardless of the biomechanical manipulation that the orthodontist might employ.

Remember that conventional but injudicious orthodontic therapy, unembellished with periodontal insight, may be hazardous to our patients' health. We have known this since the pioneering works of Zachrisson and Alnaes (1973, 1974) and Wennström *et al.* (1987, 1993). Moreover, the recent disclosures of harm that disseminating gingivitis can render (Han *et al.*, 2010) reinforce our most sobering fears. This textbook, a commendable effort by Drs Brugnami and Caiazzo, serves as an intellectual guideline of great practical merit to ameliorate these risks and impediments to efficient care. But it also lives as an evolving document that undoubtedly will increase in value as new data emerge in this "Century of the Biologist" and as orthodontists continue to evolve as dentoalveolar orthopedists.

The simple corticotomy has, throughout its long development, also ushered in a plethora of new concepts and clinical strategies that are only now becoming understood by the dental profession. This book takes the reader to a kind of "bottom-up" perspective of orthodontic practice by conjoining "optimal force" with a contrived "optimal response." Now, patients have greater options from which they may design their own personalized care as clinical practices become democratized in the Information Age. Indemnifying entities like governments and insurance companies can still proffer categorical "products." Yet, doctors are now reassured that side effects like root resorption and tissue damage are minimized while the scope of practice expands to meet 21st-century challenges. With ODC all stakeholders win.

From a more scholastic perspective, this text proffers a glimpse into a kind of biological renaissance, long in coming but destined as sovereign over art. These are dramatic leaps forward which – while bemusing to the intransigent traditionalist (Matthews and Kokich, 2013) – are, to the sensitive scientist, a fascinating trend and a compelling read. Grounded in implacably robust scientific verities, the postmodern corticotomy and its progeny – PAOO, periodontal stem cell therapy, and transmucosal perforation (perturbation) – have emerged as both a challenge to traditional orthodontic art and a solution to many of its problems. Alas, in the slow parade of scientific progress, some will always fight the tide of innovation. So Luddites and naysayers listen up.

Query. Would you buy a house from an architect who has ignored innovative civil engineering to strengthen the foundation? Of course not! And by the ancient ethical imperative, The Golden Rule, neither should we ignore the foundation of our orthodontic creations. The more immediate challenge is how to deliver the science to patients on a daily basis with practical, safe, and rewarding protocols.

This book is the roadmap to that new horizon. Specifically, the editors have assembled a worldwide consortium of scholars and translational scientists (clinicians) with a compendium of excellent cell-level science. This collection justifies a kind of orthodontic "NewThink," attractive rational algorithms that can expand the scope of the clinical biology. Further – in deference to the clinical artisan – it fortifies traditional wire bending against the ubiquitous criticism that orthodontic art lacks a cogent biological rationale (Johnston, 1990).

This "bottom-up" approach to orthodontic care does not demand radically new practices. All ODC asks of the doctor is efficient biomechanical schemes and an open mind. Yet, it is difficult to write about clinical protocols that are to be universally appealing. This is because each clinician, with limited time, wants to learn very easily how new protocols (a) have a strong basis in science, (b) can be delivered in a safe, practical, and profitable manner, and (c) will be appealing to most patients. Those elusive goals have been masterfully achieved in this textbook.

Chapters 1 and 2 provide the reader with a general overview of ODC techniques within their historical context and discuss emerging variations that are still expanding the field of SFOT. Under this rubric of all post-modern corticotomy incarnations, Professor Ferguson, one of the strongest intellectual advocates, adds an elegant and comprehensive meta-analysis of animal model research. His authoritatively provocative insights relate ODC in a way that should please both the ethereal academic and the clinical pragmatist in all of us.

In Chapter 3 Drs Mehra and Shinwari consider how PAOO and discretely selective alveolar decortication broaden the range of orthodontic therapy. They go on to contrast these innovations with traditional orthognathic surgery where ODC procedures might serve as reasonable alternatives to the inherent risks of hospitalization and major surgery.

Chapter 4 extends the applications of corticotomy even further and dovetails into the concepts of relative anchorage and piezosurgery. After this chapter the reader can better understand how piezosurgery might modify basic corticotomy techniques with so-called "one-sided" surgery described by Professors Dibart and Keser in Chapter 5.

Chapters 6, 7, and 8 give us a deeper understanding of the orthodontic–corticotomy synthesis in the context of basic science by exploring ODC as tissue engineering. It is this science that explains how judicious loading in the healing bone wound might facilitate orthodontic tooth movement and stable phenotype alteration.

Professors Melsen and Luzi in Chapter 9 explain how efficient biomechanical protocols must be deftly coordinated with surgical manipulation to effect an optimal outcome. With their artful pedagogical prose, these forward-thinking professors meld traditional wire bending art with their expertise in alveolus physiology. This culminates the biological teachings that the venerable Professor Melsen has so firmly implanted into the *Zeitgeist* of the orthodontic specialty.

In Chapter 10, Drs El-Mangoury and Mostafa investigate corticotomy-facilitated orthodontic therapy in cases of anterior open bites. Their contribution further elucidates how the parameters of traditional orthognathic surgery may need to be reconsidered in light of the nascent science that ODC promises for alveolus bone manipulation.

All these contributions have been woven into an intellectual fabric exceptionally well by the prodigious editorial efforts of Doctors Brugnami and Caiazzo. What emerges from their collaboration is the kind of book that you can place next to your office phone for quick reference between patients or read at leisure for its more profound scientific merits.

It is important to remember that the specialties of periodontics and orthodontics developed separately but are naturally indistinct in biology. They are separated only by political evolution, the microeconomic demands of private practice, and a delicate dichotomy of art and science. Yet the art of the traditional orthodontist – standing alone on ever feeble limbs – is often spoiled by delays, periodontal infection, and notoriously severe relapse. Since ODC minimizes relapse and time in treatment, it reduces the bacterial load, and thus the risks of chronic infection. In this regard, the recent revelations of significant oral–systemic interaction (Glick, 2014) make the integration of both specialties not only a biological sound decision, but also, in many respects, a professional imperative. Then why is there reluctance among recalcitrant skeptics when confronted with the word "corticotomy"?

The answer is that the science has never been fully explicated from the art in a fountainhead of clinical reports. But in this book the science is revealed. And it is widely acknowledged as *good* science (Amit *et al.*, 2012). Despite counterpoints that never fully fathom the best protocols, ODC in many forms is here to stay. The only question is: Who will define what is good science? …the patient? …the lawyer? …the managed care auditors and bureaucrats? …a government agency? This book takes the strong position that science should be defined from only one authoritative source: the scientist. And that scientist is you, doctor!

For the young orthodontist just starting to practice, this book asks a critical existential question: who are you, doctor …really? artisan or scientist? What will you choose to believe? Which path will you follow? Will you be the first among your colleagues to lead or one of the last to follow? ODC is certainly not your fathers' orthodontics. But if we are to be faithful to the promise of science, then we must be willing to embrace its bountiful harvest even when traditional art objects. Will you be the first among your colleagues to exploit this opportunity or one of the last to learn? *Quo vadis?*, young orthodontist, *quo vadis?* indeed.

The editors and contributors to this text have attempted to make the following chapters faithful to the principles of translational science, steeped in the tradition of logical positivism, yet practical in execution and healthy in its payoff for patients. So temporarily suspend disbelief while these fine contributors attempt to awaken you from complacent slumber. The 21st century is knocking at the door. Read well, practice well, and above all, as legions of dental professors worldwide would entreat, *Carpe Diem!*

Neal C. Murphy
Department of Periodontics,
Case Western Reserve University
School of Dental Medicine,
Cleveland, OH, USA
Department of Orthodontics,
Case Western Reserve University
School of Dental Medicine,
Cleveland, OH, USA

Nabil Bissada
Department of Periodontics,
Case Western Reserve University School of
Dental Medicine, Cleveland, OH, USA

Donald H. Enlow
Department of Orthodontics,
Case Western Reserve University School of
Dental Medicine, Cleveland, OH, USA

Ze'ev Davidovitch
Department of Orthodontics,
Harvard University School of
Dental Medicine, Cambridge, MA, USA
Department of Orthodontics,
Case Western Reserve University,
School of Dental Medicine,
Cleveland, OH, USA

References

Amit G, Kalra JPS, Pankaj B *et al.* (2012) Periodontally accelerated osteogenic orthodontics (PAOO) – a review. *Journal of Clinical and Experimental Dentistry*, **4** (5), e292–e296.

Glick M (ed.) (2014) *The Oral–Systemic Health Connection: A Guide to Patient Care, Quintessence*, Chicago, IL.

Han YW, Fardini Y, Chen C *et al.* (2010) Term stillbirth caused by oral Fusobacterium nucleatum. *Obstetrics and Gynecology*, **115** (2 Pt 2), 442–445.

Johnston LE Jr (1990) Fear and loathing in orthodontics: notes on the death of theory. *British Journal of Orthodontics*, 17 (4), 333–341.

Matthews DP, Kokich VG (2013) Accelerating tooth movement: the case against corticotomy-induced orthodontics. *American Journal of Orthodontics and Dentofacial Orthopedics*, **144** (1), 4–13.

Wennström JL, Lindhe J, Sinclair F *et al.* (1987) Some periodontal tissue reactions to orthodontic tooth movement in monkeys. *Journal of Clinical Periodontology*, **14** (3), 121–129.

Wennström JL, Stokland BL, Nyman S, *et al.* (1993) Periodontal tissue response to orthodontic movement of teeth with infrabony pockets. *American Journal of Orthodontics and Dentofacial Orthopedics*, **103** (4), 313–319.

Zachrisson BU, Alnaes L (1973) Periodontal condition in orthodontically treated and untreated individuals I. Loss of attachment, gingival pocket depth and clinical crown height. *Angle Orthodontist*, **43**, 402–411.

Zachrisson BU, Alnaes L (1974) Periodontal condition in orthodontically treated and untreated individuals II. Alveolar bone loss: radiographic findings. *Angle Orthodontist*, **44** (1), 48–55.

Efficiency of treatment, expanding the scope of orthodontics, and diminishing the incidence of side effects have been the focus of many clinicians and researchers for a long time. Despite corticotomy already having been described and utilized in the last century, only recently has it gained much attention. Interestingly, we have been witnessing contrasting reactions and misinterpretations about the term, the use and its indication or advantages, causing a tremendous horizontal diffusion and an extremely low vertical diffusion around the world. That is why we felt that a book entirely devoted to corticotomy or Periodontally Accelerated Osteogenic Orthodontics® was much needed.

The term. "Corticotomy" is often confused with "osteotomy." Corticotomy is the cut of the cortices and osteotomy is the cut through the entire thicknesses, including the interposed medullary bone between the cortices, potentially creating a mobilized segment of bone and teeth. The confusion was mainly created because the earlier concept of rapid tooth movement was based on bony block movement in corticotomy techniques. Paraphrasing leading author of Chapter 1, Dr Neal Murphy would say, "This kind of surgery is not intended to 'rearrange anatomical *parts*' like so many

Lego® children's toys. Parts rearrangement is within the scope of orthognathic osteotomies.

Corticotomy-facilitated therapy does not create anatomical fragments or separate 'parts.' *Corticotomies re-engineer physiology*; they seek to *re-engineer* epigenetic potential in both the basic physiology of healing and ultimate morphogenesis at the molecular level of DNA and (endogenous and grafted) stem cells." Tissue engineering is the sum of "tissue" (a collection of cells for a common purpose – cf. organ, a collection of tissues for common function; e.g., the stomach, the face, the periodontium) and "engineering" (marshaling natural forces and manipulating them to a predetermined design – cf. civil engineering turning water flow to mechanical energy by changing the design of river courses and then changing the mechanical energy of fluid dynamics, via a turbine, into the form of electrical energy before an electrical engineer manipulates it to visible wave lengths of the electromagnetic spectrum in lasers. Finally, we turn visible electromagnetic flux, dissipate it into tissue, changing the design of oral tissue and, using the osteopenia it induces, changing the form. In a much more, less ablative way, with PAOO we take the natural forces of biological wound healing and turn them into a new phenotype design). The Wilcko brothers were the first to promote that the movement does not result from repositioning of tooth–bone blocks, but rather from a cascade of transient localized reactions in the bony alveolar housing leading to bone healing, and modified the technique by adding bone grafting and drastically changing the rationale of its use. That is why we consider them the fathers of modern corticotomy.

Corticotomy-facilitated orthodontics (CFO), rapid orthodontic decrowding, modified corticotomy, alveolar corticotomy, selective alveolar corticotomy, speedy surgical-orthodontics, accelerated osteogenic orthodontics, selective alveo-lar decortication, Wilckodontics, corticotomy-assisted decompensation, augmented corticotomy, surgically facilitated orthodontic therapy, and corticotomy-enhanced intrusion are some of the names of procedures that all originate from their new approach and definition. In most of this book, PAOO and corticotomy will be used interchangeably, although the latter clearly distinguishes from the former because of bone grafting.

The use and indications. Considering corticotomy just as a method to accelerate orthodontic movement would be limitative. The most interesting effect is the osteogenic potential. When combined with bone grafting, this technique may help to expand the basal bone. This will clinically translate into at least two main positive effects: (1) more space to accommodate crowded teeth and then less extraction of healthy premolars in growing patients; (2) a thicker, more robust periodontium, which may help to prevent recessions during or after orthodontic movement. The concept can be stretched to the point that, according to Williams and Murphy, "the alveolar 'envelope' or limits of alveolar housing may be more malleable than previously believed and can be virtually defined by the position of the roots. This is the beginning of bone engineering in orthodontics, and the dental surgeons and the orthodontists should define themselves as dentoalveolar orthopedists, while embracing this new philosophy of treatment. The emphasis on bone engineering during orthodontic tooth movement promises much more than an alternative protocol to increase speed of orthodontic treatment. The orthodontists, with their surgical partners, can modulate physiological internal strains (similar to those of distraction osteogenesis in long bones) to define novel and more stable alveolus phenotypes"; this would minimize not only premolar extractions, but also orthognathic surgery morbidity (such as surgical palatal expansion, for example).

Diffusion of corticotomy. The science that studies the principle of innovation and change defines "technology transfer" as all activities leading to adoption of a new product or procedure by any group of users (http://www4.uwm.edu/cuts/bench/princp.htm).

"New" is used in a special sense, meaning any improvement over existing technologies or processes, not necessarily a chronologically recent invention. Technology transfer is not simply dissemination of information and passively awaiting its use. Technology transfer is an active term. It implies interaction between technology sponsors and users and results in actual innovation. We should also distinguish between *innovators or early adopters* and *late adopters*.

Innovators are individuals or groups who are willing to progress by adopting "new" methods, products, or practices not widely in current use. They are a key to the diffusion of innovations because they provide practical evidence that an innovation actually works, and this is important to later adopters. These users may frequently create their own innovations in response to specific problems that they face. We should also define *diffusion* (the spread of an idea, method, practice, or product throughout a social system), *horizontal transfer* (the movement of information on technology between innovators (peer-to-peer) within an organization or between similar organizations), and *vertical transfer* (the movement of information on technology from innovators to late adopters of an organization or system of organizations).

Corticotomy has been increasingly employed with great success worldwide and therefore gained a tremendous "horizontal diffusion." From South America to Africa, from the Middle East to the Far East, from Europe to North America, different groups of scientists/clinicians have been working and publishing on the subject (extensive horizontal diffusion). In contrast to this worldwide distribution, the highest percentage of orthodontists in North America are either ignoring or skeptical and fail to present it to their patients as a viable and valuable alternative (lack of vertical diffusion).

There are different reasons to explain such a difference in diffusion, other than natural resistance of people and organizations to change:

1. The innovation is not disseminated. Given that the "innovation" is truly innovative, one of the most important driving factors is the economical one. For example, most of the innovation in dentistry in the last 30 years, from implants to membranes, to clear aligners or straight wire, have been "encouraged" by suppliers and manufacturers. It's the same as in the pharmaceutical business: any revolutionary drug to cure a rare syndrome would suffer a difference in diffusion compared, for example, with Viagra® or biposphonates or statins.

2. The innovation is disseminated to the wrong people. The information is not referred to the proper person or somehow gets lost on the way.

3. The innovation is not understood by the potential user.

Most of the time this is created by a superficial knowledge of the technique or misinterpretation, lack of homogenous terminology, and underestimation of potential benefits.

We decided then to put together a "dream team" of corticotomy, with contributors from many different countries, representing directly or indirectly four of the five continents, hoping to help the application of this revolutionary technique and innovative philosophy of treatment.

Federico Brugnami and Alfonso Caiazzo

About the companion website

This book is accompanied by a companion website:

www.wiley.com/go/Brugnami/Corticotomy

The website includes:

- Demonstration videos of surgical procedures featured in the book
- PowerPoint slides of all figures and PDF versions of all tables for downloading

Corticotomy-facilitated orthodontics: Clarion call or siren song

Neal C. Murphy,[1,2] M. Thomas Wilcko,[2] Nabil F. Bissada,[2] Ze'ev Davidovitch,[1,3] Donald H. Enlow,[1] and Jesse Dashe[4]

[1] *Department of Orthodontics, Case Western Reserve University School of Dental Medicine, Cleveland, OH, USA*
[2] *Department of Periodontics, Case Western Reserve University School of Dental Medicine, Cleveland, OH, USA*
[3] *Department of Orthodontics, Harvard University School of Dental Medicine, Cambridge, MA, USA*
[4] *Department of Orthopedic Surgery, Boston University Medical Center, Boston, MA, USA*

PREFACE

All Men by nature desire knowledge.
                                                            Aristotle

This chapter attempts to create an intellectual matrix within which other contributors writing about orthodontically driven corticotomies – also known as surgically facilitated orthodontic therapy (SFOT) – find both justification and inspiration with a modicum of practicality. The corticotomy, a selective alveolus decortication (SAD) of the alveolus bone, is but one in a family of related procedures encompassed by the inchoate field of SFOT. This treatise, by the very nature of the subject, focuses more on science than orthodontic art. And that science is orthodontic (bone) tissue engineering (OTE).

Yet, the emphasis on bone engineering during orthodontic tooth movement (OTM)

promises much more than an alternative protocol or new clinical gadgetry. This chapter, in the context of an historical review, presents an evolution (and a clash) of ideas to reveal universal biologic principles. It is these principles, these transcendent truths, that should be applied to particular clinical events in a meaningful and rewarding manner. The student of SFOT should not indulge in mindless dedication to one technical recipe without understanding the specific biologic mechanisms and therapeutic objectives that define it.

The ideas and procedures of SFOT herein are increasingly being employed with great success worldwide despite the natural impediments of healthy skepticism and unintentional misrepresentation. Importantly, this global popularity is forging a new identity for those who wish to embrace it. Twenty-first-century orthodontists, periodontists and other surgeons are becoming international citizens endowed with skills and intellects of global scientists, forming a mastermind that is liberated from "brick and mortar", national, or even regional biases. We comment on that emergent event as doctors who have participated in a nascent science; we witnessed its birth, watched it develop, and remain ever fascinated by it. The contents of this book lend credence to that new identity and the authors personify the spirit of free inquiry that sustains it. Yet, in our zeal to share knowledge, we posit most humbly that we are merely the messengers.

INTRODUCTION

Conceptual issues

The title of this chapter is not a question; it is an existential choice. Because the history of the corticotomy presents thematic questions much more profound than where one should make surgical cuts, some explanation of this chapter's syntactical style is in order. The historical journey of the orthodontic specialty reflects a similar kind of thematic development replete with controversy. Throughout that rocky sojourn, two contentious themes have always emerged. The first is whether the essence of orthodontic practice is art or science. The resolution of this dichotomy is that orthodontics is neither and both. Art and science are merely two different but complementary perspectives of the world. So conflict between these two worldviews is actually quite illusory. It is resolved only by realizing that arts and sciences are merely tools, intellectual instruments with which we achieve a nobler mission: our humanitarian endeavor of caring for others. Still, the two classic perspectives always prevail and must be constantly rebalanced: humanistic art as the ends, science as the means.

The second theme, a perennial conflict between extraction and non-extraction protocols, is more philosophically relevant to our topic. One of the great advantages of SFOT is that alveolar bone can be reshaped to accommodate an idealized dental arch rather than modifying

a dentition to "inferior bone." An historical drag on this progressive trajectory is the assumption that the alveolus bone is immutable. It is not; the alveolus bone is remarkably malleable.

So, in a way, the new realization that the alveolus bone is malleable and the ability to "build a better bone" renders the extraction–expansion debate somewhat moot. With a "new biology" of orthodontics this historical debate has been rendered simplistic and false, just as epigenetics has rendered the nature–nurture debate an anachronistic dichotomy in the face of evolutionary sciences.

Our historical review cannot dictate where art ends and science begins in the mind of each orthodontist, for as every flower is beautiful, yet every flower is unique. And the sensitive orthodontist takes each individually unique "flower" to full bloom in its own season using both art and science. Likewise, one cannot dictate to every orthodontist exactly when extractions in particular should or should not be prescribed. One can only disclose a wider scope of therapeutic options, to achieve high-quality care. And, to many, quality is an event; namely, the coincidence of doctor talent with patient expectations in a universe of humanistic but rational achievement. This is the tacit mission of this textbook and its selfless contributors.

When dealing with facial esthetics the artistic imperative is undeniable and the decision to extract or not to extract reflects individual interpretations of timeless principles. Most art is intuitive. Yet even art – namely, impressions, culturally influenced in the aggregate and subjectively sensed in the individual – is not totally beyond the reach of scientific scrutiny. And, for better or worse, scientific scrutiny must always be the abiding companion of the 21st-century doctor. This is because contemporary practice, whether engaged with biological principles or indulged in psychosocial imperatives, operates in a postmodern world that demands demonstrable scientific proofs where we find them or (at least) compelling biological rationales where we can divine them. History reveals the former and justifies the latter.

In this chapter, our methods are innovative, and admittedly somewhat polemical. We do not merely report a litany of events and experimental results. We cleave existing basic science to pertinent clinical data and synthesize them with traditional protocols. This hopefully will fortify what is done right by explaining it and provide alternatives to what can go wrong by explicating errors from their historical context.

When innovative science is seen through the lens of historical context, two important revelations occur. First, sophisticated insights of nuance are clarified (e.g., bony block movement versus enhanced physiology); and second, some new ideas are revealed simply as "old wine in new bottles" (normal healing, the regional acceleratory phenomenon – see 1983: Frost and his regional acceleratory phenomenon). This chapter will undoubtedly serve some old wine, but that insight does not diminish its worth. The historical context merely legitimizes the insights as more salient and timeless.

Through the gauntlets of criticism and the civil internecine bickering that often characterizes our specialties, it is curious indeed how truth emerges. Yet it is important to note that an assiduous intellectual analysis, emancipated from the strictures of dogma, and inspired by intrepid pioneers who have preceded us, is what sets the tone for this chapter and perhaps even the textbook itself. Query: is it nobler to suffer the indignities of dogmatic tradition or bear the yoke of exciting innovation? The former is safe, but the latter is tantalizing since it unravels the nettlesome enigmas of biology.

We must choose the latter despite the fact that unraveling mysteries is politically and philosophically risky when it exposes hues of uncomfortable truth. But the explication of truth is our deontological duty, because we have the power to control the welfare of other human beings, and that duty imposes a fiduciary standard more exalted than the "treatment to the norm (average)." Axiomatic to all clinical endeavors is the view that treating patients is a privilege, not a right, and a privileged position demands excellence, not mediocrity.

Dedication

John Donne reminds us that "no man is an island, entire of itself," and this chapter is a collaborative exemplar of that reality. Yet, the exciting frontiers of oral tissue engineering herein belong to neither our venerable teachers alone nor the seasoned clinicians who wrote this chapter. Rather, the future and our efforts are dedicated to those who will enjoy a longer tenure of equity in the specialty than we. This chapter is dedicated to them: the young idealists still seeking a place in the pantheon of clinical science. *Arete*

THE NATURE OF THE PHENOMENON: INTUITED EARLY, DEFINED LATE

Diction and definitions

For the purposes of expediency and ease of reading, certain terms will depart their strict scientific definitions to be used in a liberal sense. The terms "corticotomy" and "SAD" will be used synonymously, and "mobilization" will be interchangeable with "luxation," meaning the physical jarring, fracturing, or cracking of bone. Surgically facilitated orthodontic therapy means any cutting of tissue that makes orthodontic treatment work better or faster. Other terms will submit to strict definition.

From osteotomy to corticotomy to tissue engineering

When reviewing the history of corticotomies one discovers that it originated in attempts to minimize the harsh side effects and risks of segmental osteotomy. And this history is complicated by the fact that early writers used the terms osteotomy and corticotomy synonymously. So much of the early literature is vague and prone to misinterpretation. An osteotomy starts with a linear decortication of bone and ends with a physical movement of a section of bone the way one might break a twig from the branch of a tree. Thus, "mobilization" is a kind of purposeful fracturing of bone, sometimes literally done with a mallet and chisel to move physical parts, whereas a corticotomy is limited to the initial incision to modify physiology without luxation or fracture. When studying SFOT one must keep in mind the fundamental effects and esoteric mechanisms that facilitate the phenomena.

These effects, "observed" in the mind of the surgeon during the operation, occur subclinically at the tissue and cell levels. They are less clearly defined than clinic-level gross anatomy, a level to which most orthodontists are accustomed. Therefore, new modes of thinking must occur that could not have been appreciated by the specialty's earlier advocates. However, these histological mechanisms may have been singularly intuited by John Nutting Farrer (1839–1913) as early as 1888. He was referring to orthodontic tissue effects from a "whole alveolus bone" perspective when he wrote (emphasis added):

> The softening of the socket breaks the fixedness or rigidity of the tooth leaving it comparatively easy to move, either by resorption of the tissues or by *bending of the alveolar process* or both.

Histophysiology of orthodontic-driven corticotomy

The "whole-bone perspective" is a new way of looking at alveolar bone reactions to orthodontic forces that goes beyond the narrow perspective of the periodontal ligament or a focus on the midpalatal sutures. This "NewThink" attempts to preclude retruded profile risks of extraction therapy. Williams and Murphy (2008) documented, with unequivocal biopsy images, that lingual forces can stimulate labial subperiosteal (compensatory) osteogenesis by showing samples of labial woven bone where the alveolus was expanded slowly from the lingual aspect. It should be noted, however, that any claim of permanent bone alteration with Williams and Murphy's appliances or surgical phenotype re-engineering cannot be made before 3–4 years into the retention stage when the calcification is complete to an osseous "steady state" (dynamic equilibrium). Inherent in Williams and Murphy's philosophy is the assumption that emerging esthetic standards are shifting toward "full facial" esthetics quite different from the classic retruded profile of Apollo Belvedere (Angle's esthetic standard). This philosophy is not only compelling because of his biopsy evidence of alveolus development, but also because of its natural appeal to good common sense.[1]

The osteogenic effects demonstrated by Williams and Murphy (2008) in the alveolar subperiosteal cortices in nonsurgical cases capture exactly the histophysiology of corticotomy surgeries. Surgery simply elicits the phenomenon more dramatically and faster. The theoretical concept had been alluded to previously and was most recently expanded in the excellent textbook by Melsen (2012), where it refers to a "…change in surface curvature of the alveolar walls." All contemporary orthodontists should read this most enlightened summary of basic alveolar osteology to fully understand bone strain in all patients (Verna and Melsen, 2012). This "whole-bone" perspective posits the alveolus bone, cf. alveolar "process," as a separate operative organ independent of its subjacent corpus. As the whole bone is orthodontically bent, each osteon is deformed. The "peri-orthodontic hypothesis" (Murphy, 2006) contends that this bends protein molecules and DNA, opening obscure binding sites on important molecules to elicit an epigenetic perturbation and redesigning the morphogenesis to a novel phenotype unique in alveolus in shape, mass, and volume. The value of this new perspective is that it conforms well with contemporary basic biological sciences, particularly molecular biology and epigenetics.

In this regard, alveolar subperiosteal tissue and periodontal ligament act no differently than the periosteum and endosteum respectively in any long bone (Figure 1.1).

Therefore, a lot of recent medical and basic orthopedic science can be transferred to and from alveolus bone science. This phenomenon, facilitated by corticotomy protocols, we believe may be employed to reduce the degree of clinical relapse that still plagues orthodontics after 100 years of clinical trial and error.

Standard orthodontic protocols, without surgery, cannot overcome the natural tissue "canalization" that resists phenotype change (Waddington, 1957; Siegal and Bergman, 2002; Slack, 2002; Stearns, 2002).

Cell-level orthodontics

Bone cells, and homologues in other tissues as well, sense changes in their mechanical environments, internally throughout the cytoskeleton and externally through focal adhesions to the extracellular matrix (Benjamin and Hillen, 2003; Murphy 2006; Verna and Melsen, 2012). This area of cell-level biomechanics was essentially beyond the control of most orthodontists, who relied instead on gross anatomical and clinical events to intuit cellular activity. With

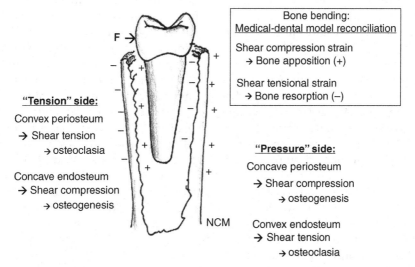

Figure 1.1 It is important to realize that SAD and particularly PAOO/AOO can change the configuration of the alveolus bone regardless of the form of the underlying maxillary or mandibular corpus. This apparently occurs by subperiosteal appositional osteogenesis stimulated by shear compression and shear tension on the facial and lingual cortices. In this respect, the periodontal ligament acts like endosteum in long bones. This realization resolves the ostensible conflict with the medical orthopedic claims that pressure is osteogenic and tension has osteoclastic effects, in contrast to the traditional orthodontic pressure–tension hypothesis that has been criticized so much in recent literature. This perspective does not deny that ischemic necrosis occurs in the periodontal ligament, but merely expands the biological concept of orthodontic histology beyond the ligament. This resorption on the so-called "pressure" side may be more related to osteogenic shear tension (–) in the cribriform plate similar to long bone homologues. On the so-called "tension" side, an increase in concavity of the cribriform plate is evident causing shear compression (+), which is osteoclastic in long bones.

the introduction of tissue engineering concepts and a revival of corticotomy-facilitated orthodontics, a new interest in cell- and tissue-level phenomena has appeared in the dawn of the 21st century.

Induced mechanical stimuli not only change the internal cytoskeleton but – by epigenetic perturbations – can determine internal stereo-biochemistry and ultimate morphogenesis. To the extent that *wound healing recapitulates regional ontogeny*, orthodontic modulation of the healing bone wound can engineer a new phenotype ideally suited for an ideal dental alignment and dental arch juxtaposition even to the point of modifying the need for orthognathic surgery. The alveolus bone, which lives, thrives and dies by virtue of its functional matrix (Moss, 1997), the dental roots, are especially responsive to therapeutic intervention in this regard because of behavioral imperatives identified by Wolff's law and Frost's "mechanostat" model (Frost, 1983).

What skeletal muscle can do to bone morphogenesis at the gross anatomical level is similar to the effects of microstrain at the cell/tissue, whether that be hypertrophy, hyperplasia, or atrophy, thus demonstrating that engineering bone morphogenesis is a threshold phenomenon; that is, too much or too little is dysfunctional. It should be remembered that the influences of mechanical stimuli at the cell and tissue levels, mechanobiology, lie not only the domain of bone alone. Indeed, the even pathoses of atherosclerotic cardiovascular disease are directly related to mechanobiological changes in vessel walls. With modern analytic methodologies and a burgeoning body of science, too extensive for the scope of this writing,[2] responses to all tissue can now be studied and actually modulated, be they integumental or neuronal, mucosal or bony. This is the essence of tissue engineering science. Thus, orthodontic scientists have a legitimate equity claim in mechanobiological fathoms as well. So, there is no reason they should not be involved considering the critical importance of their domain, the face of a human child.

The study of cell/tissue-level orthodontic therapy, especially the nature of genetic expression evident in healing bone wounds, suggests that orthodontic relapse can be seen as a simple reversion to original phenotype, regardless of the method used. That is why some SFOT has been proven to be a popular – in some cases manifestly superior (Dosanjh *et al.*, 2006a,b; Nazarov *et al.*, 2006; Walker *et al.*, 2006a,b) – and professionally acceptable adjunct to traditional orthodontic therapy. The evidence of efficacy that this innovation enjoys lends both clinical quality and stability to OTM, justifying it as a reasonable therapeutic enhancement. There are advantages and disadvantages with both conventional OTM and SFOT, and it is only fair to patients that they be made aware of all treatment alternatives. At the clinical level, SAD is termed the Periodontally Accelerated Osteogenic Orthodontics™ (PAOO) technique or the Accelerated Osteogenic Orthodontics™ (AOO)[3] technique only when a bone graft is added, and these two terms can be used interchangeably. The lead author prefers to use PAOO when there is periodontal involvement and AOO when the periodontium is healthy.

Experience suggests that, in most cases, demineralized human bone graft or viable stem cell (allograft) therapy (SCT) should provide a predictable outcome. A non-surgical derivative, trans-mucosal perforation (TMP), (Murphy, 2006) can be employed when flap surgery is not indicated in small areas with excess bony support.

A HISTORY OF THE ORTHODONTIC-DRIVEN CORTICOTOMY (OVERVIEW)

Origin of the concept

Cano *et al.* (2012), as with other authors, generally attribute the first published surgical method to facilitate orthodontic therapy to Cunningham (around 1894) after his lecture in Chicago the previous year. While having some rudimentary characteristics in common with modern corticotomies, close scrutiny of Cunningham's SFOT procedure suggests it was really a luxated segmental osteotomy. Cunningham's singular goal of making teeth move faster has since evolved to more global objectives, and variations on the corticotomy theme have spawned interesting incarnations throughout the 20th and 21st centuries in many different countries and cultures.

These variants evolved in a progression of surgical refinements designed to (a) accelerate OTM, (b) limit the quantity and pathologic potential of the inevitable bacterial load, (c) enhance stability, and (d) reduce the morbidity of orthognathic alternatives. As Cunningham's crude luxating osteotomy evolved, the term "corticotomy" emerged in the clinical lexicon with its approximate and more disciplined synonym, SAD. So both terms may be used as roughly synonymous for practical purposes.

But it should be noted that SAD with OTM will not grow new bone mass. In fact, in an adult, steady-state alveolus treatment may ostensibly slightly reduce alveolar bone mass. This is described in the non-surgical orthodontic literature as "moving bone out of the alveolar housing." So applying Cunningham's derivatives indiscriminately may indeed result in a net loss of supporting bone. This dilemma was solved by altering phenotype and creating additional bone *de novo* (Figure 1.2). Developing bone *de novo* has graced orthodontics exclusively through the prodigious efforts of many doctors in the Wilckodontics research groups, which are represented academically at Case Western Reserve University (Cleveland, OH, USA) by the second author. When grafted demineralized bone matrix (DBM)[4] (circa 1998) and viable cell allografts entered the SAD protocol, the thresholds of bone tissue engineering (Murphy, 2006) and SCT (Murphy *et al.*, 2012) were breached. This subsequently defined the dentoalveolar surgeon and orthodontist as partners in surgical dentoalveolar orthopedics and alveolar osteology.

New ideas often do not fit easily into old paradigms (Kuhn, 2012), so a new *Weltanschauung*,[5] (Freud, 1990) coined "NewThink", must be embraced to mark a clear distinction between the philosophy behind new orthodontic-driven corticotomy protocols (Pirsig's dynamic quality) and traditional orthodontic art of wire and plastic bending (Persig's static quality[6]).

The SFOT we describe here purposely executes OTM through a healing bone wound or bone graft eliciting a purposely delayed wound maturation. This occurs by perpetuating a natural bone "callus" or osteopenia until all the teeth are ideally aligned, coordinated, and detailed. This kind of surgery is decidedly *not* merely a variation of a basic surgical theme of the manner in "rearranging anatomical *parts*" like so many Lego® children's toys. Parts rearrangement is the stuff of orthognathic osteotomies. In stark contrast, the corticotomy-facilitated therapy does not create anatomical fragments or separate "parts." *Corticotomies re-engineer physiology.* Specifically SFOT, SAD, PAOO/AOO and TMP seek to *re-engineer* epigenetic potential in both the basic physiology of healing and ultimate morphogenesis at the molecular level of DNA and (endogenous and grafted) stem cells.

Early concepts: German pioneers

While Cunningham's procedure seemed bold to many American orthodontists, it soon became popular in the German scientific community. Cohn-Stock (1921), citing "Angle's method," removed the palatal bone near the maxillary teeth to facilitate retrusion of single or multiple teeth, and a host of German *Zahnartzen* followed his lead. Later, Skogsborg (1926) divided the interdental bone, with a procedure he called "septotomy," and a decade later Ascher (1947) published a similar procedure, claiming that it reduced treatment duration by 20–25%.

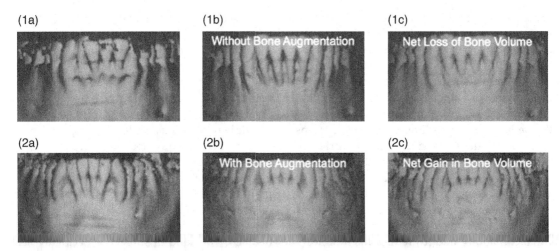

Figure 1.2 (1a) Comparison of SAD with (PAOO/AOO) and without a bone graft demonstrating the necessity for grafting when insufficient bony support is evident in adults. The figure shows the pre-treatment high-resolution computerized tomography (CT) scan (accurate to 0.2 mm) of the lower arch of a female, age 39, prior to having circumscribing corticotomy cuts performed both labially and lingually around the six lower anterior teeth. Note the arch length deficiency (overlap crowding), the pronounced crestal glabella, and the distance between the crest of the alveolus and the corresponding cemento-enamel junctions (CEJs). Clinically, the circumscribing corticotomy cuts resulted in the appearance of outlined "blocks of bone" connected by medullary bone. The total treatment time for this case was 4 months and 2 weeks with eight adjustments appointments. (1b) At 1 month retention the integrity of the outlined "blocks" of bone appears to have been completely lost and the layer of bone over the labial root surfaces appears to have vanished. In reality, this layer of bone has undergone demineralization as the result of a normal osteopenic state (RAP); the soft tissue matrix of the bone remains but is not visible radiographically. This is why radiographic assessments of expansion cases before 3–4 years in retention, while interesting in the short term, are premature for final policy conclusions. This demineralized matrix was carried into position with the root surfaces (bone matrix transportation). (1c) This shows the high-resolution CT scan at 2years and 8 months retention. Note that the layer of bone over the root surfaces has only partially reappeared due to the remineralization of the soft tissue matrix.

This suggests that there may have been a *net loss of bone volume* in this adult. In adolescents this is not seen. Owing to a greater regenerative potential there seems to be a complete regeneration of bone after SAD. (2a) This shows a high-resolution CT scan of the lower arch of a male, age 23, prior to circumscribing corticotomy cuts being performed both buccally and lingually around all of the lower teeth with a large bone graft placed over the corticotomized bone. Note the paucity of bone over the buccal root surfaces. The total treatment time was 6 months and 2 weeks with 12 adjustment appointments. (2b) At 3 months retention the labial root surfaces are now covered with an intact layer of newly engineered phenotype appropriate for the new position of tooth roots (the functional matrix of the bone).The pre-existing paucity of bone over the lingual root surfaces has been corrected in the same manner so that the roots of the teeth are now "sandwiched" between intact layers of bone both buccally and lingually. There has been a *net increase in bone volume*. (2c) At 2 years and 8 months retention the increase in the alveolar volume has been maintained. These data argue for PAOO/AOO in non-growing orthodontic patients where dental arch expansion is considered.

As good as it may appear, the scientific literature of the 20th century seems to have missed the central purpose of SFOT, SAD and PAOO/AOO, and TMP. This illustrates a social phenomenon where older, more experienced but doctrinaire, clinicians see innovation not in the context it promises, but rather in the context of the *status quo*. This is an unfortunate but common event seen best in retrospect. This bias and the lack of modern biological standards is the reason why some literature of this period is merely anecdotal, dismissive and often patently incorrect. Yet, ironically, this body of data is still cited as authoritative and used to justify specious criticisms of 21st-century dentoalveolar surgery.

1931: Bichlmayr's breakthrough – A wedge resection

After Cunningham's osteotomy publication, a series of German papers sustained the notion that outpatient surgery could be beneficial to orthodontic patients. Ironically, the original presentations of rudimentary SFOT at the turn of the 20th century languished in dusty journals and were not widely discussed in America for over half a century. However, the concepts blossomed in Europe.

Then, just before World War II, Bichlmayr (1931) described a very practical surgical procedure for patients older than 16 years to accelerate tooth movement and reduce relapse of maxillary protrusion. This was employed with canine retraction and first bicuspid extraction, by "excoriating" cortical plates of the palatal and crestal alveolus, and cortices of the extraction sites. Later, Neumann (1955), who divided the inter-radicular bone and ablated a wedge of bone palatal to the incisors meant to be retracted, would be most laudatory of Bichlmayr's work. But this praise was to be proven faint.

Important to note is that Bichlmayr probably excised significant amounts of medullary bone with his procedure. He redefined orthognathic surgery by reclassifying it into two categories: "major" (total or segmental maxillary and mandibular correction) or "minor" (interdental osteotomy or corticotomy), and was the first to described the corticotomy procedure to close diastemata (Figure 1.3). Bichlmayr's extensive wedge-shaped bone resection (*Keilfoermige Resektion*) was more extensive than the punctate and linear patterns presently employed. The latter seem more discrete and somewhat sophisticated, but the fundamentals of induced osteopenia and recalcification in retention are the same. If protracted decalcification is desired or

(a)

(b)

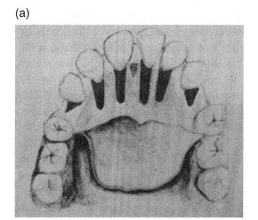 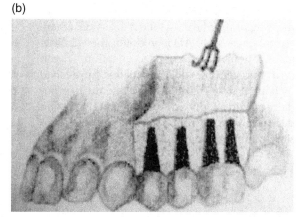

Figure 1.3 (a) Bichlmayr's representation of palatal and distal decortication. Shaded wedge-shaped areas diagram a wedge-resection (*Keilfoermige Resektion*) of alveolar cortices and probably significant medullary bone. (b) Buccal areas subjected to posterior alveolus expansion. In view of more modern revelations about the physiology of SAD it seems that Bichlmayr's aggressiveness, though done with clinical impunity, may have been somewhat superfluous. Considering the concern for buccal dehiscence and gingival recession associated with posterior dental arch expansion, a bone graft buccal to Bichlmayr's posterior corticotomies (b) may be prudent for non-growing patients.

if the degree of tooth movement is onerous (e.g., mass posterior bodily vectors), then Bichlmayr's extensive decortication is appropriate.

However, in the context of movement alone, if a simple labial tipping of mandibular incisors is desired, then a more conservative procedure, even as minor as TMPs, may work where sufficient alveolar bone is present. However, this should not be done where there is a question of bony support. Bone paucity dictates that PAOO/AOO is clearly indicated. This is why Bichlmayr's procedure is limited; not every oral site has the abundant bone of the maxillary palate. It is this wide spectrum of procedures that are presently defining the nascent clinical subspecialty of OTE.

The discerning principle of orthodontic-driven corticotomy procedures is this: the degree and duration of the necessary osteopenia is directly commensurate with the degree of induced surgical trauma, and proportional to the amount of bone density through which the teeth are moved; that is, a lot of denser bone means more decortication is needed for long tooth movement distance. It takes just as long for five 2 mm linear decortications to heal as it does two 5 mm linear decortications. Given that the comparative healing time is the same, where the sufficiency of SAD is in doubt there is little justification for timid decortication. Later, near mid-century, one can better appreciate Bichlmayr's contribution to 20th-century orthodontics with the publication of Köle (1959), who derived his work from many previous German publications, but particularly that of Bichlmayr.

1959: Köle's American debut

The seminal American work belongs to Köle because he wrote the first English-language paper describing a practical decortication of the alveolus bone to facilitate OTM. With some notable refinements, this is the basic technique that is employed today by those who promote the integration of orthodontic therapy and periodontal surgery. The Köle surgery was limited to the cortex of the dental alveolus, but subapical decortication was embellished by extending buccal and lingual cuts into the spongiosa until they communicated through the subapical medullary bone. Bucco-lingual communication is now considered unnecessarily morbid and eschewed by later SAD and PAOO/AOO protocols.

When Köle popularized corticotomy in the English literature he also promoted the so-called "bony block" hypothesis, an explanation later abandoned as the underlying physiology of SFOT became more clearly defined. He also reported buccal corticotomy in posterior inferior sectors to correct molar linguo-version and facilitate orthodontic expansion. Here, we see an emergence of physiology engineering theory as a conceptual replacement for the mechanical rearrangement models. He relied on the reduction of cortical resistance and tried to preserve the vascular supply from the trabecular bone to the teeth. Some years later this vascular issue was the focus of criticism by Bell and Levy (Verna and Melsen, 2012).

Special consideration should be made when studying this milestone contribution of Dr Köle in 1959. Where Bichlmayr indicated that he was essentially just making room for the roots by removing a physical impediment, Köle emphasized a subtle but key element. He left a thin layer of bone over the root surface in the direction of the intended tooth movement. This aspect of the root, the surface exposed to the resistance of tissue or bone, is called the root "enface" (Murphy et al., 1982). This is the area of microanatomy that we think travels with the root as a kind of "demineralized root–bone matrix transportation" tissue complex.

Köle's methods were less ablative than Bichlmayr's except for through-and-through osteotomies (cuts) made apical to the root tips of the teeth and next to the extraction sites. Köle's observations led him to surmise that the roots of the teeth were not moving through the bone, but rather the bone was moving *with* the roots of the teeth. With his technique Köle claimed to be able to complete most major movements in adults in 6–12 weeks. To illustrate how far Köle's concept has traveled, the modern incarnation of this idea can tip lower incisor teeth labially out of crowding in 4 days (Figure 1.4).

Unfortunately, Köle's interpretation of the mineralized medullary (spongiosa) bone moving with the roots of the teeth was incorrect. But in 1959 the correct scientific explanation for

(a)

(b)

(c)

(d)

Figure 1.4 The contemporary method of SAD is represented in this 23-year-old Caucasian male college student. (a) His clinical appearance, where his orthodontic treatment relapsed after losing his retainer. He presented with a chief complaint of "crooked teeth." Oral examination revealed an Angle's class I occlusion with ostensible lower incisor arch length deficiency. This is a misinterpretation, because the so-called "crowding" is actually "pseudo-crowding" due to a return of the deep bite and the restriction of space for lower incisors as they approach the maxillary incisors' cervical lingual surface. Note the relapsing dental deep bite, a musculo-skeletal phenomenon.

The patient needed treatment to be completed within a month. A full-thickness mucoperiosteal flap (c) was reflected and linear and punctate decortications (d) on the abundant labial cortex were combined with lingual TMP (trans-mucosal perforations) (e) to elicit a regional acceleratory phenomenon (RAP). A lingual hemi-circumferential fiberotomy (CSF) completed the surgical treatment. Minor interproximal enamel reduction was performed and a week later the patient presented with lower incisors well aligned (f). The treatment was maintained with a vacuum-formed plastic retainer (g). The patient reported that, "The teeth were straight in 4 days but I had to wait a week for an appointment." Such rapid tooth movement is not uncommon when simple labial tipping is facilitated by interproximal enamel reduction (stripping) and a corticotomy.

This case illustrates how a panoply of SAD procedures (PAOO/AOO, TMP, CSF, etc.) can be employed according to each individual's needs and desires. Corticotomies cannot be legitimately rendered without specific characterization of each patient's needs and preferences, an individual imperative often lost among policy-level autocrats, doctrinaire ideologues, and corporate utilization review committees who are unduly enamored by Gaussian means.

(e)

(f)

(g)

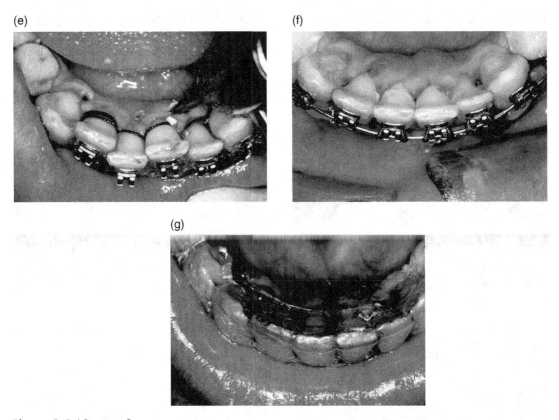

Figure 1.4 (*Continued*)

what was occurring subsequent to surgery did not yet exist. Unfortunately, this dissociation between Köle's clinical perspective and scientific reality led to confusion and contradictory rationales for over three decades. As a result of this misconception, corticotomy-based surgeries evolved mostly into buccal and lingual cuts circumscribing the entire root with little regard for the facilitating physiology. Although Köle removed the buccal and lingual plates of bone at extraction sites, there was little evidence he fathomed the principle element in altering OTM. What is critical is this: bone volume must be reduced adjacent to the root surface at the root enface; that is, *in the direction the tooth is moving*. This was not emphasized for many decades, and thus stigmatized SFOT until this misconception was cleared up by the computerized

tomography (CT) research by Professor Wilcko. Additionally, research at Loma Linda University began to bring into question the long-held notion of "bony block" movement (Anholm *et al.*, 1986; Hoff, 1986; Tetz, 1986; Ryenarson, 1987; Gantes *et al.*, 1990; Khng, 1993).

Compared with the more aggressive osteotomy protocols at the time, there was relatively little morbidity in Bichlmayr's and Köle's surgeries because luxation was not employed and the blood supply was not jeopardized. For those who subscribed to "mobilization by luxation," their patients will generally suffer more, with little or no added value. Although it would certainly be preferable to have thicker layers of bone encasing the roots of the teeth in retention, this comes later when bone grafts (PAOO/AOO) were added to corticotomy protocols.

Eventually, advances in the basic sciences would help to explain the lingering confusion and give more credence to the work of both Köle and Bichlmayr. But that would not occur until 1983 and did not reach most of the American dental profession until 2001.

1931–1965: moving parts or modulating physiology?

Kretz (1931), a contemporary of Bichlmayr, described a procedure similar to Cunningham's, creating, in effect, a therapeutic fracture of the anterior alveolus. His aggressive manipulation of bone and preoccupation with the mechanical movement of "parts" continued the kind of "Newtonian bias" orthodontics as a pure mechanical art that still haunts SFOT today and eclipses any appreciation of how physiologic alterations may be modulated. The naiveté of the surgeons using these procedures belies the insights into wound-healing sciences. And this bias, to fracture bone and then rearrange it, is evident even in Reichenbach's (1965) contribution over three decades later, which also expressed concern for iatrogenic periodontal damage.

Regarding this concern, one must certainly be adroit with a scalpel to avoid any ancillary periodontal damage. However, the benefits of SAD, PAOO/AOO, and TMP, for anyone who understands the pathogenesis of periodontitis, far outweigh any perceived risks. A number of cases over the last two decades have demonstrated that, aside from occult endodontic infection, periodontitis is not an absolute contraindication to SFOT. After flap reflection and SAD, a debrided lesion at the grafting site is no more unhealthy than that of a young child. In fact, the tissue surrounding such a debrided lesion is surfeit with a regenerative physiology and growth factors that actually facilitate phenotype changes and stem cell osteogenesis. Therefore, no resective periodontal surgery or initial therapy needs to be performed as a separate procedure before SFOT because the latter subsumes the former as long as the roots of the

teeth are fully debrided and general principles of periodontal therapy are respected.

Although seemingly naive in periodontal science, Reichenbach was very wise in concern for alveolar blood supply, because the aggressive surgery described in the article certainly poses risks. In contrast, the very purpose of a refined SAD technique is to minimize that risk and maintain as much bone vitality as possible. This is done by limiting the surgical intervention to the cortex only; this *enhances* vascularity from the spongiosa. These simple caveats will ensure that Reichenbach's concerns are honored. Unfortunately, without an empirical basis derived from controlled clinical studies, laboratory data, or conceptual sophistication (epigenetics) available, Reichenbach's misapprehensions tend to be perpetuated.

1983: Frost and his regional acceleratory phenomenon

In the late 20th-century medical orthopedic literature a new concept was emerging that would ultimately be wed to the corticotomy rationale. Frost (1983) began to educate clinicians about two biological events seen with long bone fractures, which he called the systemic phenomenon and (what concerns us) the Regional Acceleratory Phenomena, RAP. This localized trauma-induced essentially a localized trauma-induced transient osteopenia was touted as an original insight and the definitive operational entity in bone fracture healing. The concept is largely attributed to Frost, despite the fact that Kolář et al. (1965) introduced many RAP effects as early as 1965.

Frost elaborated on the concept as an acceleration of the multiple stages of natural wound healing in the long bones. He explained that RAP begins within a couple of days of the fracture (osseous wounding), usually peaks at 1–2 months, and may take 6–24 months to subside. In SFOT, OTM and TMPs can perpetuate the osteopenic state beyond 2 months. RAP provides for a dramatic acceleration in bone turnover and, in earlier stages, an increase in the number of osteoclasts that produce a significant, but transient, osteopenia, a sort of benign osteoporosis. This is a condition similar to what would be observed in hyper-parathyroidism or a simple fracture, but in the case of selective decortication (SAD) no abnormal metabolism is involved and the effect is both transient and therapeutic.

LATE MODERN PERSPECTIVES (1959–2000). CONSTRUCTIVE CONTROVERSY

1972: Bell and Levy

Bell and Levy (1972), in keeping with the *Volkgeist* of the times, published a more cynical interpretation of SFOT. Their iconoclastic approach to certain salient issues is the kind of controversy that vexes the neophyte surgeon and orthodontic students but ultimately, by intellectual conflict, results in synthesis and clarity in scientific thought. Theirs was one of many articles in about one decade that provide depth to the subject but also muddied the water by conflating simple corticotomies with osteotomy-like protocols.

This conflation obscured the important distinction between superficial cuts into the cortex of bone and deep cuts further into the spongiosa. Deep cuts indeed pose a greater risk of compromising blood supply according to animal studies, but luxated alveolar segments pose a more serious threat to the patient. In the later half of the 20th century it was unclear how deep the cuts needed to be in order to facilitate OTM and whether luxation (mobilization) was really necessary. Mobilization is a vague and variable term used as a synonym of luxation, the forcible loosening of the dentoalveolar unit

by controlled fracture of the bone. The question mobilization begs is this: is mobilization necessary to facilitate tooth movement? As we will see, the answer is probably not.

The Bell and Levy work was the first experimental animal study of 4 *Macaca mulatta* monkeys, but they used the term corticotomy as a misnomer. They described a model of simultaneous mucoperiosteal flap reflection, and interdental corticotomies with *mobilization* of all "dento-osseous segments" which, they claimed, markedly compromised the blood supply to the anterior teeth. Specifically, they described "… immediate repositioning of one- and two-tooth dento-osseous segments." They ablated excessive interradicular bone with a fissure bur, noting (emphasis added) that it should be done "…after the dental-osseous segments have been *made freely movable with an osteotome*" and warn that "Great care must be exercised to maintain a palatal soft tissue pedicle to the *mobilized segments…*"

Their histological study showed the risk of this type of procedure (full mucoperiosteal detachment plus deep cutting of medullar bone) to the vascularity of a dental pulp and surrounding medullar bone. They demonstrated distinct avascular zones that progressively recovered 3 weeks after surgery, except for the central incisor.

Referencing Köle, the authors reiterated that "…dentoalveolar segments can be readily moved bodily…" It is important to note that this "bony block" perspective is exactly the kind of misinterpretation that confuses sophisticated corticotomy with luxated osteotomies. The prejudice is noted further in the Bell and Levy article when the authors claim the rationale for "corticotomy" is vague and that circulation based on "pedicled cortical bone to a relatively small amount of spongy alveolar bone would *presumably* imperil circulation to the mobilized dental segment" (emphasis added).

Bell and Levy express legitimate concerns for safety with the mobilized osteotomies, but transferring that concern for corticotomies is illogical and untenable. It is ironic that the authors also claim that, theoretically, the corticotomy could "… have a destructive effect on the periodontium." By its very definition the corticotomy part of their protocol refers to the *cortex*, and only an indiscrete surgeon could jeopardize the periodontal anatomy. Even where inadvertent periodontal tissues are breached, the regenerative potential of the organ – in the absence of infection – is robustly regenerative. In the modern definition of corticotomy the periodontal anatomy is explicitly excluded for SAD, PAOO/AOO, and TMP. When thus protected it is precisely the root–periodontal ligament–demineralized cribriform plate complex that seems to move, rendering luxation and mobilization absolutely unnecessary. Bell and Levy, it seems, criticized a clinical straw man.

What is actually surprising in their article is the degree of normal healing given the ablative nature of their surgery. They note, "postoperative healing in all animals was uncomplicated." Histological evaluation demonstrated avascular zones at the site of decortications, but all the other vasculature maintained its normal course. The authors claimed that the roots were "traumatized" but failed to elaborate on the specific sense of the term. All surgeries "traumatize" to some degree, and with corticotomies that is precisely the therapeutic objective; that is, controlled therapeutic "trauma." Technically and biologically speaking, a therapeutic "trauma" is the same physical mechanism that normally strengthens muscle tone in weightlifters and elicits healing in wound debridement.

At 3 weeks the bony cuts showed noticeable evidence of repair. This observation gives evidence of normal clinical behavior. It is significant because with any OTM, a 2–3-week post-surgical latent period is encountered after which the OTM is accelerated. By 9 weeks the authors noted "complete healing in the posterior corticotomy sites." In their discussion the surgeons make a most revealing observation about the cause of "excessive tissue damage". They stated,

> ….immediate mobilization of each dental alveolar segment probably compounded the injury by producing complete interdental osteotomies in certain areas.

We would contend that the mobilization of the segments was not merely a compounding factor but indeed the *sine qua non* of any serious injury and that SAD *per se* will produce normal tissue healing after measured precise, discretely targeted, and conservative cuts limited to bone cortices. This contention is based largely on the work of later research (Twaddle, 2001; Fulk, 2002; Hajji, 2002; Machado, 2002a,b; Kasewicz *et al.*, 2004; Skountrianos *et al.*, 2004; Ahlawat *et al.*, 2006; Dosanjh *et al.*, 2006a,b; Nazarov *et al.*, 2006; Oliveira *et al.*, 2006; Walker *et al.*, 2006a,b), which investigated both the clinical behavior and the tissue science in much greater depth. Particularly impressive in this paroxysm of scholastic excellence was the study of the rat model (Ferguson *et al.*, 2006; Sebaoun *et al.*, 2006, 2008), an even more difficult specimen to work with than the rhesus monkey. These researchers showed histological sections that clearly demonstrate normal tissue changes with corticotomy without luxation or deep cuts into the spongiosa.

Bell and Levy, from a clinical perspective, may indeed have genuinely worried about irreversible damage. That is understandable and laudable. However, they did not document permanent damage; and since ischemia or any kind of normal healing can be seen as temporarily "destructive," it appears that the authors also committed a logical error common to many clinical investigators. They pathologized normal variations. Without replicable empirical data, fully displayed, clinical impressions, for better or worse, must be taken as less compelling than "hard science."

Wherever this error is committed it over-states authors' cases and undermines their credibility. The wise writer knows that very few universals can be legitimately defended in clinical biology. It seems that the Bell and Levy article merely achieved a consecration of bias and documentation that any overly aggressive surgery is risky. To their credit, however, the authors discussed the thoughtful idea of a two-staged procedure reflecting the palatal flap and labial flaps 5 weeks apart. Moreover, it must be acknowledged that Bell and Levy made a significant contribution about how alveolar bone heals, despite their vague and confusing overstatements about what should be done.

1975: Düker's redemption

After, Bell and Levy's article demonstrated lux-ation and questioned whether the risk was worth the benefit, other exceptional articles on corticotomy were published that presented a solution to this quandary with lucid simplicity. Düker (1975) replicated Köle's work more exactly in dogs, moved an incisor segment 4 mm in 8–20 days, and concluded that neither the periodontal attachment nor the pulps of teeth demonstrated significant injury. In fact, he stated correctly but vaguely that, "…weakening

in the bone by surgery and consequent ortho-dontic treatment reduces these dangers."

The authors seem to have grasped the central concept of SFOT but expressed the rationale too ineloquently for immediate implementation. This limited scope still haunts the literature today, since many commentators, often uniniti-ated, feel a surgically induced and transient osteopenia is too effete and temporary for prac-tical use. This myopic perspective misappre-hends a critical central element of SFOT; that is, to induce constant internal bone strain by effi-cient, judicious tooth movement designed to perpetuate the osteopenia state.

Düker published his elegant study of the corticotomy in six male beagle dogs by using injections of "plastoid" (presumably a viscous polymer) into the gingival vasculature (Figure 1.5). He demonstrated that little to no changes occurred after corticotomy with the Köle style. Rearrangement of the teeth within a short time after corticotomy damaged neither the pulp nor the periodontal ligament. Yet, he supported the idea of preserving the marginal crest bone in relation to interdental cuts. He also proposed that linear cuts should always leave at least 2 mm of the alveolar crestal bone untouched.

The author warned rather naively that there may be an increased risk of periodontal damage

(a)

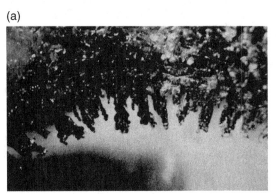

(b)

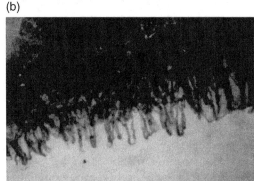

Figure 1.5 Marginal gingival vascular "agglomeration" (loosely organized masses) of capillaries (a) are dem-onstrated keeping the structural integrity intact with only mild atrophic appearance (b), which could easily be a processing artifact caused by a drop in blood pressure when the animals were exsanguinated upon sacrifice. *Source:* Düker (1975). Reproduced with permission of Elsevier.

(a)   (b)   (c)

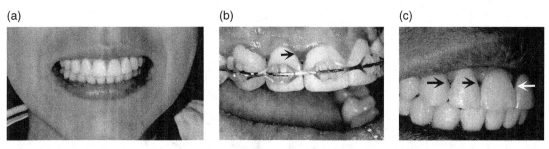

Figure 1.6 Despite an excellent 9-month class II treatment outcome (a) this patient objected to the open embrasures (b,c) at the lateral incisor (black arrows) contrasting with the central incisors' embrasure (white arrow) filled with healthy gingival tissue. The embrasure opening was caused by dehydration of a mucoperiosteal flap during a protracted surgical procedure. Good surgery is "swift, sure, and clean." Indications of gingival slough were evident in the first post-operative appointment (arrow in b).

in cases in which the interradicular space is less than 2 mm. This paean to the obvious is germane where one fears damage to root surfaces but cannot be extrapolated too far. Given contemporary knowledge about infectious periodontitis, SAD and PAOO both include the debridement of infectious accretions during the surgical procedure and therefore constitute a kind of surgical periodontal debridement themselves. This is both harmless and helpful. While surgical misadventures can adversely affect the patients' periodontal health, infection mismanagement is a greater threat to the integrity of the periodontal organ than the cuts of a skilled surgeon as long as the periodontal anatomy is preserved. The simple mucoperiosteal flap surgery itself can have salutary effects, in that the singular reflection alters redox potential of the bacterial niche, making it relatively unsupportive of anaerobic infection.

In summary, Düker's article is instructive in three major ways. First, he efficiently dismissed fears of vascular damage with credible photographic evidence. Second, citing previously underreported German authors, he intimated that American literature was deficient, a subtle criticism with which we agree. Third, he noted that the corticotomies were made short of the marginal alveolus and attributes the benign side effects of corticotomy to this forbearance. It is this last notation that should be

addressed more deeply. In our experience, carrying the corticotomy to the marginal crest of the alveolus is acceptable if no physical ablation of the periodontal ligament is made and the periodontal anatomy is otherwise healthy. Nonetheless, this is a legitimately debatable issue.

Sometimes, cases of post-operative recession and papillary atrophy create unaesthetic open labial embrasures (Figure 1.6). However, wherever periodontal structures are intact and healthy tissue appears after periodontal flap reflection, inattentive authors may commit a *post hoc* fallacy,[7] inaccurately attributing the "black triangle" appearance of open embrasures to the surgery rather than pre-existing periodontal attachment loss obscured by arch length deficiencies. In contrast to exceptional cases such as the case in Figure 1.6, the underlying cause of spontaneous open embrasures is usually preexisting and undiagnosed marginal periodontal disease, not the surgery itself. When periodontal disease is present and the surgeon wishes to avoid opening labial embrasures, the sub-crestal limits of the interproximal linear decortication should be maintained in the mass of attached gingiva apical to the osseous crest (Figure 1.7). Full-thickness flaps can be elevated after a sub marginal incision that preserves the alveolar crest and interdental papillae. Where no periodontal attachment loss

(a)

(b)

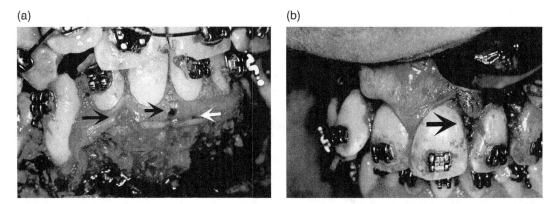

Figure 1.7 Demonstration of how contemporary alveolar tissue engineering can employ a constellation of techniques to facilitate "smile engineering" by applying TMPs (black arrows), submarginal initial incisions (white arrow) to preserve the structural integrity of the alveolar crest, and aggressive linear and punctate decortication (blue arrow). Each technique can contribute to a composite, wholly *orchestrated* manipulation of alveolus bone physiology inducing a transient therapeutic osteopenia with stem cell "targetting". Allogeneic stem cell grafting, and alveolus mass augmentation (PAOO/AOO) for use with accelerated and traditional but efficient biomechanical protocols.

(a)

(b)

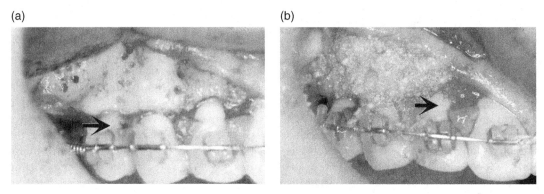

Figure 1.8 Where crestal alveolar bone is to be avoided, a sub-marginal initial incision can be made as indicated to keep the crestal bone and interdental papilla (arrows) untouched. Contrast this timid decortication with the aggressive decortications of 1.7(a). The degree of osteopenia and OTM acceleration is directly commensurate with the degree of decortication, and experience will allow an accurate, albeit subjective, sense of "how much is enough." When in doubt, there is little justification for timidity. *Source:* Mihram and Murphy (2008). Reproduced with permission of Elsevier.

is evident, the surgeon can reflect flaps with impunity in the labial esthetic zone as long as the supporting lingual half of the lingual papilla remains intact.

However, where periodontitis is active and esthetics is not an issue, opening embrasures actually indicates a rational, prudent treatment plan and should be encouraged by combining traditional ostectomy and osteoplasty with the linear decortication. Thus, the admonition that SAD and AOO should not be performed in the presence of "infection" is imprecise and misleading; submarginal incisions bypass crestal defects (Figure 1.8).

(a)

(b)

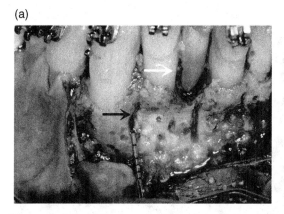
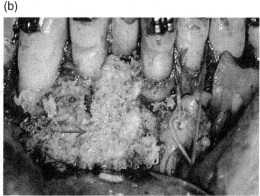

Figure 1.9 Simultaneous treatments of an infrabony defect and PAOO. (a) A periodontal defect (white arrow) after linear and punctate decortication for accelerated OTM. Note, depth of decortication (black arrow) approximates 3 mm the thickness of the labial cortex. Decortication was designed to simultaneously liberate endogenous stem cells from the medullary bone and induce a transient osteopenia to accelerate the rate of tooth movement. This demonstrates that PAOO can be combined with conventional periodontal surgical pocket reduction and that bone grafting can serve the dual purpose of creating a new bony phenotype and regenerating new periodontal attachment. *Source:* UniversityExperts.com. Used with permission. (b) The use of exogenous Stem Cell Therapy in conjunction with PAOO. Blue arrow indicates viable allogeneic stem cell graft. *Source:* UniversityExperts.com. Used with permission.

Certainly when bone grafts are used, in either PAOO or AOO, no active periapical lesions or untreated periodontitis should be present as the bone grafts or stem cells are placed. But when flaps are reflected for orthodontic purposes and the opportunity presents for traditional marginal alveolar bone management (infrabony pocket decortication, ostectomy, osteoplasty, or bone grafting,), pocket reduction and regeneration should be included in the surgical treatment plan (Figure 1.9).

To neglect this important service would constitute an error of omission and a logical *non sequitur*. Given that full disclosure of pathosis is *de rigueur* (and a legal imperative) in any healthcare venue, it can even be considered ethically untenable to overlook periodontal health. Ignoring periodontitis renders lesions vulnerable to exacerbation during accelerated orthodontic therapy because moving teeth in the presence of active periodontitis can pump supragingival pathogens subgingivally, accelerating the permanent loss of supporting periodontal attachment and creating problematic vertical defects.

Despite the subapical through-and-through transverse cut in the alveolus, no pulpal or alveolar necrosis was evident in Düker's model (Figure 1.10). The distinguishing characteristic in Düker's procedure was the absence of luxation (mobilization). So the results of Düker's beagle dog study sufficiently confirm that luxation provides little advantage to SFOT and only invites, as correctly feared, an untreatable ischemic necrosis.

1978: Generson – The open bite

Three years after Düker published his article, Generson *et al.* (1978) applied corticotomy to the treatment of apertognathia (anterior open bite). The authors' concern for the possibility of compromising the blood supply to the teeth was settled when the authors make a point that "the bony cuts were made only through the cortex." So, articles on simple decortications of the alveolus begin, with Generson *et al.*, to

(a)   (b)

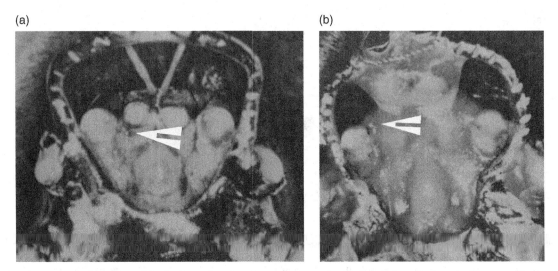

Figure 1.10 The arrows indicate the wake of tooth movement in the adult male beagle dogs before (a) and after (b) SFOT. This successfully accelerated movement suggests that a pedicle-based osteotomy (which risks both pulpal and alveolar necrosis) is unnecessary for SFOT, thus allaying the fears expressed by Bell and Levy (1972). The figures (a) and (b) suggest that a tipping motion resulted in 4 mm movement in 8–20 days. *Source:* Düker (1975). Reproduced with permission of Elsevier.

suggest that through-and-through osteotomies connecting linear decortications, like luxations, are superfluous.

Generson *et al.* applied the decortication concept and initiated orthodontic force 3 days after surgery. This is significant, because some authorities generally recommend a 2-week hiatus between surgery and the initiation of tooth movement. In contrast, the senior author has been initiating tooth movement with fixed brackets and a 0.018″ or round nickel–titanium archwire immediately after tying the last suture.

What is more significant in Generson *et al.*'s work is their description of the open bite. Again, we see a conflation of concepts where Generson *et al.* stated that their Case 1 exhibited "…no skeletal abnormality." Apertognathia is a dento-skeletal abnormality that may or may not reflect a similar spatial abnormality in the skeletal corpus subjacent to the alveolus bone. However, the surgeons did not present a cephalometric tracing or numerical parameters defining the underlying dysplasia of the

skeletal corpus. An insufficient overbite is called "dental open bite" and may or may not be combined with aberrant overjet, and a dentoalveolar open bite can appear with a normal mandibular plane angle. Consequently, the reader must presume that the patient presented with the kind of dento-alveolar anterior open bite often caused by thumbsucking during the transitional dentition.

This contrasts with a *skeletal* open bite caused by an excess posterior maxillary vertical dimension. This is measured by the mandibular plane angle which is formed by the inferior border of the mandible *vis à vis* a Frankfort horizontal reference plane. As a rough guideline, skeletal open bites and skeletal deep bites begin with great deviations of the angle above and below 26° respectively.

The excess vertical dimension of the posterior maxilla, caused either by aberrant craniofacial growth or extrusion of the maxillary molars, causes a posterior–inferior autorotation of the mandible at the temporomandibular joint and often requires orthognathic surgical correction.

The dental open bite, in contrast, is quite amenable to anterior alveolus elongation by SAD as long as the inferior elongation, a kind of distraction osteogenesis of the maxillary anterior alveolus, does not create an unaesthetic gingival display.

The distinction between a "skeletal open bite" and "dental open bite" is critical, and it is unfortunate that Generson et al. did not even produce a facial photograph for their article. In "dolichocephalic open bites" characteristic of a "long face syndrome," indiscriminate use of a corticotomy to elongate the maxillary alveolus can be just as ill-coceived as when orthognathic surgery is used for simple dental open bites. Both facial forms can produce unaesthetic results, pejoratively referred to as a "gummy smile." So, cephalometric analysis and photographic documentation are critical in these cases.

The authors published a post-operative photograph of the treated apertognathia, but the outcome displays an insufficient residual overbite and overjet. This documents the notorious potential for "vertical problems" (skeletal deep bites and open bites) to relapse.

Many fundamental musculo-skeletal deformities are clearly beyond the reach of dentoalveolar SAD. So, it may be unrealistic to expect corticotomy procedures to correct some skeletal dysplasias, and yet an alteration of the alveolus form may indeed provide sufficient clinical camouflage for them.

It would be helpful if a twin study were possible to directly compare the treatment of apertognathia with selective decortication versus LeForte procedures. In the absence of a comparative study it seems the corticotomy, while displaying some relapse potential when unretained, offers less biological cost (surgical morbidity) with presumably equally satisfactory results. So it seems that in some cases of apertognathia the corticotomy may be the first treatment of choice. However, in any case, a cephalometric analysis is still de rigueur when counseling the patient for any SFOT that might alter the vertical dimension of occlusion.

Interesting in this regard is the publication by Oliveira et al. (2006). In this article the authors describe a case of an apparent skeletal open bite that was treated to an excellent clinical outcome in only 4 months using corticotomy without orthognathic surgery. This outcome, which would normally involve major in-patient surgery, confirms that any proposal for orthognathic surgery may need to consider corticotomy-type surgery as a singular alternative or at least an adjunctive therapy. Relevant to this point, 2 years later Generson et al. ended their article with the statement that, indeed, "...corticotomy has a place in the armamentarium of the orthognathic surgeon."

1976: Merrill and Pedersen

Merrill and Pedersen (1976) resurrected the role of iconoclast when they investigated SFOT further for "immediate repositioning" of "dental-osseous elements." Ironically, after claiming to document the safety of the osteotomy and immediate repositioning of the dentoalveolar complex, the authors said that some unspecified complications had occurred, but were not sufficient to condemn the procedures. Based on our experience, these complications may well have been papillary slough, ecchymosis, or pain, all the hallmark of limited experience, naive clinical management, and serendipity.

Even more controversially, they stated that a corticotomy "...has not proved to be a successful method... in our hands...," adding that "...resistance by cortical bone has little to do with the reaction of teeth to force..." and "...little if any time is saved when classical corticotomy is used..." This intemperate conclusion stands in sharp contrast to recent controlled studies, by orthodontists and periodontists, that have demonstrated stunning efficacy, comfort, and safety with SAD, PAOO/AOO, TMP, and SCT. So, in the long history of literature on this subject, to some extent the Merrill and Pedersen article must be considered an aberration.

Conceptually, the most common cause of such tepid endorsements or unsubstantiated statement of difficulties is a failure to understand either the malleability of the alveolus or the need for managed strain in the spongiosa. This strain must be episodically induced with bi-weekly clinical adjustments in order to perpetuate the therapeutic osteopenic state. The strain must not induce resonance in the bone. That would cause premature recalcification, a return to steady-state physiology, and complicate the therapy. The well-designed perpetuation of decalcification produces a bone state similar to the relatively decalcified status of a malunion or a therapeutic site in long bone distraction osteogenesis.

When the RAP is thus perpetuated, the orthodontic clinician has sufficient time to adapt to interruptions and inefficiencies in their clinical biomechanics treatment. Yet even when the RAP dissipates (usually due to poor patient compliance or outright patient negligence) it may be resurrected with periodic and benign TMP of the alveolus (refer to Figure 1.4e). Thus, an optimal osteopenia, engineered intelligently, can be maintained almost indefinitely. Even though Merrill and Pedersen offer no one-to-one comparisons or quantitative data to substantiate their claim, relying solely on the disclaimer that results were limited "…in our hands…," they suggested a meaningful alternative.

Repeating the beliefs of Bell and Levy, they posit that two surgeries could be performed sequentially, first on the buccal aspect and then on the lingual side of the alveolus to provide collateral circulation for each surgery. A vascular anastomosis was proposed as the theoretical connection from the contra-lateral mucoperiosteal tissue that was not reflected. They also suggested that a 0.25 mm thin blade is preferred to a Stryker saw (0.80 mm) if safety for the adjacent roots is considered. We propose that a high-speed irrigated no. 2 or no. 4 round bur is the instrument of choice for precision and control (see Figure 1.4d).

In defense of Merrill and Pedersen, SAD limited to the labial alveolar cortex is a reasonable variant where the surgeon may wish to facilitate simple labial movement and wants to maintain a copious blood supply from the lingual aspect. Bear in mind, however, that the facilitating osteopenia is commensurate with the degree of therapeutic surgical "trauma" to the alveolus, and reflection of both a facial and lingual mucoperiosteal flap – even for simple labial movement – may contribute greater stability via more dissipated decalcification. Still, since the relative merits of a two-staged protocol are largely a matter of a surgeon's style, it would be too presumptuous to endorse or condemn such a procedure categorically.

1987–1974 Rynearson's revelation, Yaffe's physiology

Rynearson (1988) made a meaningful contribution to dentoalveolar surgery that even he may not have appreciated. He tested Köle's hypothesis that, under orthodontic force, teeth in a corticotomy-treated segment move as a tooth–bone unit. Utilizing implanted radiopaque pins and bone labeling, he found no evidence of movement of the cortical plates and concluded that the corticotomy procedure, albeit efficacious, did not effect a mechanical movement of a tooth–bone unit, but rather elicited a facilitation of normal physiologic tooth movement metabolism. The fallacy of "bony block" movement was finally beginning to be challenged, at least for space-closing procedures. However, the exact cell- and molecular-level mechanism responsible for the facilitated tooth movement was still an enigma.

Seven years later Yaffe et al. (1994) added a very important clue to unraveling that mystery by reporting a robust RAP response in the jaw bone of rats to a simple mucoperiosteal flap reflection. They documented not only massive decalcification of the alveolar bone, but also a widening of the periodontal ligament space. The demineralized zone was observed as early as 10 days, and the alveolar bone returned to control levels 120 days after surgery. The authors also suggested that RAP might be responsible for tooth mobility and bony dehiscence formation where the bone was thin. Although Yaffe *et al.*'s research did not include tooth movement, in terms of our understanding today this is an ideal explanation for facilitated tooth movement. That is to say, a thin layer of bone, ahead of the movement vector, will demineralize, leaving the soft tissue matrix of the cribriform bone to be carried with the root surface into the desired positioning. The term used for this phenomenon is *bone matrix transportation.*

1985: Mostafa – Limited objective therapy

Mostafa *et al.* (1985) diagrammed a surgical–orthodontic technique to treat overerupted maxillary molars showing that corticotomy could be used for one or two tooth segments. It was a Köle-like decortication localized to the alveolus of one tooth, an extruded molar.

They reported a survey of 15 patients, noting that only the cortex was incised with a surgical bur and osteotome. No explanation was made about the specific nature of the surgery. Further, no statistical analysis or even photographs were presented. It was noteworthy, however, that the authors found a single-tooth procedure helpful. As discussed below, the same issue was debated between Kim *et al.* (2009) and Murphy (2010) as late as 2010 and is helpful as pre-prosthetic SAD.

1987: Goldson and Reck

Goldson and Reck (1987) reported a similar surgical–orthodontic treatment of malpositioned cuspids. They reported on the use of a bur and osteotome combination to completely separate the dentoalveolar segment through both the buccal cortex and medullary bone. A blood

supply from the collateral sources in the adjacent mucoperiosteum was apparently sufficient for this procedure, which went deeper than today's SAD. Although one may need to induce a thorough osteopenia, there are reasonable limits. For example, osteopenia usually needs to be induced only within 2–3 mm of the teeth to be moved.

Suya and the Asian connection

Suya (1991) stimulated significant academic interest in Asia (Chung *et al.*, 2001; Hwang and Lee, 2001; Kim and Tae, 2003) for nearly two decades.

As doctors collaborated in the USA, Chung *et al.* (2001) in Asia also reported a decortication-assisted orthodontic method. Also, Hwang and Lee (2001) introduced a technique for intrusion of overerupted molars, using a combination of decortication and magnets. Kim and Tae (2003) moved teeth facilitated by decortication, referring again to the phenomenon as "distraction osteogenesis," and citing it as a "new paradigm in orthodontics." They removed part of the cortical bone, which resulted in "a speedy rate" compared with "conventional" OTM. They noted that intrusive movements were without side effects, such as root resorption or periodontal breakdown, and reaffirmed other colleagues' observations that corticotomy procedures were actually clinically superior to conventional orthodontic methods.

Park *et al.* (2006) and Kim *et al.* (2009) reported an interesting technique that is often contrasted with flap reflection methods. Although it does not allow the surgeon to visualize periodontal pathosis, and may indeed exacerbate pre-existing lesions if not executed with precision, it is noteworthy. These talented clinicians successfully used a method of surgical incision called "corticision," wherein a reinforced scalpel is used as a thin chisel to separate the interproximal cortices trans-mucosally, without a surgical flap reflection. This trans-mucosal incisional manipulation, similar in effect to TMP of alveolar bone, minimizes mor-bidity but may fail to recruit significant RAP, which occurs simply with mucoperiosteal flap reflection as reported by Yaffe et al. in 1994. Also, the corticision is designed merely to accelerate tooth movement, not to redesign underlying bony phenotype. Nonetheless, used prudently in cases without periodontal prob-lems, the corticision appears to have earned a place in clinical practice as a legitimate and meaningful SAD modification.

Suya's paper reintroduced a refinement of Köle's work into the American mind with a report on "corticotomy-facilitated orthodon-tics." His contentions were well received because it demonstrated that conservative intervention could yield dramatic results, and he substanti-ated that opinion by reporting his experiences in over hundreds of patients. Importantly, he also did not connect the buccal and labial incisions, like Köle, but relied purely on linear interproxi-mal decortication. Although Suya contended that the facilitated tooth movement was the result of "bony block" movement, we now know that the style of decortication, divots, lines, or other patterns is irrelevant. Only the sum total of therapeutic trauma is significant. Suya's refine-ment of Köle's methods has essentially set the standard for decortication procedures that fol-lowed in the post-modern era.

1986: Anholm and the Loma Linda investigation

Following communications with prior vision-aries, periodontists and orthodontists collabo-rated in the first major university studies of the phenomenon at Loma Linda University in 1986 (Anholm et al., 1986; Hoff, 1986; Tetz, 1986; Rynearson, 1987; Gantes et al., 1990; Khng, 1993), and some elaboration of their work is fitting.

Preeminent in this collaboration is the work of Anholm et al. (1986). Sobered by minor attach-ment loss, the orthodontists on the team were

cautious in their praise of corticotomy-facili-tated treatment in a male patient. While the attachment loss was not clinically significant, it is often noted in some cases, but not related directly to SAD or PAOO/AOO, as a proximal association. Some ostensible attachment loss will sometimes occur if the periodontal (muco-periosteal) flap is reflected for too long, and thus dehydrated (see Figure 1.6(b)). Another source of error is the failure to completely debride the surgical site of infective detritus. The surgery should be "sterile, sure, and swift." Most other examples of presumptive attachment loss are usually due to undiagnosed previous periodon-titis. This misinterpretation of side effects is common in poorly educated orthodontists, who overemphasize the art of clinical biomechanics to the detriment of life science, and argues that better education in principles of periodontal sci-ence and bacteriology should be incorporated in orthodontic educational curricula.

1990: Gantes et al. To pool or not to pool?

The issues of root resorption and potential periodontal damage were substantially dis-missed in an excellent article by Gantes et al. (1990). They treated five patients, 21–32 years old, with Suya's protocol and a removal of cor-tices adjacent to an extraction site, and the original intent of the research was only to mea-sure attachment level changes. They observed accelerated OTM, some mild root resorption, but no significant loss of attachment or loss of root vitality. The issue of root resorption was subsequently dismissed by later controlled studies, which finally revealed that SAD and PAOO/AOO, done correctly, indeed produced less root resorption than conventional nonsur-gical protocols. By this time it was well under-stood that a regional osteopenia offers less physical resistance to root movement.

The Gantes et al. article can be disappointing to neophyte orthodontists and surgeons because they reported that, even when the buccal and lingual cortical plates were removed at the extraction sites, the mean overall treatment times were still only 14.8 months in comparison with 28.3 months for the control group. The authors then questioned the practicality of the corticotomy because of increased complexity, the frequency of patient visits, and chair-time being approximately the same as conventional orthodontic treatment. So the authors seriously saw very little practical benefit to the patient.

One can agree with this assessment if surgery is eschewed by a patient who has no concerns for the protracted therapy time in conventional orthodontic protocols. However, the increasing risk of root resorption and bacterial load virulence has always loomed as a dark shadow over conventional therapy, and SFOT offers a reasonable solution to this threat. So, despite doctor disdain, the corticotomy in this regard is done for patient safety not doctor convenience. Moreover, the ostensible lack of significant time savings in Gantes *et al.*'s work appears to be a misinterpretation when one takes a closer look at these raw data. This deep

analysis also reveals a common but startling hidden trend in commercial-based literature and a more profound schism of epistemological perspective in our profession.

It is said that "The devil is in the details", and the article by Gantes *et al.* provides a good example of that pithy truth. Overall, the authors' "data pooling" may represent an accurate, albeit highly diverse, sample of "what walks into the office," but it obscures a very important fact. Assuming *arguendo* the questionable axiom that the authors' five patients accurately reflect the nature of the patient population, then indiscriminate application of corticotomy would indeed render little practical advantage. But, as applied scientists, orthodontists must be more discriminating and identify clinically significant subsets of the general heterogeneous population.

So, setting aside the data of "outlier" of patient no. 1 as nonrepresentative, it is entirely legitimate to interpret the Gantes *et al.* clinical observations in an entirely different manner. When the extreme data are dropped as nonrepresentative, a new picture emerges (Table 1.1)

Table 1.1 Reanalysis of the Gantes *et al.* (1990) data.

Patient type		Treatment time (months)		Time saved (months)	Reduction (%)
		With corticotomy	Without corticotomy		
1.	Brachy[a,b]	20	24	4	16.7
2.	Brachy	Indeterminate data			
3.	Brachy	11	28	17	60
4.	Bracy	12	35	23	65
5.	Meso	16	16	26	38

Source: Gantes *et al.* (1990). Used with permission.
The table shows that, in general, we can expect in most cases of SFOT to reduce treatment time by 40–60%. This is not true if the outlier, patient number 1, is included in pooled data. The decision to drop outliers from data is a controversial heuristic issue in quantitative research, but is often easier for seasoned clinicians. The decision determined by researchers familiar with the subject being studied and determining if such an outlier represents central tendency of the sample universe of data.
[a] Data for patient number 1 can legitimately be discarded as outliers.
[b] Brachycephalic refers to a "low (small) mandibular plane angle facial phenotype, skeletal dysplasia). Brachycephalic class II, division 2 malocclusions belong to a class by themselves. They are musculo-skeletal phenomena, a subset of malocclusion not within the universe of dentoalveolar pathosis and should not be conjoined with the standard universe of patients seeking therapy. This "data pooling" is a very common experimental design problem even in National Institutes of Health studies of arteriosclerotic cardiovascular disease and cancer research.

that indicates the corticotomy can be of significant advantage to doctors and patients alike. The existential question is, will the orthodontist choose to discriminate subsets?

Each philosophical approach – (a) pooling to reflect a heterogeneous clinical universe or (b) discriminating subset analysis to more precisely predict our clinical outcomes – has its proponents. The first is less accurate but convenient; the latter is precise but arduous. Arguing against discrimination one can say that all decisions are practically 50/50, and neither patients nor doctors alike can make such fine probabilistic discriminations. (So why try?) This is the rationale of the orthodontist-as-artist. The other perspective is that of the orthodontist-as-scientist, presuming that a reductionist approach will indeed allow more robust forecasting of an empirical event in fields of future uncertainly; that is, precise prediction.

This chapter argues for discrimination because such an analytical approach has characterized the orthodontic field since Angle discriminated three basic malocclusion classes in the sagittal plane. Beyond tradition, however, it is wise to discriminate subclasses of data to explicate nuance that otherwise might compromise the quality of clinical outcomes. Finally, reductionist thought is what scientists do, and thus justifies itself. Yet, in the entrepreneurial class of clinicians in open societies the choice is ultimately a matter of independent and often arbitrary professional standards. Those who choose subset discrimination are in good company for a number of reasons that involve a branch of scientific epistemology too tedious to argue here. Suffice it to say that one is compelled to agree with Popper (2002) on falsification as the most exalted test of universal truth, not independent corroboration or, worse, collaboration.

The Gantes *et al.* article still remains as a milestone in the evolution of corticotomy development, even though the outlier case

may have been caused by inefficient biomechanics, effete surgery, complicating medical issues, or idiosyncratic individual biodiversity. There is still a great deal of variance of style among surgical procedures, and contemporary protocols are still developing. So, some "failure" is always predictable. It is worth noting that a 95% confidence interval in biological research is merely another way of saying that one time in 20 (5%) we are wrong. This is why the research of Gantes *et al.* was valuable: it lent a note of caution, and that alone is clinically significant.

Their research also revealed a significant deficiency in the conceptual organization of orthodontically driven corticotomies in that generation. This deficiency, of course, has been addressed and rectified in subsequent publications. Worldwide, clinicians and academic researchers have found that the corticotomy works quite well where its limitations, so well defined by the excellent scholarship of Loma Linda University, are realized and avoided.

A twentieth-century summary

In retrospect, from the work of Bichlmayr and Köle to the turn of the new century, it becomes obvious that thinning of the alveolar volume in the direction of the tooth movement is a critically important consideration in the protocols of any orthodontic-driven corticotomy procedure. When one applies this nuanced philosophy to the surgical preparations, it becomes much easier to keep the entire OTM treatment times under 10 months except in cases of severe class III skeletal dysplasias.

The majority of treatment times range from 6 to 8 months with class I and mild class II malocclusions. Independent clinicians have documented that severe posterior crossbites and anterior open bites may be treated successfully in about 10–12 months. With the use of *ortho-pedic* forces (e.g., jack screws), space closing alone could be accomplished in 3–4 weeks, and with orthodontic forces one should reasonably expect a treatment duration of 10–12 weeks.

As the century closed, the specialty of dentoalveolar surgical orthodontics was reaching the end of clinical art and the beginning of a long scientific journey. Scientific specialists remained reasonably skeptical but undaunted because, with the consistently gratifying clinical results around a shrinking world, their collective confidence continued to grow.

TWENTY-FIRST-CENTURY PIONEERS

The entry of academics

By 2007, collaboration among clinicians and researchers at Case Western Reserve University and St, Louis and Boston universities (Twaddle, 2001; Hajji, 2002; Fulk, 2002; Machado *et al.*, 2002a,b; Kasewicz *et al.*, 2004; Skountrianos *et al.*, 2004; Ahlawat *et al.*, 2006; Dosanjh *et al.*, 2006a,b; Ferguson *et al.*, 2006; Nazarov *et al.*, 2006; Oliveira *et al.*, 2006; Sebaoun *et al.*, 2006, 2008; Walker *et al.*, 2006a,b) resulted in significant documentation of the SAD efficacy with disciplined university-level studies. Clinical researchers resolved once and for all much of the contention among the earlier clinicians by subjecting the SAD to detailed analysis and rigorous standards of evidence-based science. This is important because it positioned corticotomy procedures at the exalted level of university-based analysis and the kind of controlled experimentation it demands. At the time, these early 21st-century studies of SAD and PAOO were unparalleled; in retrospect their findings seem epochal.

PAOO/AOO and tissue engineering

Wilcko and co-workers (Wilcko *et al.*, 2001, 2003, 2008, 2009a,b, 2012) described an innovative strategy of combining the corticotomy with alveolar grafting in a technique referred to as the AOO technique or the PAOO technique. Initially, these protocols combined fixed orthodontic appliances, labial and palatal/lingual corticotomies, bone-thinning ostectomies at extractions sites and other selected areas, and particulate bone grafting materials. The introduction of PAOO/AOO marked a particular quantum leap into 21st-century tissue engineering and the tantalizing dynamics of biological nonlinear complexity (see Bak, P in Recommended reading). This is because these techniques engineer novel genetic expression and morphogenesis[8] that seems to account for the stability of the outcome.

Tooth movement with the PAOO/AOO techniques was typically initiated sometime during the week preceding the surgery and every 2 weeks thereafter by activation of the orthodontic appliance. The resultant the creation of bone *de novo* was a revelation. Prior to this observation it was considered axiomatic that one "…cannot grow bone on a flat surface." Yet PAOO/AOO did just that.

The first publication by Wilcko and co-workers was preceded by 8 years of research and development on humans, which began by performing corticotomy surgeries without bone grafting on both young adolescents and adults. Prior to this research, corticotomy-based surgeries were only recommended for individuals 18 years of age or older following the cessation of growth. As a part of their research protocols, high-resolution hospital-based surface CT scans were performed on their patients both pre- and post-treatment.

The high-resolution surface CT scans showed what appeared to be a demineralization–remineralization process at work. The Drs Wilcko first suggested that this was consistent with Frost's (1983) RAP. The most rapid movement was most highly correlated with the thinnest volumes of bone attached to the periodontal ligament (attachment apparatus). This is what inspired the hypothesis that a demineralized matrix was seemingly transported with the root surface and available for remineralization following the cessation of tooth movement. The remineralization process, when completed in the adolescent, seemed to reestablish the original bony (native) architecture usually within 2–3 years. In the adult, however, the remineralization process, when complete, seemed to result in a net loss in bone volume and mass if particulate bone grafts were not included in the surgical procedure (PAOO/AOO).

Wilcko and co-workers have repeatedly referred to this phenomenon as "bone matrix transportation," and it is that phenomenon that effects a consistent 300–400% increase in tooth movement rate when combined with efficient biomechanical protocols. These evidence-based studies replicated those of Köle and Bichlmayr and substantiated the merits of SFOT with more sophistication than the prior clinical reports achieved by trial, error, and speculation.

It is important to note that if a tooth is being moved through a large volume of bone it is likely that only about a 30% increase in movement efficiency will be realized. This is consistent with the many findings of others throughout the last two decades. For example, even when RAP is employed, the bodily translation of a tooth through the long axis of the alveolus will typically only allow for about a millimeter of movement per month when no significant entry into interproximal medullary bone is made (Iino et al., 2006).

What the corticotomy-derived procedures are not

The PAOO technique[9] was proven to be a very efficient orthodontic protocol with a predictable and safe in-office surgical component. It was demonstrated in many independent cases that patient care could be completed in one-third to one-fourth the time required for traditional orthodontics, and borderline orthognathic cases could be improved or even precluded entirely. It is important to note that, through the research, two salient functions of PAOO/AOO were repeatedly emphasized. The newest developments of SFOT continue to define new horizons for orthodontists, periodontists, and oral/maxillofacial surgeons alike, but they are not variants of orthognathic surgery. The latter is a rearrangement of basal bone parts rather than a re-engineering of alveolus bone physiology with endogenous biochemical and exogenous load applications. Yet, this modest manipulation of the alveolus bone with PAOO/AOO and other surgical interventions serves two basic functions: (a) facilitated tooth movement and (b) an increase in the alveolar volume. Alluded to above, this dualism deserves some elaboration.

Facilitated tooth movement

The facilitated tooth movement can be maximized as RAP provides a dramatic decrease in bone density (mass per unit volume). SAD must maintain a thin layer of bone over the root enface, the surface in the direction of the intended tooth movement. This thin layer of bone can readily undergo amplified demineralization as a result of a surgically stimulated RAP, and the resulting soft demineralized tissue matrix of the bone carried with the root surfaces (demineralized bone matrix transportation) can remineralize during retention. This remineralization process is fairly complete in the adolescent, but only partially complete in the adult. That is to say, in the absence of alveolar augmentation there may be a net loss in bone volume in the adult that justifies the bone graft with DBM or stem cells (see Figure 1.2) allografts to compensate for matrix deficiency (e.g., iatrogenic gingival recession) during mechanotherapy.

Increasing the alveolar volume

The increased alveolar volume is accomplished by placing a relatively large mass of resorbable particulate bone grafting material or stem cell allograft between an intact elevated periosteum and the opposing denuded alveolus. The main intent is to increase the likelihood of having the roots of the teeth "sandwiched" between intact buccal and lingual plates of bone. Maintaining the continuity of the periosteum is critical in maximizing the volume of this new bone. Pre-existing dehiscences and fenestrations can be eliminated (Figure 1.11), but only where

(a)   (b)

(c)   (d)

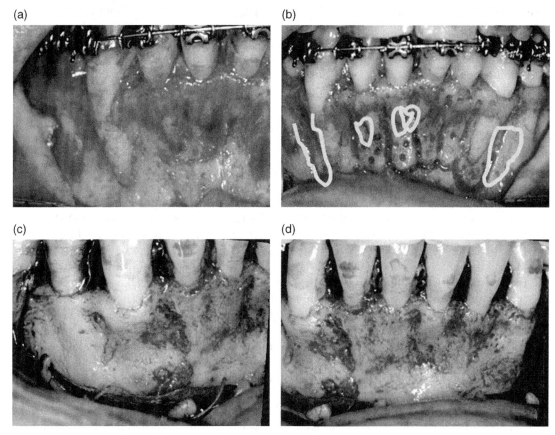

Figure 1.11 Demonstration that PAOO/AOO can create healthy alveolar bone in a steady state that lasts indefinitely. The bony dehiscence on the patient lower right canine in (a) and the fenestrations, outlined with light blue in (b) are sufficiently ensconced in bone even after 8 years (c,d). This is understandable since the procedure takes advantage of epigenetic restructuring of morphogenesis during healing by using the roots of the teeth as the functional matrix (see Moss (1997)) for new phenotype formation. This exemplifies how healthy, stable alveolus bone can be created *de novo* with the PAOO/AOO protocol. Previous to this demonstration it was believed by many periodontists that alveolar bone could not be "grown on a flat surface." This opinion is generally correct and precludes complete alveolus regeneration in the absence of orthodontic-induced strain. The combination of bone grafting, decortication, and induced strain suffice to overcome epigenetic buffering. Courtesy of Wilckodontics, Inc.

there is still vital root surface apical to the epithelial attachment (junctional epithelium). The ability to increase the alveolar volume makes it feasible to dramatically increase the envelope of motion, minimize gingival recession, reduce relapse, reduce the need for tooth extractions, minimize the risks of some orthognathic surgery, soften the acute angle of the labiomental fold, and reshape facial appearance ("face morphing") as an applied epigenetic event (Hochedlinger and Plath, 2009).

Special elaboration should be made about PAOO/AOO. In the growing child or adolescent the robust regenerative potential is evidenced by copious bony support of the teeth even in arch length deficiencies. Yet, in the older adolescent and adults there is often a net tissue loss when SAD is performed without bone graft supplementation. Figure 1.2 illustrates this phenomenon most clearly. Figure 1.2-1a demonstrates a pre-treatment high-resolution CT scan (accurate to 0.2 mm) of the lower arch of a female, age 39, prior to having circumscribing corticotomy cuts performed both labially and lingually around the six lower anterior teeth. Note the arch length deficiency (overlap crowding), the pronounced crestal glabella, and the distance between the crest of the alveolus and the corresponding cemento-enamel junctions. Clinically, the circumscribing corticotomy cuts resulted in the appearance of outlined "blocks of bone" connected by medullary bone.

The total treatment time for this case was 4 months and 2 weeks with eight adjustment appointments. Figure 1.2-1b shows that, at 1 month retention, the integrity of the outlined blocks of bone appears to have been completely lost and the layer of bone over the labial root surfaces appears to have vanished. In reality this layer of bone has undergone demineralization as the result of the normal osteopenic state (RAP); the soft tissue matrix of the bone remains but is not visible radiographically. This demineralized matrix was carried into position with the root surfaces (bone matrix transportation).

Figure 1.2-1c shows the high-resolution CT scan at 2 years and 8 months retention. Note that the layer of bone over the root surfaces has only partially reappeared due to the remineralization of the soft tissue matrix. This suggests that there has been a *net loss of bone volume* in this adult. In adolescents this is not seen. Owing to a greater regenerative potential, there seems to be a complete regeneration of bone after SAD.

Figure 1.2-2a, again a high-resolution CT scan of the lower arch, this time of a male, age 23, prior to circumscribing corticotomy cuts being performed both buccally and lingually around all of the lower teeth with a large bone graft placed over the corticotomized bone. Note the paucity of bone over the buccal root surfaces. The total treatment time was 6 months and 2 weeks with 12 adjustment appointments. At 3 months retention Figure 1.2-2b shows the labial root surfaces are now covered with an intact layer of newly engineered phenotype appropriate for the new position of tooth roots (the functional matrix of the bone).The pre-existing paucity of bone over the lingual root surfaces has been corrected in the same manner so that the roots of the teeth are now "sandwiched" between intact layers of bone both buccally and lingually. There has been a *net increase in bone volume*. At 2 years and 8 months retention, Figure 1.2-2c shows the increase in the alveolar volume has been maintained.

In the years around 2006 the Ferguson research group made great strides in documenting the science behind corticotomy procedures, which should inspire others. They characterized the RAP as amplified metabolic modeling of the alveolus adjacent to the SAD. The intensified anabolic activity in the rat appears to be increased by 150% at 3 weeks. This increase represents about a two- to threefold greater anabolic modeling activity in the spongiosa compared with same-animal contralateral controls. This same year, Sebaoun *et al.* (2008) reported a 200% multiple of spongiosa catabolic activity and a 400% increase in osteoblastic activity at 3 weeks in the rat model. It was concluded that this effect represents the normal physiologic mechanism at the molecular level which quite adequately explains rapid OTM.

This emphasis on biochemical analysis evokes speculation about possible pharmaceutical manipulations to elicit so-called "optimal bone response." Optimal response is now the natural complement of any dialogue about optimal force. The fact that it may be done with pharmaceutical manipulation in situ is not only intriguing, but also, by reports of the Ferguson research group,[10] both proven in principle and justified by evidence.

The researchers of SAD, PAOO/AOO, TMP, and various other corticotomy incarnations have shown that it is important to maintain a strict, technique-sensitive protocol if one wishes to avoid a wide variance in clinical outcomes. While variance is inevitable, and indeed the fountainhead of creative progress, variance and occasional untoward events can be minimized by strict adherence to protocols that have been proven to protect patients and doctors. Undocumented facsimiles may not work as well as the evidence-based original described herein as it has evolved and is taught at university-standard institutions.

The post-modern consortium of dental scientists has convincingly demonstrated the very limited distance to which RAP extends from the point of surgical entry (approximately 2–3 mm in conservative surgery). Another advantage that analytical science lends to orthodontics is the concept of "enhanced relative anchorage." This is a term reserved for the development of differential anchorage advantages incurred when the treated segment of the dentition is rendered more mobile, thus enhancing the established anchorage units, *relatively*.

Following the realization that the facilitated tooth movement was an amplification of normal physiologic tooth movement metabolism, researchers attempted to rapidly close bicuspid extraction spaces without removing the interradicular bone around the extraction

socket (buccal and lingual cortices). This attempt met relative failure, demonstrating that the cortices were indeed a source of anchorage strain and tooth movement resistance. The space closure alone was requiring nearly 7 months, and the overall treatments took over 1 year to complete.

What had begun at American universities as treating moderate malocclusion faster has blossomed within two decades into predictable protocols for the successful treatment of very complicated cases and ushered in the compelling science of tissue engineering and SCT. The treatment planning can at first seem daunting, and sometimes requires different sets of diagnostic parameters (even to the threshold of life itself (Gibson *et al.*, 2010), and, indeed, even new ways of thinking. But with a much better understanding of alveolar bone osteology, the new depth of orthodontic science has expanded the horizons of both orthodontics and periodontics and fostered their development into sophisticated multidisciplinary specialty options.

ORTHO-INFECTION HYPOTHESIS FOR GINGIVAL RECESSION

A credible discussion of any clinical practice is painfully incomplete without addressing the potential for irreversible tissue damage by oral infection. The fact that therapy may be accelerated also implies that the emergence of pernicious side effects may also be accelerated. Periodontal infections are endemic, and we operate in a bacterial stew of pathogens and commensal microorganisms. The bacterial biofilm in which they thrive can be modified, but this habitat cannot be eliminated. So, its effect on treatment must be acknowledged and constantly modulated. Knowing how the bacterial niche created by orthodontic appliances interacts with orthodontic therapy gives us insight into side effects that are predictable in the aggregate but *not necessarily foreseeable in the particular*. Thus, a kind of universally precautionary protocol must always be maintained, and every patient must be informed of untoward bacterial events.

Usually, the orthodontist cannot act without some significant compromise of the supporting structures; periodontal impunity is the exception, not the rule. For example, Waldrop (2008) has pointed out that over 50% of adolescents may have permanent damage to soft gingival tissue, and we have known for nearly four decades that about 10% will demonstrate permanent damage to the alveolus bone (attachment apparatus) (Zachrisson and Alnaes, 1973). Permanent damage to the soft tissues (hyperplasia) is easily rectified by periodontal flap surgery. But when gingivitis progresses to periodontitis, with the loss of the first bone cell, the tissue dynamic is no longer a steady state; it is progressive and self-perpetuating.

However, one area of tissue dynamics has been placed at the feet of orthodontists unfairly. Gingival recession (bony and soft tissue dehiscence) is one example of a self-perpetuating bony pathosis, referred to in orthodontic parlance by the unfortunate term "runner." But this particular phenomenon is mischaracterized as an effect of orthodontic therapy which pushes a tooth outside of its "alveolar housing." This is a mistaken notion. Djeu *et al.* (2002), among others (Artun and Krogstad, 1987; Wennstrom *et al.*, 1987; Ruf *et al.*, 1998; Artun and Grobety, 2001), showed that there is no correlation between specific types of OTM and gingival recession, while others consider such movement a mucogingival threat (Dorfman, 1978; Hollender *et al.*, 1980; Genco, 1996), or at least a contestable issue (Melsen, 2012). So any discussion of corticotomy-like procedure involves the issue of mucogingival stress, bony dehiscences, and gingival recession.

A thorough review of the scientific literature suggests that an indeterminate variable in many of the studies of gingival recession and OTM is the quantity and quality of bacterial biofilm (plaque) accumulations and the host's local/systemic resistance. So, from an etiological and logical epistemological perspective indeed, a strong case can be made that the proximate cause of "runners" may not even involve OTM at all. Aleo *et al.* (1974) noted that bacteria endotoxins can inhibit fibroplasia. So, one may hypothesize that, when tooth movement requires fibroplasia to adjust phenotype for compensatory gingival adaptation, the compensatory soft tissue generation can be inhibited by patient noncompliance. Where OTM is increasingly viewed as a commodity the risk to patient welfare is increased by the contributory negligence of the dental "consumer."

Thus, although gingival recession cannot be correlated with OTM, the attachment loss it reflects can indeed be directly attributed to patient negligence. So any "cause" by orthodontists can only be attributed to acts of behavioral omission, not acts of therapeutic commission. In other words, OTM may be, in some cases, a necessary cause (contributory factor), but it appears as neither a proximate cause nor a *sine qua non* in all cases. The categorical assertion that "orthodontics tooth movement 'causes' gingival recession" is without compelling scientific basis and assumes the status of a clinical wives' tale. A new, better substantiated, and logical orthodontic-infection hypothesis posits that "runners are caused by germs." The take-home message is this: practicing corticotomy-facilitated orthodontic therapy without some management and disclosure of the risk of infection is tantamount to practicing in a wooden structure without a fire extinguisher.

CONCLUSIONS

This treatise purposely evokes controversial issues in a historical context to give the thoughtful clinician pause for reflection in a meaningful dialectic. The dialectical progression, borne of controversy and its consequent explication of important nuance, continue today through the *Sturm und Drang* of daily practice. When kept legitimate it is the stuff of progress; when abused it invites intellectual corruption. That difference is decided by the earnest professional men and women, elevating daily observations and opinions to that higher level of intellectual abstraction where universal truth abides. What is heartening to any progressive orthodontist is that this moderate and collegial dissonance can deliver practical clinical outcomes and enriching professional insights. With the artists' intuitions and the scientists' cold, redoubtable truths, it is the clinician as the frontline soldier who must sort out all the proverbial wheat from the sophistic chaff, all on behalf of the patient. That is our mission, our duty, and our privilege.

It is incumbent on all students of dentofacial orthopedics to actualize their full potential if this technique is to be realized. As specialists, we need to continually strive for perfection knowing full well that we will never achieve it. To quote Professor Colin Richman, "The PAOO™ technique is not for unschooled amateurs."[11] But challenge is why good students become scientists.

Art, while endlessly enchanting, can all too often parade as pseudo-intellectualism. The artist's mind runs free but undisciplined. Then, like a random walk, it ultimately leads us nowhere but where we started. Proffering an enriching grace to the human condition, the artist's brush, especially drawn untrue over the face of youth, cannot be erased if wrong. By contrast, the disciplined journey through the rigors of logical and scientific scrutiny leads to greater certitude, health, and predictable success. For the certitude we seek, science must be universal and timeless, reassuring us that, whenever we employ it, we may find a safe and steady path, literally into the human genome itself.[12]

True, it cannot be denied that at times many clinical imperatives of scientific truth require an artistic embellishment. This is indeed evident in the literature of orthodontic-driven corticotomy procedures. Still, it is within the firmament of science where fragile individual expressions of clinical art bloom under the aegis of predictable competence. Thus, in the grander schemes of the dental specialties, we posit that all SFOT will be enriched and fortified, in the dawn of oral tissue engineering. Rathbun's and Gantes' (personal communication, 2013) cautions in this regard are particularly sage. In retrospect, they remind us that treatments of young patients and short durations make careful treatment planning a critical clinical imperative; there is no substitute for assiduous scholarship. This is why constant tooth movement or the liberal use of periodic TMP is important, and an adroit orchestration of many modalities is needed to define the master clinician.

This, we contend, complementing the art of traditional biomechanics, is a clarion call to progress, not a siren song. SFOT protocols are destined neither to founder on the shoals of fatuous novelty nor fall ensnared in clinical disappointment. They shall find enrichment through the following chapters as our esteemed and dedicated colleagues take us on a journey toward an exciting future. And that personal future, liberated from the minions of corporate leviathans, untethered from the mindless morass of autocratic statists, renders individually and collectively a bountiful province for each of us to define in our clinical practice. The rhetorical question that this sojourn entreats is: "Will we choose to?"
Quo Vadis

AN AFTERWORD FOR ACADEMIC LEADERS

Twentieth-century orthodontist educators have the comfortable option of continuing the standard model of orthodontic tissue dynamics, essentially a 1901–1911 dogma, but that is fraught with significant risks to clinical identity and patient safety. The fate of the new generation of orthodontists can lie within a greater vision, one of biological engineering that transcends the venerable art of wire bending. On a practical level, traditional wire bending art, in the age of evidence-based dentistry, may fade into an interesting anachronism as straight-wire biomechanics becomes commoditized in the hands of nonspecialists.

Tissue engineering, in contrast, does not lend itself to commoditization. Therefore, new orthodontists, heirs apparent and champions of the specialty, have an existential choice upon graduation from their training: will they become corporate minions, distributing a mere commodity of short-order smiles, plebian artisans, or applied tissue engineers, thinking independently to bring the best science to each individual patient.

As this brief history lesson has demonstrated, time carries us to new vistas often only dreamed about or hinted at by previous generations. Sometimes these vistas are presaged in other specialty literature or in discussions of other subjects, or ironically even from nonacademic sources. It is only the thorough scholar who will pick up such nuances. Then, the future arrives at our doorstep whether we like it or not. The challenge is to separate transient fashion from tidal change.

Orthodontic-driven corticotomy procedures subsumed by the entire promise of SFOT is tissue engineering and it is not going away; the question is whether curricular innovations will go along with it. Defining new frontiers has always been the credo for the orthodontic specialty, but that legacy will endure only by the younger generation of orthodontists who wish to supplement the mantle of clinical artist with surgical dentofacial orthopedics. This "NewThink," like the existential choice of personal optimism, can define both the specific nature of each case and the specialty in general.
Carpe diem!

Notes

1 "Give the adolescent an adult smile he can grow into, not an adolescent smile he will grow out of" (Williams MO, personal communication, 2013).
2 See Recommended reading.
3 Both the AOO technique and the PAOO technique are patented and trademarked by Wilckodontics, Inc. Erie, PA, USA. The acronym PAOO is generally used by the lead author when AOO candidates present periodontal issues.
4 Also known as demineralized freeze-dried bone allograft.
5 *Weltanschauung* (worldview) is a term used by educational psychologists and refers to the phenomenon by which the psyche interprets and adapts to a novel environment. Freud (1990: 195) said it is "…an intellectual construction which gives a unified solution of all the problems of our existence in virtue of a comprehensive hypothesis, a construction, therefore, in which no question is left open and in which everything in which we are interested finds a place." This plays an important part in the acculturation process for SFOT, which some academic institutions are precluded from inculcating due to intransigent socio-political commitments.
6 See Pirsig R in Recommended reading.
7 *Post hoc ergo propter hoc* (after this therefore because of this).
8 Wound healing recapitulates regional ontogeny (Murphy, 2006).
9 Both the AOO technique and the PAOO technique are patented and trademarked by Wilckodontics, Inc. Erie, PA, USA. The acronym PAOO is generally used by the lead author when AOO candidates present periodontal issues.
10 Donald J Ferguson DMD, MSD and his academic protégés made significant contributions to accelerated OTM and the nascent science of oral tissue engineering from his research facilities at St Louis University and

Boston University. After this prodigious independent corroboration he was appointed Dean of the European University College of the United Arab Emirates.

11 Assistant Clinical Professor, Georgia Health Sciences University, Augusta, GA, USA. Personal communication, 2013.

12 23andme, Inc. Mountain View, CA USA, www.23andme.com.

References

Ahlawat A, Ferguson DJ, Wilcko WM *et al.* (2006) Influence of DI on orthodontic outcomes following selective alveolar decortication. ADEA/AADR/CADR, Orlando, FL, March 8–11, abstract 0779.

Aleo JJ, DeRenzis FA, Farber PA *et al.* (1974) The presence and biologic activity of cementum-bound endotoxin. *Journal of Periodontology*, **45** (9), 672–675.

Anholm JM, Crites DA, Hoff R *et al.* (1986) Corticotomy-facilitated orthodontics. *Journal of California Dental Association*, **14** (12), 7–11.

Artun J, Grobety D (2001) Periodontal status of mandibular incisors after pronounced orthodontic advancement during adolescence: a follow-up evaluation. *American Journal of Orthodontics and Dentofacial Orthopedics*, **119**, 2–10.

Artun J, Krogstad O (1987) Periodontal status of mandibular incisors following excessive proclination: a study in adults with surgically treated mandibular prognathism. *American Journal of Orthodontics and Dentofacial Orthopedics*, **91**, 225–232.

Ascher F (1947) Zur Spaetbehandlung der Prognathie des Oberkiefers. *Deutsche Zahnarztliche Zeitschrift*, **2**, 218–226.

Bell WH, Levy BM (1972) Revascularization and bone healing after maxillary corticotomies. *Journal of Oral Surgery*, **30**, 640–648.

Benjamin M, Hillen B (2003) Mechanical influences on cells, tissues and organs – 'mechanical morphogenesis'. *European Journal of Morphology*, **41** (1), 3–7.

Bichlmayr A (1931) Chirurgische Kiefer-orthopaedie und das verhalten des Knochens und der Wurzelspitzen nach derselben. *Deutsche Zahnaerztl Woschenschrift*, **34**, 835–842.

Cano J, Campo J, Bonilla E *et al.* (2012) Corticotomy-assisted orthodontics. *Journal of Clinical and Experimental Dentistry*, **4** (1), e54–e59.

Chung KR, Oh MY, Ko SJ (2001) Corticotomy-assisted orthodontics. *Journal of Clinical Orthodontics*, **35**, 331–339.

Cohn-Stock G.(1921) Die Chirurgische immediatregulierung der Kiefer Speziell die Chirurgische Behandlung der Prognathie. *Vierteljahrsschrift fur Zahnheilkunde*, **37**, 320–354.

Cunningham G (1894) Methode sofortiger regulierung von Anomalenz Oesterreichisch–Ungarische. *Vierteljahrsschrift Zahnheilkd*, **10**, 455–457.

Djeu G, Hayes C, Zawaideh S (2002) Correlation between mandibular central incisor proclination and gingival recession during fixed appliance therapy. *Angle Orthodontics*, **72** (3), 238–245.

Dorfman HS (1978) Mucogingival changes resulting from mandibular incisor tooth movement. *American Journal of Orthodontics*, **74**, 286–297.

Dosanjh MS, Ferguson DJ, Wilcko WM *et al.* (2006a) Orthodontic outcome changes during retention following selective alveolar decortication. ADEA/AADR/CADR, Orlando, FL, March 8–11, abstract 0768.

Dosanjh MS, Ferguson DJ, Wilcko WM *et al.* (2006b) Orthodontic outcome changes during retention following selective alveolar decortication. *Journal of Dental Research*, **85** (Spec Iss A), abstract 0768.

Düker J (1975) Experimental animal research into segmental alveolar movement after corticotomy. *Journal of Maxillofacial Surgery*, **3** (2), 81–84.

Ferguson DJ, Sebaoun J-D, Turner JW *et al.* (2006) Anabolic modeling of trabecular bone following selective alveolar decortication. *Journal of Dental Research*, **85** (Spec Iss A), abstract 0786.

Freud S (1990) *New Introductory Lectures on Psycho-Analysis, The Standard Edition. Complete Psychological Works of Sigmund Freud* (ed. J Strachy), Norton, New York, NY.

Frost HM (1983) The regional acceleratory phenomenon: a review. *Henry Ford Hospital Medical Journal*, **31**, 3–9.

Fulk L (2002) Lower arch decrowding comparing corticotomy-facilitated, midline distraction and conventional orthodontic techniques. Master's thesis, St Louis University, St Louis, MO, USA.

Gantes B, Rathbun E, Anholm M (1990) Effects on the periodontium following corticotomy-facilitated orthodontics: case reports. *Journal of Periodontology*, **62**, 234–238.

Genco RJ (1996) Current view of risk factors for periodontal diseases. *Journal of Periodontology*, **67**, 1041–1049.

Generson RM, Porter JM, Zell A *et al.* (1978) Combined surgical and orthodontic management of anterior open bite using corticotomy. *Journal of Oral Surgery*, **36**, 216–219.

Gibson DG, Glass JI, Lartigue C *et al.* (2010) Creation of a bacterial cell controlled by a synthesized genome. *Science*, **329** (5987), 52–56.

Goldson L, Reck VJ (1987) Surgical-orthodontic treatment of malpositioned cuspids. *Journal of Clinical Orthodontics*, **21**, 847–851.

Hajji SS (2002) The influence of accelerated osteogenic response on mandibular decrowding. Master's thesis, St Louis University, St Louis, MO, USA.

Hochedlinger K, Plath K (2009) Epigenetic reprogramming and induced pluripotency. *Development*, **136**, 509–523.

Hoff RE (1986) Corticotomy-facilitated orthodontic treatment in adults: a report of two cases. Master's thesis, Department of Orthodontics, School of Dentistry, Loma Linda University, Loma Linda, CA, USA.

Hollender L, Ronnerman A, Thilander B (1980) Root resorption marginal bone support and clinical crown length in orthodontically treated patients. *European Journal of Orthodontics*, **2**, 197–205.

Hwang HS, Lee KH (2001) Intrusion of over-erupted molars by corticotomy and magnets. *American Journal of Orthodontics and Dentofacial Orthopedics*, **120**, 209–216.

Iino S, Sakoda S, Miyawaki S (2006) An adult maxillary protrusion treated with corticotomy-facilitated orthodontics and titanium miniplates. *Angle Orthodontics*, **76**, 1074–1082.

Kasewicz MJ, Ferguson DJ, Wilcko WM (2004) Characterization of tooth movement in corticotomy-facilitated, non-extraction orthodontics. *Journal of Dental Research*, **83** (Spec Iss A), abstract 1289.

Khng PFM (1993) A non-human primate model for evaluating a fenestration corticotomy technique. Master's thesis, Department of Orthodontics, School of Dentistry, Loma Linda University, Loma Linda, CA, USA.

Kim S-C, Tae K-C (2003) Corticotomy and intrusive tooth movement. *Korean Journal of Orthodontics*, **33** (5), 399–405.

Kim SJ, Park YG, Kang SG (2009) Effects of corticision on paradental remodeling in orthodontic tooth movement. *Angle Orthodontics*, **79** (2), 284–291.

Kolář J, Babicky A, Vrabec R (1965) *The Physical Agents and Bone.* Czechoslovak Academy of Sciences, Prague.

Köle H (1959) Surgical operations of the alveolar ridge to correct occlusal abnormalities. *Oral Surgery, Oral Medicine, Oral Pathology*, **12**, 515–529.

Kretz R (1931) *Die chirurgische Immediatregulierung der Prognathie.* Deutsche Zahnheilkunde in Vorträgen, Issue 81, Thieme, Leipzig.

Kuhn TS (2012) *The Structure of Scientific Revolutions*, University of Chicago Press, Chicago, IL.

Machado I, Ferguson DJ, Wilcko WM (2002a) Root resorption following orthodontics with and without alveolar corticotomy. *Journal of Dental Research*, **81**, abstract 2378.

Machado IM, Ferguson DJ, Wilcko WM *et al.* (2002b) Reabsorción radicular despues del tratamiento ortodoncico con o sin corticotomia alveolar. *Review Venezuela Orthodontics*, **19**, 647–653.

Melsen B (2012) *Adult Orthodontics*, Wiley–Blackwell, London.

Merrill RG, Pedersen GW (1976) Interdental osteotomy for immediate repositioning of dental-osseous elements. *Journal of Oral Surgery*, **34**, 118–125.

Mihram ML, Murphy NC (2008) The orthodontist's role in 21st century periodontic-prosthodontic therapy. *Seminars in Orthodontics*, **14** (4), 272–289.

Moss ML (1997) The functional matrix hypothesis revisited. 2. The role of an osseous connected cellular network. *American Journal of Orthodontics and Dentofacial Orthopedics*, **112** (2), 221–226.

Mostafa YA, Tawfik KM, El-Mangoury NH (1985) Surgical-orthodontic treatment for overerupted maxillary molars. *Journal of Clinical Orthodontics*, **19**, 350–351.

Murphy NC (2006) In vivo tissue engineering for the orthodontists: a modest first step, in *Biologic Mechanisms of Tooth Eruption, Resorption and Movement* (eds Z Davidovitch, J Mah, S Suthanarak), Harvard Society for the Advancement of Orthodontics, Boston, MA, pp. 385–410 (available at www.University Experts.com).

Murphy NC. (2010) Accelerated osteogenic orthodontics [Letter to Editor]. *American Journal of Orthodontics and Dentofacial Orthopedics*, **137** (1), 2–3.

Murphy NC, de Alba JA, Chaconas SJ *et al.* (1982) Experimental force analysis of the contraction utility arch wire. *American Journal of Orthodontics*, **82** (5), 411–417.

Murphy NC, Bissada NF, Davidovitch Z *et al.* (2012) Corticotomy and stem cell therapy for orthodontists and periodontists: rationale, hypotheses and protocol, in *Integrated Clinical Orthodontics* (eds V Krishnan, Z Davidovitch), Blackwell, Oxford.

Nazarov AD, Ferguson DJ, Wilcko WM *et al.* (2006) Improved orthodontic retention following corticotomy using ABO objective grading system. *Journal of Dental Research*, **85** (Spec Iss A), abstract 2644.

Neumann D (1955) Die Bichlmayrsche keilresektion bei der kieferothopaedischen Spaetbehandlung. *Fortschritte der Kiefer- und Gesichts-Chirurgie*, **1**, 205–210.

Oliveira K, Ferguson DJ, Wilcko WM *et al.* (2006) Orthodontic stability of advanced lower incisors following selective alveolar decortication. ADEA/AADR/CADR, Orlando, FL, March 8–11, abstract 0769.

Park Y-G, Kang S-G, Kim S-J (2006) Accelerated tooth movement by corticision as an osseous orthodontic paradigm. *Journal of Kinki-Tokai Orthodontic Society*, **41** (1), 62.

Popper K (2002) *The Logic of Scientific Discovery*, Routledge, New York, NY.

Reichenbach E (1965) Die chirurgische Behandlung des offenen Bisses. Cited by Mohnac AM (1965) Surgical correction of maxillo-mandibular deformities. *Journal of Oral Surgery*, **23**, 393–407.

Rynearson RD (1987) A non-human primate model for studying corticotomy-facilitated orthodontic tooth movement. Master's thesis, Department of Orthodontics, School of Dentistry, Loma Linda University, Loma Linda, CA, USA.

Rynearson RD (1988) A nonhuman primate model for studying corticotomy-facilitated orthodontic tooth movement. *American Journal of Orthodontics and Dentofacial Orthopedics*, **94** (6), 528.

Ruf S, Hansen K, Pancherz H (1998) Does orthodontic proclination of lower incisors in children and adolescents cause gingival recession? *American Journal of Orthodontics and Dentofacial Orthopedics*, **114**, 100–106.

Sebaoun JD, Ferguson DJ, Kantarci A *et al.* (2006) Catabolic modeling of trabecular bone following selective alveolar decortication. *Journal of Dental Research*, **85** (Spec Iss A), abstract 0787.

Sebaoun J-D, Kantarci A, Turner JW *et al.* (2008) Modeling of trabecular bone and lamina dura following selective alveolar decortication in rats. *Journal of Periodontology*, **79** (9), 1679–1688.

Siegal ML, Bergman A (2002) Waddington's canalization revisited: developmental stability and evolution. *Proceedings of the National Academy of Sciences of the United States of America*, **99**, 10528–10532.

Skogsborg C (1926) Die permanente Fixierung der Zähne nach orthodontischer Behandlung. *Vierteljahrsschrift fur Zahnheilkunde*, **4**, 278.

Skountrianos HS, Ferguson DJ, Wilcko WM *et al.* (2004) Maxillary arch de-crowding and stability with and without corticotomy-facilitated orthodontics. *Journal of Dental Research*, **81**, abstract 2643J.

Slack JM (2002) Conrad Hal Waddington. The last renaissance biologist? *Nature Reviews/ Genetics*, **3**, 889–895.

Stearns SC (2002) Progress on canalization. *Proceedings of the National Academy of Sciences of the United States of America*, **99** (16), 10229–10230.

Suya H (1991) Corticotomy in orthodontics, in *Mechanical and Biological Basics in Orthodontic Therapy* (eds E Hosl, A Baldauf), Huthig Buch Verlag, Heidelberg, pp. 207–226.

Tetz DF (1986) Active treatment time and incisor root resorption of malocclusions treated with corticotomy-facilitated orthodontics vs. non-corticotomy treatment. Master's thesis, Department of Orthodontics, School of Dentistry, Loma Linda University, Loma Linda, CA, USA.

Twaddle BA (2001) Dentoalveolar bone density changes following accelerated osteogenesis. Master's thesis, St Louis University, St Louis, MO, USA.

Verna C, Melsen B (2012) Tissue reaction, in *Adult Orthodontics* (ed. B Melsen), Wiley-Blackwell, Oxford, pp. 80–92.

Waddington CH (1957) *The Strategy of the Genes: A Discussion of Some Aspects of Theoretical Biology*, Allen & Unwin, London.

Waldrop T (2008) Gummy smiles: the challenge of gingival excess: prevalence and guidelines for clinical management. *Seminars in Orthodontics*, **14** (4), 260–271.

Walker E, Ferguson, DJ, Wilcko WM *et al.* (2006a) Orthodontic treatment and retention outcomes following selective alveolar decortication. ADEA/AADR/CADR, Orlando, FL, March 8–11, abstract 0770.

Walker E, Ferguson DJ, Wilcko WM *et al.* (2006b) Orthodontic treatment and retention outcomes following selective alveolar decortication. *Journal of Dental Research*, **85** (Spec Iss A), abstract 0770.

Wennstrom JL, Lindhe J, Sinclair F *et al.* (1987) Some periodontal tissue reactions to orthodontic tooth movement in monkeys. *Journal of Clinical Periodontology*, **14**, 121–129.

Wilcko WM, Wilcko MT, Bouquot JE, Ferguson DJ (2001) Rapid orthodontics with alveolar reshaping: Two case reports of decrowding. *Int J Periodontics Restorative Dent*, **21** (1), 9–19.

Wilcko WM, Ferguson DJ, Bouquot JE, Wilcko MT (2003) Rapid orthodontic decrowding with alveolar augmentation:case report. *World J Orthodont*, **4** (3), 197–205.

Wilcko MT, Wilcko WM (2009) Single Surgery comprehensive gingival grafting utilizing palatal donor tissue. *Journal of Implantology and Advanced Clinical Dentistry*, **1** (6), 29–45.

Wilcko MT, Wilcko WM (2011) The Wilckodontics Accelerated Osteogenic Orthodontics (AOO) technique: an overview. *Orthotown*, (July–August), 36–48.

Wilcko MT, Wilcko WM, Omniewski KB *et al.* (2009a) The Periodontally Accelerated Osteogenic Orthodontics (PAOO) technique: efficient space closing with either orthopedic or orthodontic forces. *Journal of Implantology and Advanced Clinical Dentistry*, **1** (1), 45–63.

Wilcko MT, Wilcko WM, Pulver JJ *et al.* (2009b) Accelerated Osteogenic Orthodontic technique: a 1-stage surgically facilitated rapid orthodontic technique with alveolar augmentation. *Journal of Oral and Maxillofacial Surgery*, **67** (10), 2149–2159.

Wilcko MT, Wilcko WM, Bissada NF (2008) An evidence-based analysis of periodontally accelerated orthodontic and osteogenic techniques: a synthesis of scientific perspectives. *Seminar in Orthodontics*, **14** (4), 305–316.

Williams MO, Murphy NC (2008) Beyond the ligament: a whole-bone periodontal view of dentofacial orthopedics and falsification of universal alveolar immutability. *Seminars in Orthodontics*, **14** (4), 246–259.

Yaffe A, Fine N, Binderman I (1994) Regional accelerated phenomenon in the mandible following mucoperiosteal flap surgery. *Journal of Periodontology*, **65** (1), 79–83.

Zachrisson B, Alnaes L (1973) Periodontal condition in orthodontically treated and untreated individuals. I. Loss of attachment, gingival pocket depth and clinical crown height. *Angle Orthodontics*, **43**, 402–411.

Recommended reading

Alberts B, Johnson A, Lewis J, *et al.* (2012) *Molecular Biology of the Cell*, 5th edn, Garland Science, New York, NY.

Bak, P (1999) *How Nature Works: The Science of Self-Organized Criticality*, Copernicus Springer Verlag, New York, NY.

Bilezikian JP, Raisz LG, Martin TJ (eds) (2008) *Principles of Bone Biology*, 3rd edn, Academic Press, San Diego, CA.

Lanza R, Langer R, Vacanti J. (2013) *Principles of Tissue Engineering*, 4th edn, Elsevier, Boston, MA.

Pirsig RM (1991) *Lila: An Inquiry into Morals*, Bantam Press, London.

Waddington CH (1957) *The Strategy of the Genes*, 1st edn, George Allen & Unwin, London.

Accelerated tooth movement following alveolar corticotomy: Laboratory canine model evidence

Donald J. Ferguson

European University College, Dubai Healthcare City, UAE

ACCELERATED TOOTH MOVEMENT

One of the biological constraints in orthodontics is the amount of time it takes to resolve malocclusion. A reduction in active treatment time would logically mean that teeth would need to move faster. Treatment times for nonextraction and extraction orthodontic treatment strategies respectively average 23.8 years and 28.1 years, according to Buschang *et al.* (2012), and corticotomies increase the rates of tooth movement and decrease treatment duration. Long *et al.* (2013) evaluated the effectiveness of five interventions on accelerating orthodontic tooth movement, including low-level laser therapy, corticotomy, electrical current, pulsed electromagnetic fields, and dentoalveolar or periodontal distraction; corticotomy was judged as safe and able to accelerate orthodontic tooth movement.

It is well established that tooth movement rate is, in part, a function of alveolar bone density (Verna *et al.*, 2000), and that tooth movement is accelerated under conditions of low bone density. Bone densities change regularly as bone renews itself. Roberts *et al.* (2004) contrasted the process of bone renewal for cortical and trabecular bone; cortical bone requires an activation that initiates resorption (cutting cones) followed by formation (filling cones) in a couple sequence; that is, remodeling, otherwise known as secondary osteon formation. Trabecular bone is thin, which sustains a simpler process; that is, modeling, wherein stimulus activation can result in either apposition or resorption. The milieu of orthodontic tooth movement is trabecular bone modeling with the exception of the thin cortical lamina dura surrounding each tooth root.

Orthodontic clinicians understand that tooth movement results from alveolar bone resorption and formation, and that application of a biomechanical force results in a shift in cell population dynamics within the periodontal

---

Orthodontically Driven Corticotomy: Tissue Engineering to Enhance Orthodontic and Multidisciplinary Treatment,
First Edition. Edited by Federico Brugnami and Alfonso Caiazzo.
© 2015 John Wiley & Sons, Inc. Published 2015 by John Wiley & Sons, Inc.
Companion Website: www.wiley.com/go/Brugnami/Corticotomy

ligament (PDL). Until sufficient osteoclasts and osteoblasts have accumulated within the PDL, tooth movement after initial force application is limited to the width of the PDL space; this 3–5-week "lag" phase dissipates as PDL cell populations supportive of tooth movement have accumulated and hyalinization has diminished (Von Böhl and Kuijpers-Jagtman, 2009).

Orthodontic researchers understand "bone turnover" as a phrase describing the dynamics of a living osseous tissue that by nature is compensatory and adaptive. The research methods for the study of bone turnover include histomorphometry; that is, quantitative analysis of the physical size and shape (form) of bone. "Bone turnover" is a histomorphometric expression that includes anabolic (apposition) and catabolic (resorption) bone changes that occur and an appraisal of the varying degrees and relative amounts of mineral salts, namely calcium, present or absent.

Alveolar demineralization or decreased alveolar bone density leads to increased tooth movement rate (Verna et al., 2000). Reduction of the availability of calcium metabolite (i.e., calcium manipulation either pharmacologically or through diet), results in greater tooth movement rate and scope (Midgett et al., 1981; Goldie and King, 1984; Engström et al., 1988; Verna and Melsen, 2003).

CORTICOTOMY

Corticotomy is the intentional cutting of only cortical bone leaving intact the medullary vessels and endosteum and was first cited in the professional dental literature in the late 1800s to correct malocclusion. Alveolar decortication has evolved during the past decade, gathering noteworthy attention of orthodontic clinicians and academicians. After lying fallow for the previous half century, interest in the corticotomy concept was rekindled by Köle's (1959) journal publication describing interproximal corticotomy combined with subapical

through-and-through osteotomy in the rapid treatment of an openbite patient. Seminal technique changes since Köle include corticotomy-only (without subapical osteotomy) in the orthodontic treatment of two apertognathia patients (Generson et al., 1978), and blending augmentation bone grafting with corticotomy-only in combination with orthodontics treatment (Wilcko et al., 2001).

For 5 years following the Wilcko et al. (2001) publication, only a few corticotomy articles appeared in the professional literature (Chung, 2001; Chung et al., 2001; Ferguson et al., 2001; Hwang and Lee, 2001; Owen, 2001; Ferguson, 2002; Wilcko et al., 2003; Iseri et al., 2005; Germec et al., 2006; Iino et al., 2006).

Anecdotal accounts of accelerated tooth movement following corticotomy abound in the literature. But it was not until 2007 that evidence based upon controlled experimentation became available describing post-corticotomy rapid tooth movement. Corticotomy experiments in laboratory animals prior to 2007 focused on tissue responses (Düker, 1975), but tooth movement rate or magnitude were not study variables until after 2006.

Since 2007, interest in alveolar decortication as a technique to enhance the rate of tooth movement increased notably (Fischer, 2007; Kanno et al., 2007; Lee JK et al., 2007; Moon et al., 2007; Wilcko MT et al., 2007, 2009; Lee W et al., 2008; Nowzari et al., 2008; Oliveira et al., 2008; Park et al., 2008; Wilcko WM et al., 2008; Akay et al., 2009; Chung et al., 2009; Dibart et al., 2009, 2010; Ferguson, 2009; Kim SH et al., 2009; Kim S-J et al., 2009a,b; Murphy et al., 2009; Roblee et al., 2009; Spena et al., 2007; Wang et al., 2009; Hassan et al., 2010b; Choo et al., 2011; Keser and Dibart, 2011; Kim et al., 2011). Moreover, two alveolar corticotomy literature reviews were published in regional journals (AlGhamdi 2010; Hassan et al., 2010a) and one in an international journal (Long et al., 2013). Ten of the more recent experimental publications have included data on tooth movement as a study variable in human and/or animal subjects with additional information on the biology of alveolar bone change dynamics (Cho *et al.*, 2007; Iino *et al.*, 2007; Kim SH *et al.*, 2009; Mostafa *et al.*, 2009; Cohen *et al.*, 2010; Sanjideh *et al.*, 2010; Aboul-Ela *et al.*, 2011; Baloul *et al.*, 2011; Iglesias-Linares *et al.*, 2011; Safavi *et al.*, 2012).

ACCELERATED TOOTH MOVEMENT IN LABORATORY ANIMALS

The validity of bone research in laboratory animals depends upon the choice of the animal model (Buschang *et al.*, 2012). Rogers (1993) points out that there are at least three characteristics of an animal model: (1) convenience, (2) relevance (comparability to the human condition), and (3) appropriateness (a complex of other factors that make a given species the best for studying a particular phenomenon). As long as the limitations of a specific animal are candidly addressed by the investigator, experimental data can lead to a valid understanding of the effects on corticotomy-induced bone loss on the human skeleton.

It is clear that bone composition in some species more closely resembles human bone composition than others (Jee and Yao, 2001). Aerssens *et al.* (1998) compared cortical bone composition, density, and quality in bone samples derived from seven vertebrates that are commonly used in bone research: human, dog, pig, cow, sheep, chicken, and rat. Large interspecies differences were observed in all analyses of cortical bone; rat bone was most different, whereas canine bone best resembled human bone. Trabecular bone density and mechanical testing analyses also demonstrated large interspecies variations; human samples showed the lowest bone density and fracture stress values, and porcine and canine bone best resembled the human samples. In summary, of all species examined by Aerssens *et al.*, the bone composition of the dog most resembles that of human bone.

Ten refereed journal articles have been published after 2006 with precision measurement of experimental and control tooth movement following alveolar corticotomy from which amount and rate of tooth movement could be ascertained (Table 2.1).

Seven of the 10 investigations used dog as the laboratory model, two studies used the rat (Baloul *et al.*, 2011; Iglesias-Linares *et al.*, 2011), and there was one human study (Aboul-Ela *et al.*, 2011). The type of alveolar cortical bone injury was by surgical bur in all but one project, which used a scalpel (Kim SH *et al.*, 2009) and which was excluded from further consideration. Translation-type tooth movement following extraction was the prospective design of all studies except three; one was buccal tipping (Iglesias-Linares *et al.*, 2011) in rats, a second was mesial tipping (Baloul *et al.*, 2011) in rats, and a third was dental distraction (Cohen *et al.*, 2010) in dogs. Dental distraction or distraction osteogenesis articles were not considered.

ACCELERATED TOOTH MOVEMENT IN THE CANINE LABORATORY MODEL

Canine study description and design

Given the fact that bone of the canine laboratory animal best resembles the human condition, five dog investigations utilizing bur injury for corticotomy were isolated for further consideration and data pooling (Table 2.2).

Cho *et al.* (2007) utilized two beagles in the longitudinal examination of mesial movement of the upper and lower third premolars after extraction of all second premolars followed by 4 weeks of post-extraction healing. Corticotomy technique included upper and lower full-thickness flaps and 12 cortex non-perforating "dots" with a no. 2 round bur into the buccal and lingual cortical plates in the right maxillary and mandibular quadrants in a split-mouth design.

Table 2.1 Tooth movement following alveolar decortication injury is represented by 10 evidence-based, refereed, professional journal articles through to May 2013. All investigations include measurements of accumulated and/or rate of tooth movement and provide experimental and control data typically in a split-mouth design. One study is in humans (Aboul-Ela et al., 2011) and the remainder used either laboratory dogs or rats.

First author	Subjects	Article title	Journal details	Injury type	Tooth movement type	Data type
Cho	Dog	The effect of cortical activation on orthodontic tooth movement	Oral Dis **13**: 314–319, 2007	Bur buc-ling with flap / Split mouth	Tipping Up3 after ext Up2 / Translate Lp3 after ext Lp2	Longitudinal
Iino	Dog	Acceleration of orthodontic tooth movement by alveolar corticotomy in the dog	AJODO **131**: 448e1–8, 2007	Bur buc-ling with flap / Split mouth	Translate Lp3 after ext Lp2	Cross-sectional
Mostafa	Dog	Comparison of corticotomy-facilitated vs standard tooth-movement techniques in dogs with miniscrews as anchor units	AJODO **136**: 570–577, 2009	Bur buccal with flap / Split mouth	Tipping Up1 after ext Up2	Cross-sectional
Kim	Dog	Effects of low-level laser therapy after corticision on tooth movement and paradental remodeling	Lasers Surg Med **41**: 524–533, 2009	Scalpel buc-ling / No flap / Split mouth	Translate Up2 after ext Up1	Longitudinal
Sanjideh	Dog	Tooth movements in foxhounds after one or two alveolar corticotomies	EJO **32**: 106–113, 2010	Bur buc-ling with flap / Split mouth	Translate Up3 after ext Up2 / Translate Lp2 after ext Lp3	Longitudinal
Cohen	Dog	Effects of increased surgical trauma on rates of tooth movement and apical root resorption in foxhound dogs	Orth Craniofac Res **13**: 179–190, 2010	Bur buccal with flap / Remove labial cortex / Split mouth	Distract Up2 after ext Up1	Longitudinal

First author	Model	Title	Reference	Surgical technique	Movement	Study design
Baloul	Rat	Mechanism of action and morphologic changes in the alveolar bone in response to selective alveolar decortication-facilitated tooth movement	AJODO **139**: S83–101, 2011	Bur buc-ling with flap Split mouth	Tipping – non-extract	Cross-sectional
Aboul-Ela	Human	Miniscrew implant-supported maxillary canine retraction with and without corticotomy-facilitated orthodontics	AJODO **139**: 252–259, 2011	Bur buccal with flap Split mouth	Translate Up2 after ext Up1	Longitudinal
Iglesias-Linares	Rat	The use of gene therapy vs. corticotomy surgery in accelerating orthodontic tooth movement	Orth Craniofac Res **14**: 138–148, 2011	Bur buc-ling with flap Split mouth	Tipping – non-extract	Cross-sectional
Safavi	Dog	Effects of flapless bur decortications on movement velocity of dogs' teeth	Dent Res J **9**: 783–789, 2012	Bur buccal no flap Corticotomy monthly split mouth	Translate Up2 after ext Up1	Longitudinal

Table 2.2 Five investigations of tooth movement following alveolar decortication utilizing the canine laboratory model are summarized by author and year, dog type, sample size and data type, time after extraction and tooth movement (TM) force used, corticotomy surgery details, tooth movement type, anchorage and appliance used, measurement, location and frequency.

First author Year	Type dog (sample = n) Data type	Extraction healing TM force	Corticotomy surgery details	TM type	Anchorage + appl	Measurement Location Frequency
Cho (2007)	Beagle (n=2) Longitudinal	4 weeks healing Up3 mesial – 150 g Lp3 mesial – 150 g	Flap + non-perf cortex "dots" 12 holes injury – #2 rd bur Buccal–lingual	Tipping Up3 after ext Up2 Translate Lp3 after ext Lp2	U canine L canine + slot guide	Digital vernier caliper Gingival margins Weekly for 8 weeks
Iino (2007)	Beagle (n=12) Cross-sectional	16 weeks healing Lp3 mesial – 51 g	Flap + vert & horizontal cuts 1 mm wide – #009 fissure bur Buccal–lingual	Translate Lp3 after ext Lp2	L canine Bands + fixed tube	Caliper & radiograph Protocone tip Lp3 Superimposed tracing Weeks 1, 2, 4, 8
Mostafa (2009)	Non-purpose-bred (n=6) Cross-sectional	Immediate Up1 distal – 400 g	Flaps + vert & horizontal cuts and 8–10 holes – #2 rd bur Extract site buccal cortex	Tipping Lp1 after ext Lp2	Miniscrew Lp1 cervical lig. tie	Boley gauge Notched cervical crown Weekly for 5 weeks
Sanjideh (2010)	Foxhound (n=5) Longitudinal	Immediate Up3 mesial – 200 g Lp2 distal – 200 g	Flaps + cuts around root #702 tapered fissure bur Buccal to Up3 Buccal–lingual to Mn ext site	Translate Up3 after ext Up2 Translate Lp2 after ext Lp3	Teeth Bonds + fixed tube	Digital caliper & radiograph Implant bone markers Lp2 mesial tube to Lc tip Up3 mesial tube to Uc tip Days 10, 14, 28, 42, 56
Safavi (2012)	German (n=5) Longitudinal	Immediate Up2 mesial – 150 g Lp2 mesial – 150 g	Flapless + holes thru attached Pointed tungsten carbide bur 25 penetrations 2 mm deep Buccal to p2 and extract site	Tipping Up2 after ext Up Tipping Lp2 after ext Lp1	Miniscrew Up2 cervical lig tie Lp2 cervical lig tie	Digital caliper Marks on p2s & canines Months 1, 2, 3

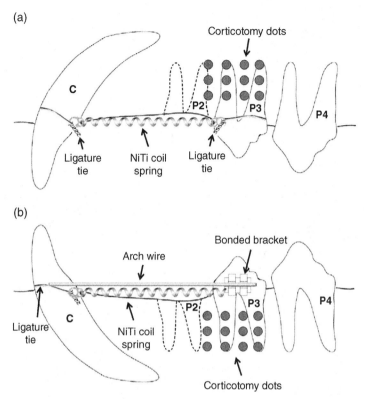

Figure 2.1 Cho *et al.* (2007) used 150 g nickel–titanium closed coil springs placed 4 weeks after extraction of upper and lower second premolar (P2) and affixed to maxillary third premolars and canines with ligature ties around the cervical crowns. Corticotomy technique consisted of 12 dots buccal and lingual to the third premolars (P3) using a no. 2 round bur. The mandibular orthodontic appliance differed from the upper and was comprised of a 0.017 × 0.025 mm² stainless steel guide wire from mandibular canine (C) sliding through an orthodontic bracket bonded to the mandibular third premolar (P3).

The third premolars were protracted into the extraction site with 150 g nickel–titanium closed coil springs using adjacent teeth as anchorage; upper third premolars were tipped and lower third premolars were tipped-translated with a "guide-wire and slot" device (Figure 2.1). Measurements were made weekly with a vernier caliper at the cervical–gingival margins of teeth adjacent to extraction site.

Iino *et al.* (2007) used 12 adult beagle dogs in the cross-sectional evaluation of mesial movement of lower third premolars after extraction of the mandibular second premolars and 16 weeks of post-extraction healing. Corticotomy technique included lower full-thickness flaps and

no. 009 fissure bur to make horizontal subapical and vertical interproximal cuts perforating the alveolar cortex buccal and lingual to the lower third premolar in a split-mouth design. The third premolars were protracted into the extraction site with 0.5 N (51 g) nickel–titanium closed coil springs using adjacent teeth as anchorage; lower third premolars were translated mesially with a fixed band-and-tube cemented appliance (Figure 2.2). Measurements were made at 1, 2, 4 and 8 weeks from radiographs taken using a standardized format. Radiographs were superimposed on the fourth premolar and measured between the tips of protocone of the third premolar on the tracing; error of method was 0.02 mm.

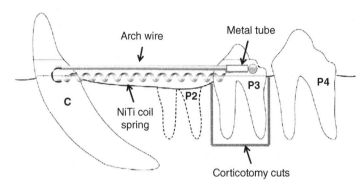

Figure 2.2 Iino *et al.* (2007) orthodontic appliance comprised of 1.0 mm wire soldered to mandibular canine (C) orthodontic band with other end sliding freely through a 1.14 mm metal tube on mandibular third premolar (P3). Mandibular third premolars were moved mesially with 51 g nickel–titanium closed coil springs 16 weeks after extraction of lower second premolar (P2). Corticotomy technique was two vertical and one subapical horizontal cut 1 mm wide buccal and lingual using no. 009 fissure bur. Adapted from Iino *et al.* (2007).

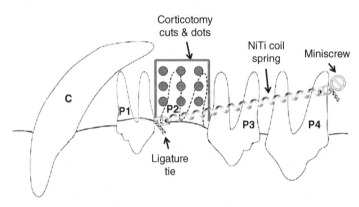

Figure 2.3 Mostafa *et al.* (2009) moved maxillary first premolars (P1) distally with an orthodontic appliance comprised of 400 g nickel–titanium closed coil springs placed immediately after extraction of upper second premolar (P2) and affixed to upper P1 and a miniscrew placed between roots of the fourth premolar (P4) and first molar. Corticotomy technique immediate post-extraction consisted of one horizontal and two vertical cuts and 8–10 dots buccal-only to the second premolar (P2) extraction site using a no. 2 round bur.

Mostafa *et al.* (2009) used six dogs that were not purpose-bred in the cross-sectional evaluation of distal movement of upper first premolars after extraction of the maxillary second premolars and immediate corticotomy. Corticotomy technique included upper full-thickness flaps and a no. 2 round bur to make two vertical and one subapical cut, and 8–10 perforations of the buccal alveolar cortex adjacent to the extraction site (not the upper first premolar) in a split-mouth design. The upper first premolars were tipped into the extraction site with a 400 g nickel–titanium closed coil spring anchored to 1.2 mm diameter miniscrews placed between roots of upper third premolar and first molars. Appliance for upper first premolars consisted of a hook fashioned from a heavy ligature wire secured around the cervical portion of the upper first premolar crown (Figure 2.3). Direct intraoral measurements were made weekly for 5 weeks from crown notches placed cervically on upper first and third premolars with a Boley gauge to the nearest 0.1 mm.

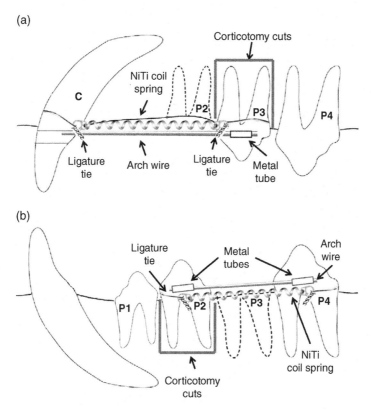

Figure 2.4 Sanjideh *et al.* (2010) moved maxillary third premolars (P3) mesially and mandibular second premolars (P2) distally. Orthodontic appliance in both arches was comprised of bonded 0.045-inch headgear tube and 0.040-inch guiding round wire combined with 200 g nickel–titanium closed coil springs. Maxillary P3 protraction was accomplished with springs ligated with steel ties to maxillary canine and third premolars; mandibular P2 retraction was accomplished by ligating springs across the extraction site to fourth premolar (P4) and first molar (not shown). Corticotomy technique in both arches consisted of one horizontal and two vertical cuts using a no. 703 tapered-fissure bur. Buccal-only cuts were made surrounding the maxillary P3 immediately after extraction of maxillary second premolar (P2); buccal and lingual cuts were made surrounding P2 immediately after extraction of lower P3.

Sanjideh *et al.* (2010) used five foxhound dogs in the longitudinal appraisal of mesial movement of upper third premolar and distal movement lower second premolars after extraction of the maxillary second and mandibular third premolars and immediate corticotomy. Full-thickness flaps were made followed by corticotomy cuts with a no. 703 tapered-fissure bur buccal-only to maxillary third premolar and both buccal and lingual surrounding the mandibular second premolar in a split-mouth design. A 0.045-inch diameter headgear tube was soldered to bracket bases and an appliance was bonded to the lower second and fourth premolars as well as the upper third premolar. Premolars were translated along a 0.040-inch stainless steel round wire using 200 g nickel–titanium closed coil spring forces calibrated every 2 weeks and stretched from hooks fashioned from heavy ligature wire and secured around the cervical portion of the upper third premolar and canine crowns as well as the lower second premolar and the combined lower first molar and fourth premolar crowns (Figure 2.4). Direct intraoral measurements were made with a

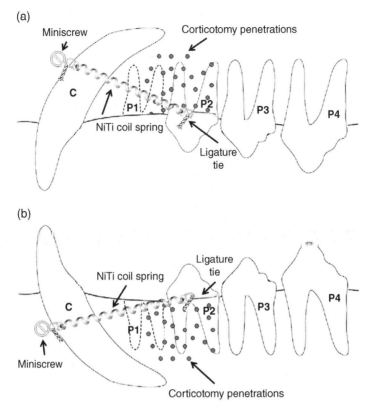

Figure 2.5 Safavi *et al.* (2012) protracted maxillary and mandibular second premolars (P2) with an orthodontic appliance comprised of 200 g nickel–titanium closed coil springs placed immediately after extraction of upper first premolar (P1) and steel ligature tied to upper and lower P2 and to a miniscrew placed anterior to the canine (C). Corticotomy technique was flapless with 25 penetrations drilled through attached gingival buccal to P2 and P1 extraction site using a pointed tungsten carbide bur in a slow-speed handpiece.

digital caliper on post-corticotomy days 10, 14, 28, 42, and 56 from fixed appliance tubes to the canine cusp tips of the respective dental arch. Control data were available only from the lower dental arch. Both maxillary quadrants had initial buccal flaps and corticotomies; one randomly selected quadrant had a second buccal flap surgery and corticotomy after 28 days.

Safavi *et al.* (2012) employed five German dogs in the longitudinal appraisal of mesial movement of upper and lower second premolars after extraction of the first premolars and immediate flapless corticotomy. Corticotomy was performed directly through the attached

gingival with a pointed carbide bur in a slow-speed handpiece; 25 penetrations were made buccal to second premolars and extraction sites in a split-mouth design. Forces was applied with 200 g nickel–titanium closed coil springs from hooks fashioned from heavy ligature wire and secured around the cervical portion of the second premolars stretched to miniscrew implants placed mesial to canines (Figure 2.5). Direct intraoral measurements were made with a digital caliper on post-corticotomy months 1, 2 and 3 from 1 mm pointed holes placed in the canine and second premolar crowns. Corticotomies were repeated at the end of months 1 and 2.

Canine tooth movement data

The only controlled experimental evidence in humans of accelerated tooth movement following corticotomy was reported by Aboul-Ela *et al.* (2011). The purpose of this study was to clinically evaluate miniscrew implant-supported maxillary canine retraction with corticotomy-facilitated orthodontics. The sample consisted of 13 adult patients with class II, division 1 malocclusion and increased overjet requiring maxillary first premolar extractions, with subsequent retraction of the maxillary canines. Corticotomy-facilitated orthodontics was randomly assigned to one side of the maxillary arch at the canine–premolar region, and the other side served as the control. Using miniscrews as anchorage, canine retraction was initiated via closed nickel–titanium coil springs applying 150 g of force per side. Among the variables examined over a 4-month follow-up period was rate of tooth movement. Average daily rate of canine retraction was significantly higher on the corticotomy side than the control side by two times during the first 2 months after the corticotomy surgery. This rate of tooth movement declined to only 1.6 times higher in the third month and 1.06 times higher by the end of the fourth month.

Because the canine laboratory animal best resembles the conditions of human bone, data from the five canine investigations were pooled and analyzed. All five publications met the following criteria: (1) decortication by surgical bur, (2) reliable measurement technique for gathering accumulated tooth movement, (3) data available for both experimental and control, and (4) data available at the end of weeks 1, 2, 3, and/or 4 weeks from either tabular or graphical formats. For all five studies, a split-mouth study design was used, thereby reducing selection, assignment, and reporting biases, and methodologies were judged sound; measurement reliability testing was reported for only two of the studies (Iino *et al.*, 2007; Sanjideh *et al.*, 2010).

Data from the five publications were collated according to weekly accumulated tooth movement and rate of tooth movement at end of weeks 1, 2, 3, and/or 4 (Table 2.3). Descriptive statistics (means) were either extracted directly from the article narrative or tables or estimated from the graphical display; standard deviations were provided in only one of the publications (Safavi *et al.*, 2012). Tooth movement data were extracted only when corresponding control data were provided. Only data following alveolar corticotomy were selected, and not data related to dental distraction or distraction osteogenesis.

Because the published weekly and/or monthly mean value data represented small sample sizes, nonparametric statistical testing was utilized; Wilcoxon signed-rank testing for paired samples was used to compare pooled experimental and pooled control side data (Table 2.4; Figure 2.6). Significant differences for accumulated tooth movement at 2, 3, and 4 weeks were observed by factors of 1.9, 1.9, and 2.3 respectively. Tooth movement rate comparisons revealed significant differences during weeks 2 and 4 by factors of 2.0 and 3.7 respectively.

TOOTH MOVEMENT PARADIGMS: PERIODONTAL LIGAMENT CELL-MEDIATED VERSUS SPONGIOSA OSTEOPENIA

The prevailing, dominant tooth movement paradigm in orthodontics is modeled on a PDL cell-mediated process (Krishnan and Davidovitch, 2006, 2009). Laboratory research related to alveolar decortication suggests another tooth movement paradigm, because rapid/greater tooth movement following injury to cortical bone cannot be explained solely by the PDL model. A tooth movement model that explains what happens following alveolar

Table 2.3 Tooth movement data was extracted and collated from five investigations using the canine as laboratory animal. Experimental data without corresponding control data and data unrelated to corticotomy-only or control were ignored. Extracted data are summarized by author, dog type, and sample size (*n*), timing of data collection, accumulated and rate of tooth movement for both experimental and control sites.

First author (Dog type = n)	Timing (days)	Accumulated tooth movement				Rate of tooth movement			
		Experimental		Control		Experimental		Control	
Cho		Exp-U	Exp-L	Ctl-U	Ctl-L	Exp-U	Exp-L	Ctl-U	Ctl-L
(Beagle = 2)	7	0.6	0.6	0.6	0.3	0.6	0.6	0.6	0.6
	14	1.2	1.15	0.85	0.55	0.6	0.55	0.25	0.25
	21	1.4	1.95	0.95	0.55	0.2	0.8	0.1	0.0
	28	2.5	2.15	0.95	0.55	1.1	0.2	0.0	0.0
Sanjideh		Exp-U/2	Exp-L	Ctl-U/2	Ctl-L	Exp-U/2	Exp-L	Ctl-U/2	Ctl-L
(Foxhound = 5)	14	—	0.6	—	0.25	—	0.6	—	0.25
	28	—	1.5	—	0.75	—	0.9	—	0.5
Mostafa		Experimental		Control		Experimental		Control	
(Non-purpose bred = 6)	7	2.00		0.92		2.00		0.92	
	14	3.30		1.80		1.30		0.88	
	21	4.25		2.33		0.96		0.53	
	28	4.67		2.33		0.42		0.00	
Iino		Experimental		Control		Experimental		Control	
(Beagle = 12)	7	0.8		0.4		0.8		0.4	
	14	1.3		0.5		0.5		0.1	
	21	1.7		0.8		0.4		0.3	
	28	2.2		0.9		0.5		0.1	
Safavi		Experimental		Control					
(German = 5)	28	2.17		1.35					

decortication is a paradigm unfamiliar to the orthodontic community; that is, a spongiosa or trabecular bone mediated tooth movement process involving transient osteopenia and swings in alveolar bone density (Ferguson and Makrami, 2013).

It is well established that tooth movement rate is, in part, a function of alveolar bone density (Verna *et al.*, 2000) and that tooth movement is accelerated under conditions of low bone density. Rapid tooth movement following alveolar decortication is made possible because the injury to alveolar cortical bone results in a healing response that reduces trabecular and lamina dura bone density and thereby reduces the resistance to tooth movement. The healing response has been characterized by Frost (1981, 1983, 1989a,b) as regional

Table 2.4 Results of Wilcoxon signed-rank testing for paired samples for all data. Note that the experimental side was significantly higher for accumulation (*) of tooth movement (TM) at the end of 2, 3 and 4 weeks and significantly higher in rate (^) of tooth movement during weeks 2 and 4.

	Variable	N	Mean	SD	z-value	Significance
Accumulated TM	Experimental – week 1	4	1.00	0.67		
	Control – week 1	4	0.55	0.27	1.83	0.146
	Experimental – week 2	5	1.51	1.04		
	Control – week 2	5	0.79	0.60	2.21	0.028*
	Experimental – week 3	4	2.32	1.30		
	Control – week 3	4	1.16	0.80	2.02	0.035*
	Experimental – week 4	7	2.48	1.01		
	Control – week 4	7	1.17	0.59	2.37	0.001*
TM rate	Experimental – week 1	4	1.00	0.67		
	Control – week 1	4	0.63	0.21	1.60	0.242
	Experimental – week 2	5	0.71	0.33		
	Control – week 2	5	0.35	0.30	2.21	0.000^
	Experimental – week 3	4	0.59	0.35		
	Control – week 3	4	0.23	0.23	1.76	0.121
	Experimental – week 4	5	0.62	0.37		
	Control – week 4	5	0.12	0.22	2.37	0.031^

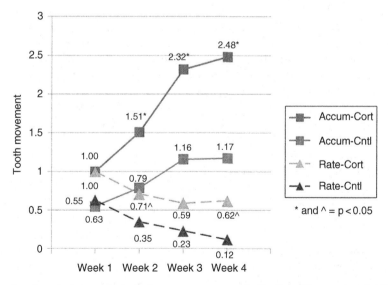

Figure 2.6 Results of pooled data analysis demonstrate accumulation (in millimeters – solid line) and rate (in millimeters/week – dashed line) of tooth movement. The corticotomy group showed significantly ($p < 0.05$) greater tooth movement accumulation (*) at end of weeks 2, 3, and 4 and greater rate (^) during weeks 2 and 4. Cort: alveolar corticotomy plus tooth movement; Cntl: tooth movement without alveolar corticotomy; * and ^ signify probability <0.05.

acceleratory phenomena (RAP), a transient process including a reduction in the mineral content of bone but without a reduction in bone matrix volume. The RAP response is directly related and proportional to injury magnitude and proximity (Ferguson and Makrami, 2013).

It has been clearly demonstrated that the anabolic and catabolic activities required for tooth movement occur following a shift in cell dynamics in response to applied biomechanical forces. Orthodontic force application results in compression of the PDL followed by a lag or arrest phase of about 2 weeks; clinically apparent tooth movement occurs after the arrest phase when appropriate numbers of osteoblasts and osteoclasts have accumulated. Under conditions of orthodontic tooth movement, cell-free hyalinization is nearly impossible to avoid; it is the PDL hyalinization process that is used to explain the tooth movement arrest or lag phase as well as a process that precedes external root resorption (Ren *et al.*, 2003; Von Böhl and Kuijpers-Jagtman, 2009). Hyalinization is eliminated or substantially reduced following alveolar corticotomy (Cho *et al.*, 2007; Mostafa *et al.*, 2009).

The following concepts accurately explain accelerated and greater tooth movement following alveolar corticotomy:

1. Injury to cortical bone invokes a rapid (hours to days) modeling (change in bony surfaces) of mostly trabecular bone and lamina dura immediately adjacent to the injury (Lee *et al.*, 2008; Sebaoun *et al.*, 2008; Milne *et al.*, 2009; Wang *et al.*, 2009). While cortical bone is certainly affected by the injury, response of the cortices to that injury is slower (weeks to months) compared with trabecular bone (hours to days). Hence, the structure function of bone is served by the integrity of the cortices (slow turnover via remodeling or secondary osteon formation) while the metabolic function of bone is served by the rapid release (rapid turnover via modeling) of vital metabolites, especially calcium, from the trabecular bone (Ferguson and Makrami, 2013).

2. Alveolar demineralization leads to increased tooth movement rate and amount. Reduction of the availability of calcium metabolite (i.e., calcium manipulation either pharmacologically or through diet) results in greater tooth movement rate and scope (Verna and Melsen, 2003). There is a transient reduction of alveolar bone density following corticotomy, and remineralization is slowed while teeth are moving within the alveolus (Ferguson and Makrami, 2013).

3. Following alveolar corticotomy, the demineralized bone matrix is transported with the tooth movement; as soon as tooth movement is arrested or malocclusion is resolved, the alveolus remineralizes (Ferguson *et al.*, 2007; Wilcko *et al.*, 2009). The bone matrix transport concept is consistent with histomorphometric observations of the alveolar osseous tissues as a function time after alveolar decortication. The mineralized fraction of alveolar trabecular bone reduces considerably following decortication, and the integrity of the PDL and lamina dura literally disappears from view when assessed histologically. However, when the alveolus is allowed to remineralize, the integrity of the PDL and lamina dura reappears (Lee *et al.*, 2008; Sebaoun *et al.*, 2008; Wang *et al.*, 2009).

References

Aboul-Ela SM, El-Beialy AR, El-Sayed KM *et al.* (2011) Miniscrew implant-supported maxillary canine retraction with and without corticotomy-facilitated orthodontics. *American Journal of Orthodontics and Dental Orthopedics*, **139**, 252–259.

Aerssens J, Boonen S, Lowet G *et al.* (1998) Interspecies differences in bone composition, density and quality: potential implication for *in vivo* bone research. *Endocrinology*, **139**, 663–670.

Akay MC, Aras A, Günbay T *et al.* (2009) Enhanced effect of combined treatment with corticotomy and skeletal anchorage in open bite correction. *Journal of Oral and Maxillofacial Surgery*, **67**, 563–569.

AlGhamdi AST (2010) Corticotomy facilitated orthodontics: review of a technique. *Saudi Dental Journal*, **22**, e1–e5.

Baloul SS, Gerstenfeld LC, Morgan EF *et al.* (2011) Mechanism of action and morphologic changes in the alveolar bone in response to selective alveolar decortication-facilitated tooth movement. *American Journal of Orthodontics and Dental Orthopedics*, **139**, S83–S101.

Buschang PH, Campbell PM, Ruso S (2012) Accelerating tooth movement with corticotomies: is it possible and desirable? *Seminars in Orthodontics*, **18**, 286–294.

Cho K-W, Cho S-W, Oh C-O *et al.* (2007) The effect of cortical activation on orthodontic tooth movement. *Oral Diseases*, **13**, 314–319.

Choo H-R, Heo H-A, Yoon H-J *et al.* (2011) Treatment outcome analysis of speedy surgical orthodontics for adults with maxillary protrusion. *American Journal of Orthodontics and Dental Orthopedics*, **140**, e251–e262.

Chung KR (2001) Speedy orthodontics, in *Textbook of Speedy Orthodontics* (ed. KR Chung), Jeesung, Seoul.

Chung KR, Oh MY, Ko SJ (2001) Corticotomy-assisted orthodontics. *Journal of Clinical Orthodontics*, **35**, 331–339.

Chung K-R, Lee B-S, Lee W (2009) Speedy surgical orthodontic treatment with skeletal anchorage in adults: sagittal correction and open bite correction. *Journal of Oral Maxillofacial Surgery*, **67**, 2130–2148.

Cohen G, Campbell PM, Rossouw PE *et al.* (2010) Effects of increased surgical trauma on rates of tooth movement and apical root resorption in foxhound dogs. *Orthodontic and Craniofacial Research*, **13**, 179–190.

Dibart S, Sebaoun JD, Surmenian J (2009) Piezocision: a minimally invasive, periodontally accelerated orthodontic tooth movement procedure. *Compendium of Continuing Education in Dentistry*, **30**, 342–344.

Dibart S, Surmenian J, Sebaoun JD, Montesani L (2010) Rapid treatment of Class II malocclusion with Piezocision: two case reports. *International Journal of Periodontics and Restorative Dentistry*, **30**, 487–493.

Düker J (1975) Experimental animal research into segmental alveolar movement after corticotomy. *Journal of Maxillofacial Surgery*, **3**, 81–84.

Engström C, Granström G, Thilander B (1988) Effect of orthodontic force on periodontal tissue metabolism: a histologic and biochemical study in normal and hypocalcemic young rats. *American Journal of Orthodontics and Dental Orthopedics*, **93**, 486–495.

Ferguson DJ (2002) Risk, rate and stability of corticotomy-assisted orthodontics. *Orthodontics Select*, **3**, 1–4.

Ferguson DJ (2009) Rapid orthodontics following alveolar decortication and grafting. *Journal of Taiwanese Orthodontic Society*, **2**, 31–47.

Ferguson DJ, Makrami SB (2013) Rapid orthodontics following alveolar decortication: why the resistance? *Journal de Parodontologie & d'Implantologie Orale*, **32**, 121–129.

Ferguson DJ, Wilcko MW, Wilcko TM (2001) Accelerating orthodontics by altering alveolar bone density. *Good Practice*, **2**, 2–4.

Ferguson DJ, Wilcko MW, Wilcko TM (2007) Selective alveolar decortication for rapid surgical–orthodontic correction of skeletal malocclusion, in *Distraction Osteogenesis of the Facial Skeleton* (eds WH Bell, CA Guerrero), BC Decker, Inc., Hamilton, Ontario.

Fischer TJ (2007) Orthodontic treatment acceleration with corticotomy-assisted exposure of palatally impacted canines. *Angle Orthodontics*, **77**, 417–420.

Frost HM (1981) The regional accelerated phenomenon. *Orthopedic Clinics of North America*, **12**, 725–726.

Frost HA (1983) The regional acceleratory phenomena: a review. *Henry Ford Hospital Medical Journal*, **31**, 3–9.

Frost HM (1989a) The biology of fracture healing. An overview for clinicians. Part I. *Clinical Orthopedics and Related Research*, **248**, 283–293.

Frost HM (1989b) The biology of fracture healing. An overview for clinicians. Part II. *Clinical Orthopedics and Related Research*, **248**, 294–309.

Generson RM, Porter JM, Zell A *et al.* (1978) Combined surgical and orthodontic management of anterior open bite using corticotomy. *Journal of Oral Surgery*, **36**, 216–219.

Germec D, Giray B, Kocadereli I *et al.* (2006) Lower incisor retraction with a modified corticotomy. *Angle Orthodontics*, **76**, 882–890.

Goldie RE, King GJ (1984) Root resorption and tooth movement in orthodontically treated, calcium-deficient, and lactating rats. *American Journal of Orthodontics*, **85**, 424–430.

Hassan AH, Al-Fraidi AA, Al-Saeed SH *et al.* (2010a) Corticotomy-assisted orthodontic treatment: review. *Open Dental Journal*, **4**, 159–164.

Hassan AH, Al-Ghamdi AT, Al-Fraidi AA *et al.* (2010b) Unilateral cross bite treated by corticotomy-assisted expansion: two case reports. *Head and Face Medicine*, **6**, 1–9.

Hwang H, Lee K (2001) Intrusion of over-erupted molars by corticotomy and magnets. *American Journal of Orthodontics and Dental Orthopedics*, **120**, 209–216.

Iglesias-Linare A, Moreno-Fernandez AM, Yanez-Vico R *et al.* (2011) The use of gene therapy vs. corticotomy surgery in accelerating orthodontic tooth movement. *Orthodontics and Craniofacial Research*, **14**, 138–148.

Iino S, Sakoda S, Miyawaki S (2006) An adult bimaxillary protrusion treated with corticotomy-facilitated orthodontics and titanium miniplates. *Angle Orthodontics*, **76**, 1074–1082.

Iino S, Sakoda S, Ito G *et al.* (2007) Acceleration of orthodontic tooth movement by alveolar corticotomy in the dog. *American Journal of Orthodontics and Dental Orthopedics*, **131**, 448.e1–448.e8.

Iseri H, Kisnisci R, Bzizi N *et al.* (2005) Rapid canine retraction and orthodontic treatment with dentoalveolar distraction osteogenesis. *American Journal of Orthodontics and Dental Orthopedics*, **127**, 533–541.

Jee WSS, Yao W (2001) Overview: animal models of osteopenia and osteoporosis. *Journal Musculoskeletal and Neuronal Interactions*, **1**, 193–207.

Kanno T, Mitsugi M, Furuki Y *et al.* (2007) Corticotomy and compression osteogenesis in the posterior maxilla for treating severe anterior open bite. *International Journal of Oral and Maxillofacial Surgery*, **36**, 354–357.

Keser EI, Dibart S (2011) Piezocision-assisted Invisalign® treatment. *Compendium of Continuing Education in Dentistry*, **32**, 46–51.

Kim HS, Lee YJ, Park YG *et al.* (2011) Histologic assessment of the biological effects after speedy surgical orthodontics in a beagle animal model: a preliminary study. *Korean Journal of Orthodontics*, **41**, 361–371.

Kim SH, Lee KB, Chung KR *et al.* (2009) Severe bimaxillary protrusion with adult periodontitis treated by corticotomy and compression osteogenesis. *Korean Journal of Orthodontics*, **39**, 54–65.

Kim S-J, Park Y-G, Kang S-G (2009a) Effects of corticision on paradental remodeling in orthodontic tooth movement. *Angle Orthodontics*, **79**, 284–291.

Kim S-J, Moon S-U, Kang S-G, Park Y-G (2009b) Effects of low-level laser therapy after corticision on tooth movement and paradental remodeling. *Lasers in Surgery and Medicine*, **41**, 524–533.

Köle H (1959) Surgical operation on the alveolar ridge to correct occlusal abnormalities. *Oral Surgery Oral Medicine Oral Pathology*, **12**, 515–529.

Krishnan V, Davidovitch Z (2006) Cellular, molecular, and tissue level reactions to orthodontic force. *American Journal of Orthodontics and Dental Orthopedics*, **129**, 469.e1–469.e32.

Krishnan V, Davidovitch Z (2009) On a path to unfolding the biological mechanisms of orthodontic tooth movement. *Journal of Dental Research*, **88**, 597–608.

Lee JK, Chung KR, Baek SH (2007) Treatment outcomes of orthodontic treatment, corticotomy-assisted orthodontic treatment, and anterior segmental osteotomy for bimaxillary dentoalveolar protrusion. *Plastic and Reconstructive Surgery*, **120**, 1027–1036.

Lee W, Karapetyan G, Moats R et al. (2008) Corticotomy-/osteotomy-assisted tooth movement micro-CTs differ. *Journal of Dental Research*, **87**, 861–867.

Long H, Pyakurel U, Wang Y (2013) Interventions for accelerating orthodontic tooth movement: a systematic review. *Angle Orthodontics*, **83**, 164–171.

Midgett RJ, Shaye RS, Fruge JF (1981) The effect of altered bone metabolism on orthodontic tooth movement. *American Journal of Orthodontics*, **80**, 256–262.

Milne TJ, Ichim I, Patel B et al. (2009) Induction of osteopenia during experimental tooth movement in the rat: alveolar bone remodelling and the mechanostat theory. *European Journal of Orthodontics*, **31**, 221–231.

Moon CH, Wee JU, Lee HS (2007) Intrusion of overerupted molars by corticotomy and orthodontic skeletal anchorage system. *Angle Orthodontics*, **77**, 1119–1125.

Mostafa YA, Fayed MM, Mehanni S (2009) Comparison of corticotomy-facilitated vs standard tooth movement techniques in dogs with miniscrews as anchor units. *American Journal of Orthodontics and Dental Orthopedics*, **136**, 570–577.

Murphy N, Wilcko MT, Wilcko WM et al. (2009) Periodontal accelerated osteogenic orthodontics: a description of the surgical technique. *Journal of Oral and Maxillofacial Surgery*, **67**, 2160–2166.

Nowzari H, Yorita FK, Chang HC (2008) Periodontally accelerated osteogenic orthodontics combined with autogenous bone grafting. *Compendium of Continuing Education in Dentistry*, **29**, 200–206.

Oliveira DD, de Oliveira BF, de Araújo Brito HH et al. (2008) Selective alveolar corticotomy to intrude overerupted molars. *American Journal of Orthodontics and Dental Orthopedics*, **133**, 902–908.

Owen AH III (2001) Accelerated Invisalign treatment. *Journal of Clinical Orthodontics*, **35**, 381–385.

Park WK, Kim SS, Park SB et al. (2008) The effect of cortical punching on the expression of OPG, RANK, and RANKL in the periodontal tissue during tooth movement in rats. *Korean Journal of Orthodontics*, **38**, 159–174.

Ren Y, Maltha JC, Kuijpers-Jagtman AM (2003) Optimum force magnitude for orthodontic tooth movement: a systematic literature review. *Angle Orthodontics*, **73**, 86–92.

Roberts WE, Huja S, Roberts JA (2004) Bone modeling: biomechanics, molecular mechanisms, and clinical perspectives. *Seminars in Orthodontics*, **10**, 123–161.

Roblee RD, Bolding SL, Landers JM (2009): Surgically facilitated orthodontic therapy: a new tool for optimal interdisciplinary results. *Compendium of Continuing Education in Dentistry*, **30**, 264–275.

Rodgers JB, Monier-Faugere MC, Malluche H (1993) Animal models for the study of bone loss after cessation of ovarian function. *Bone*, **14**, 369–377.

Safavi SM, Heidarpour M, Izadi SS et al. (2012) Effects of flapless bur decortications on movement velocity of dogs' teeth. *Journal of Dental Research*, **9**, 783–789.

Sanjideh PA, Rossouw PE, Campbell PM et al. (2010) Tooth movements in foxhounds after one or two alveolar corticotomies. *European Journal of Orthodontics*, **32**, 106–113.

Sebaoun JD, Turner JW, Kantarci A et al. (2008) Modeling of trabecular bone and lamina dura following selective alveolar decortication in rats. *Journal of Periodontology*, **79**, 1679–1688.

Spena R, Caiazzo A, Gracco A et al. (2007) The use of segmental corticotomy to enhance molar distalization. *Journal of Clinical Orthodontics*, **41**, 693–699.

Verna C, Melsen B (2003) Tissue reaction to orthodontic tooth movement in different bone turnover conditions. *Orthodontic and Craniofacial Research*, **6**, 155–163.

Verna C, Dalstra M, Melsen B (2000) The rate and the type of orthodontic tooth movement is influenced by bone turnover in a rat model. *European Journal of Orthodontics*, **22**, 343–352.

Von Böhl M, Kuijpers-Jagtman AM (2009) Hyalinization during orthodontic tooth movement: a systematic review on tissue reactions. *European Journal of Orthodontics*, **31**, 30–36.

Wang L, Lee W, Lei DL *et al.* (2009) Tisssue responses in corticotomy- and osteotomy-assisted tooth movements in rats: histology and immunostaining. *American Journal of Orthodontics and Dental Orthopedics*, **136**, 770.e1–770.e11.

Wilcko MT, Wilcko WM, Marquez MG (2007) The contribution of periodontics to orthodontic therapy, in *Practical Advanced Periodontal Surgery* (ed. S Dibart), Blackwell, Ames, IA.

Wilcko MT, Wilcko WM, Pulver JJ *et al.* (2009) Accelerated osteogenic orthodontics technique: a 1-stage surgically facilitated rapid orthodontic technique with alveolar augmentation. *Journal of Oral and Maxillofacial Surgery*, **67**, 2149–2159.

Wilcko WM, Wilcko MT, Bouquot JE *et al.* (2001) Rapid orthodontics with alveolar reshaping: two case reports of decrowding. *International Journal of Periodontics and Restorative Denistry*, **21**, 9–19.

Wilcko WM, Ferguson DJ, Bouquot JE *et al.* (2003) Rapid orthodontic decrowding with alveolar augmentation: case report. *World Journal of Orthodontics*, **4**, 197–205.

Wilcko WM, Wilcko MT, Bissada NF (2008) An evidence-based analysis of periodontally accelerated orthodontic and osteogenic techniques: a synthesis of scientific perspectives. *Seminars in Orthodontics*, **14**, 305–316.

Corticotomy-facilitated orthodontics: Surgical considerations

Pushkar Mehra and Hasnain Shinwari

Department of Oral and Maxillofacial Surgery, Boston University
Henry M. Goldman School of Dental Medicine, Boston, MA, USA

INTRODUCTION

Alveolar arch crowding is the most common manifestation of a dental malocclusion. Correction of dental malocclusions has been shown to improve periodontal health and psychosocial status (Rusanen *et al.*, 2010). The conventional orthodontic approach for resolution of dental crowding involves either extraction of selected teeth (often bicuspids) or alternative mechanics like expansion, interproximal stripping, and/or angulation modifications using nonsurgical orthodontic treatment alone. Generally speaking, mild to moderate crowding in most cases can be managed without extraction of teeth, but moderate to severe cases are usually best treated with dental extractions. Adult orthodontics is becoming very popular, and an increasing number of adults in recent years are undergoing orthodontic treatment. Duration and cost of the treatment still remain the biggest challenges for the orthodontic field in the current era relative to treatment of adults. Typical orthodontic treatment ranges from 1 to 2 years, which requires continuous compliance and expense from the patient's perspective for a considerable period of time. The duration and management of comprehensive orthodontic treatment for adults is significantly longer than for adolescents (Vig *et al.*, 1990). Thus, it is only likely that many potential orthodontic patients either decline or discontinue the treatment due to their changing social and financial situations.

Decreasing the time for tooth movement has been the focus of many clinicians and researchers for a long time. For the last few decades, investigators have recommended many unique treatment modifications with an aim to reduce the overall treatment time. Introduction of newer minimally invasive, predictable surgical techniques (e.g., distraction osteogenesis, alveolar bone corticotomies) has been the main focus of many clinicians for the past century (Frost, 1983, 1989a,b). This chapter will discuss one such surgical technique: selective alveolar decortication (SAD) or corticotomy.

SAD is a relatively new technique in the dental literature. However, documentation of the original concept in orthopedics literature

Orthodontically Driven Corticotomy: Tissue Engineering to Enhance Orthodontic and Multidisciplinary Treatment,
First Edition. Edited by Federico Brugnami and Alfonso Caiazzo.
© 2015 John Wiley & Sons, Inc. Published 2015 by John Wiley & Sons, Inc.
Companion Website: www.wiley.com/go/Brugnami/Corticotomy

dates back to the early 19th century. SAD refers to intentional surgical disruption of alveolar cortical bone that aims to reduce the resistance that native bone can offer towards orthodontic dental movement, thereby making orthodontic treatment more rapid. Many modifications of this basic technique have evolved in the field of dentistry over the last few years, and different authors have changed the terminology as per their own preferences (e.g., corticotomy, Wilckodontics®, corticotomy-facilitated orthodontics, accelerated osteogenic orthodontics, and Piezocision® to name a few).

In the orthodontic literature, the term "corticotomy" is vaguely defined and is often confused with "osteotomy." Strictly speaking, the corticotomy procedure refers to a surgical technique in which a cut is made into the buccal and/or lingual cortical plates that surround the tooth without completely going through both cortices; as a result, the teeth will be present in an alveolar bone segment connected to other adjacent teeth and structures only through the medullary bone. In contrast, an osteotomy is defined as complete cuts though the entire thicknesses of both buccal and lingual cortical plates and the interposed medullary bone, potentially creating a mobilized segment of bone and teeth. Osteotomies, theoretically, may have a higher incidence of complications, such as ischemic necrosis of the bone segment, wound dehiscences at the osteotomy site, and devitalization of the teeth adjacent to the osteotomy sites.

HISTORICAL BACKGROUND

The technique to accelerate tooth movement (alveolar corticotomy) was first introduced by Köle (1959). It was believed that, by creating blocks of bone with vertical buccal and lingual corticotomies and apical horizontal osteotomy connecting cuts, segments of bone with the embedded teeth could be moved rapidly. However, owing to the invasive nature of

Köle's technique, it was never widely accepted. In early 1990s, Suya (1991) revised Köle's technique with the "substitution of a subapical horizontal corticotomy cuts in place of the horizontal osteotomy cut beyond the apices of the teeth" and published a clinical study that showed good results. The concept of "regional acceleratory phenomenon" (RAP) was introduced by an orthopedist, Dr Henry Frost who proposed that intentional injury to the cortical bone results in a modification of the bone metabolism, leading to a transient state of osteopenia described as RAP. The RAP mechanism potentiating tissue healing was shown to occur in the mandible as well (Yaffe et al., 1994).

The Wilcko brothers in 2000 reintroduced and later perfected this combined surgical–orthodontic therapy with an innovative technique of combining corticotomy surgery with alveolar grafting. They initially termed their technique Accelerated Osteogenic Orthodontics™ (AOO) and more recently changed the terminology to Periodontally Accelerated Osteogenic Orthodontics® (PAOO®) (Wilcko et al., 2001). This technique entails comprehensive fixed orthodontic appliances in conjunction with full-thickness flaps and labial and lingual corticotomies around teeth to be moved. In addition, particulate bone graft is also applied directly over the bone cuts and the flap sutured in place. Tooth movement is initiated at least 1 week before the surgery and every 2 weeks thereafter by activation of the orthodontic appliance. The Wilcko's were the first to demonstrate that the movement does not result from repositioning of tooth–bone blocks, but rather from a cascade of transient localized reactions in the bony alveolar housing leading to bone healing. The earlier concept of the rapid tooth movement was based on bony block movement in corticotomy techniques including buccal and lingual vertical and sub-apical horizontal cuts circumscribing the roots of the teeth. Current research has proven that the rapid tooth movement after corticotomy is facilitated by RAP, described as accelerated bone turnover and decreased regional bone density (Wilcko *et al.*, 2001).

BIOPHYSIOLOGIC CONSIDERATIONS

An injury of any type initiates healing by perturbing some of the surviving local cells, sensitizing them so that they can respond better to specific local and systemic messengers and stimuli. Injury also releases local biochemical and biophysical messengers that make cells respond and help to determine how they should respond. The bone remodeling basic multicellular unit (BMU) first produces osteoclasts that remove preexisting hard tissue and then produces osteoblasts that replace it with well-oriented lamellar bone in the stereotypical activation–resorption–formation sequence. Bone resorption and bone formation occur in tandem in the remodeling process. This coupling mechanism has been postulated as a means by which bone is neither lost nor gained during repair. At the end of healing, when the stimulus to RAP resolves, the BMU activation declines to normal, remodeling spaces fill back with new bone, and osteopenia disappears.

The initial response of bone to a traumatic injury is by a biologic state called RAP characterized by a transient increase in bone turnover and a decrease in trabecular bone density (Frost, 1983). This localized burst of tissue remodeling is also witnessed after a surgical osteotomy or a fracture (Shih and Norrdin, 1985). Alveolar corticotomy is a surgical intervention limited to cortical bone that is incorporated into orthodontic treatment plan to facilitate the treatment of complex occlusal problems (Köle, 1959). It generates the localized RAP at the site of injury (Wilcko *et al.*, 2001) due to which bone regenerates faster than the normal regional regeneration process. This faster regeneration is due to the enhanced stages of bone healing which could be as fast as 2–10 times that of normal physiologic healing

(Frost, 1983). A localized and reversible decrease in mineral bone density or osteopenia that begins with the initial stage of RAP and diminishes with the end of RAP is responsible for the faster tooth movement. Locally induced osteopenia weakens the trabeculae of the alveolar bone, and this lesser resistance subsequently leads to the rapid movement of teeth (Sebaoun *et al.*, 2008). Once orthodontic tooth movement is completed, an environment is created that favors alveolar remineralization. The effect of RAP begins within 2–3 days of injury and reaches its peak at 1–2 months. This effect lasts usually for 4 months, but may take 6–24 months to completely subside (Wilcko *et al.*, 2003).

Indications

1. Decreasing the duration of orthodontic treatment in patients who are undergoing conventional, nonsurgical orthodontic therapy (treatment of dental malocclusions with orthodontics alone) (see Chapters 4–6).
2. Expanding the alveolar basis, therefore reducing the need for premolar extractions and strengthens the periodontium, lowering the risk for periodontal damage during and after treatment (see Chapter 7).
3. Selectively altering the differential anchorage among groups of teeth, hastening and facilitating the movement of teeth that have to be moved and diminishing the countereffect in the teeth that should not be moved (see Chapter 6–8).
4. As a tool in multidisciplinary treatment, including managing of partial edentulism in adult and growing patients (see Chapter 8).
5. Modifying the lower third of the face (see Chapters 6 and 7).
6. Adjunctive measure in facilitating treatment of impacted teeth (see Chapter 6).
7. Decreasing the duration of pre-operative orthodontic treatment in patients undergoing conventional, combined surgical–orthodontic

therapy (treatment of skeletal malocclusions with orthognathic surgery).

8. Alternative to orthognathic surgery for combined surgical–orthodontic management of select dentoskeletal malocclusions.

9. Salvage technique for the management of post-orthognathic, occlusion-related complications.

10. Management of clinically refractory orthodontic dental conditions.

Contraindications

These are similar to those for any minor oral surgery or periodontal surgery procedures, especially when related to conditions affecting systemic health and illness (cardiac, endocrine, musculoskeletal, etc.). Additionally, SAD may be contraindicated in certain local disease states, such as active periodontitis or systemic conditions (e.g., uncontrolled osteoporosis). It may also have an increased complication rate in patients who have a history of use of certain medications (e.g., nonsteroidal anti-inflammatotory drugs, immunosuppressive medications, steroids, bisphosphonates) and radiation therapy to the maxillofacial region.

Advantages

1. Minimally invasive surgery:
   i. Decreased post-operative discomfort (compared with orthognatic surgery such as surgically assisted rapid palatal expansion (SARPE)).
   ii. Minimal complications.
2. Eliminates the need for dental extractions in many patients.
3. Improved post-surgical outcomes:
   i. Less root resorption during active orthodontic movement due to decreased resistance of cortical bone.
   ii. Improved quantity and quality of periodontium; more bone support due to the addition of bone graft.

4. Decreased duration of treatment:
   i. Orthodontic treatment;
   ii. Total treatment time;
   iii. Decrease of length-related side effects of orthodontics due to plaque accumulation, such as decay and periodontal disease.
5. Ability to perform surgery in an office setting:
   i. Improved efficiency;
   ii. Decreased costs;
   iii. No requirement for hospitalization.

SURGICAL TECHNIQUE

Pre-operative considerations

Medical and surgical history should be obtained and considerations for surgery are similar to routine indications and clearance for intraoral dentoalveolar procedures. A panoramic radiograph is recommended to evaluate the maxillary sinus, nasal cavities, and other skeletal and dental structures from a general perspective. Full-mouth periapical X-rays are recommended to evaluate root proximity and other structures, such as periodontal health and status, lamina dura, and so on. Cone beam computed tomography scans are becoming widely popular and have the benefit of a precise evaluation of the thickness of buccal and lingual cortical plates and their intimate relationship to the roots of teeth, besides giving all the information that plain films would give.

Orthodontic appliances are placed approximately 1–2 weeks week prior to the surgery. Standard brackets, arch wires, and normal orthodontic force level can be used. Surgery is performed in an office setting with or without sedation, depending on patient and doctor preference. The surgical armamentarium required is similar to any intraoral, minor dentoalveolar surgical, or implant surgery procedure (hand instruments, rotary instrumentation, piezoelectric module, bone graft materials, sutures, etc.). Local anesthetic with vasoconstrictor should be infiltrated buccally/labially and palatally at least 7 min prior to incision to maintain optimal hemostasis. Use of appropriate antibiotics with adequate oral flora coverage (oral amoxicillin or clindamycin) and oral chlorhexidine rinse is recommended prior to surgery. These are usually started approximately 1 h prior to the procedure and continued for 1–2 weeks post-operatively.

Incision design

A no. 15 Bard–Parker surgical blade is used on a suitable scalpel handle and held at a slight angle to the teeth. For four quadrant cases, a smooth continuous stroke is made in the gingival sulcus from first molar to first molar crossing the midline in one arch. A vertical releasing incision can then be made behind the first molar. Vertical incisions are not recommended in the anterior region because of esthetic reasons. Although some cases can be performed with only sulcular incisions, vertical releases ensure increased access and ease of flap reflection, and may especially be indicated for those practitioners who are less experienced with surgical procedures. The authors also recommend that, in the anterior midline region, the incision be designed in a manner that avoids incising the triangular papilla on the labial mucosa between the central incisors (papilla-sparing incision) (Figure 3.1a). The above-mentioned incision design is indicated for conventional surgery; many other modifications have been proposed including vertical separate incisions for piezoelectric instrumentation (Figure 3.1b). These modifications are beyond the scope of this chapter and will be described in Chapter 5.

Flap reflection and exposure

The reflection of a full-thickness mucoperiosteal flap is carried out next. The sharp end of a no. 9 Molt's periosteal elevator or Woodson is slipped underneath the papilla in the area of the incision and is turned laterally to reflect the papilla away from the underlying bone (Figure 3.2). This technique is then utilized for the remainder of the flap, extending laterally. Care should be exercised not to damage any of the neurovascular bundles exiting the bone and stay subperiosteal so as not to disturb deeper

(a)

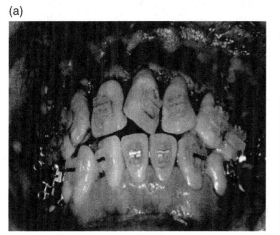

(b)

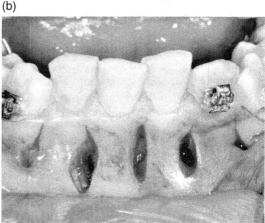

Figure 3.1 (a) A sulcular incision has been made around the necks of the individual teeth in the areas to be decorticated. The flap has been reflected apically to demonstrate bone exposure. (b) Modified incisions have been proposed by some authors, especially using piezoelectrical instrumentation. This photograph depicts five vertical incisions in the areas where piezoelectric instrumentation would be used to decorticate the bone in the interdental regions.

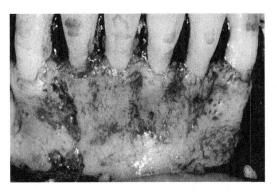

Figure 3.2 A full-thickness mucoperiosteal flap has been reflected exposing the anterior mandible, which is the area to be decorticated. Care should be taking while reflecting this flap, as many areas may have bony dehiscence and root exposures and overzealous instrumentation may cause complications such as root resorption. Flaps should be retracted with standard instrumentation, such as Seldin, Minnesota, or other retractors.

muscle attachments. After this initial reflection of the free edge of the flap, the broad end of the periosteal is often then used to reflect the entire mucoperiosteal flap, and this exposes the alveolar housing and bone plates (Figure 3.2). This technique assures an atraumatic, hemostatic reflection of the mucoperiosteal flap.

Once the flap has been reflected, a Seldin, Minnesota, or similar retractor should be used subperiosteally to hold the flap to its reflected position and maintain adequate exposure and protection for soft tissues. Clinicians should be careful not to force the retractor into the soft tissue flap, but instead place tissue retractors firmly against the bone.

Corticotomy/surgical decortication

Selective alveolar decortication is conventionally performed on buccal and lingual/palatal bone plates using rear-vented high-speed, rotary surgical instrumentation and carbide burs under copious saline irrigation (Figure 3.3a). Adequate irrigation is essential to minimize intraoperative

thermal bone damage and optimize postoperative bone healing. Any fine surgical bur of choice can be used to perform thorough decortication all over the area. Recently, piezoelectric instrumentation (Figure 3.3b) has also been used to perform decortication and demonstrated to be effective by some clinicians. However, at the time of publication of this material, the short- and long-term efficacy in causing comparable RAP to conventional surgery and the predictability of clinical outcomes is unknown and has not been widely studied or reported.

Decortication refers to surgical violation of the cortex and purposeful entry into medullary bone. The specific design or type of decortication (e.g., holes, lines, grooves, any geometrical figure) is not relevant (Figure 3.3c). Entry into medullary bone is a prerequisite, and this is verified by evidence of bleeding in the decortication sites. Care should be taken to stop 2–3 mm short of the alveolar crest (Figure 3.3d), as violation of this area can cause complications with soft tissue esthetics and loss of periodontal support. The clinician must also respect other vital anatomic structures, such as maxillary sinus, inferior alveolar nerve canal, and dental roots, which could be damaged by overzealous instrumentation. Care should be taken not to injure the anterior loop of the inferior alveolar nerve that could extend several millimeters (6 mm loop) mesial to the mental foramen and is usually positioned just beneath the buccal cortical plate in this region. Additional cortical perforation can be made at selected, safe areas to increase blood supply to the graft material. The decortication performed is interdentally in vertical fashion paralleling the roots. Many a time, owing to dental crowding, roots have very close proximity to each other, and thus extreme caution must be exercised in order to avoid iatrogenic damage.

Bone grafting

The use of bone grafting is controversial. Some practitioners use it universally on all cases, whereas others do not recommend its use in

(a)

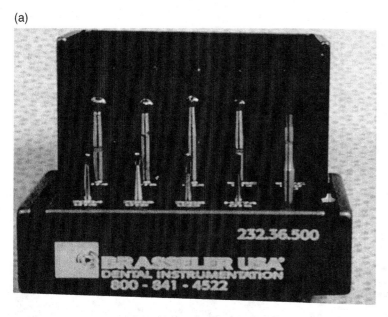

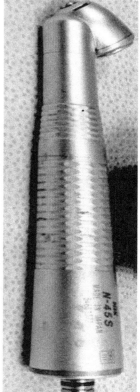

(b)

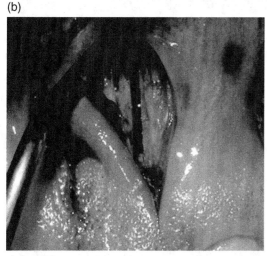

Figure 3.3 (a) Any appropriate rear-vented handpiece and surgical/dental bite burs can be used to perform decortication effectively. The rear air venting of the handpiece is important to prevent subcutaneous emphysema. (b) Piezoelectric instrumentation has been used to make an interdental cut into the medullary bone through a vertical incision in the maxillary quadrants. (c) Any geometrical pattern is effective for decortication, as long as the cortex is surgically violated and entry into medullary bone accomplished. Bleeding from the surgical sites typically ensures that medullary bone has been entered. This figure demonstrates various shapes in the form of lines versus dots and/or combination procedures that are all effective for SAD. (d) Decortication has been performed in both the maxillary and mandibular quadrants in two different patients. Care is taken to avoid performing decortication in the alveolar crest area, and it is recommended that the clinician preserves 1–2 mm of bone in this area to prevent bone resorption and gingival recession (arrows). Figure courtesy of Dr. Donald Ferguson and Dr. Ruben Figueroa.

(c)

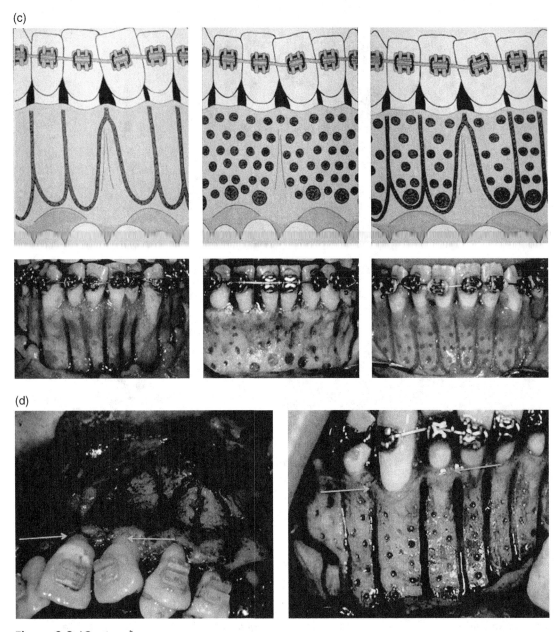

(d)

Figure 3.3 (Continued)

any case. Still others recommend using a bone graft to augment the alveolus if there are areas of dehiscence of roots and also if the native bony cortical plates are thin (<2 mm thickness on a cone beam computed tomography scan).

We recommend the use of a particulate bone graft in all cases as we feel it promotes bone healing and, in our experience, improves the clinical and radiographic appearance of the soft and hard tissues of the periodontium.

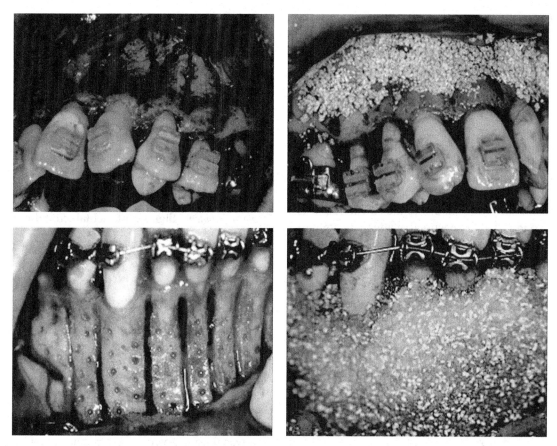

Figure 3.4 When indicated, bone grafting of the alveolus is performed with particulate bone grafts. Some clinicians prefer soaking the graft with antibiotic solution, but this is not mandatory. The maxillary quadrant has been bone grafted with bovine bone graft and the mandibular quadrant has been grafted with demineralized human freeze-dried bone. Approximately 0.5–1 cm³ of particular bone graft is required for each tooth-bearing segment. Care should be taken not to overpack, as this could compromise a tension-free closure of the soft tissues overlying the decortication and grafted areas.

If grafting is elected, any US Food and Drug Administration-approved, good-quality bone grafting material sourced from a reputable tissue bank can perhaps be used. We recommend use of either human freeze-dried bone or bovine allografts, and have found both to be successful and comparable in clinical outcomes. Grafting material is placed over the exposed decorticated area directly without any membrane use (Figure 3.4). Approximately 0.5–1 cm³ of particulate graft material is required for each tooth-bearing segment that is decorticated.

Care should be taken not to place an excessive amount of bone graft volume as it may interfere with proper flap repositioning and suturing.

Closure

Once the above surgical steps have been completed, the flap is then returned to its original position and reapproximated with resorbable sutures (3-0 or 4-0 vicryl or chromic gut are commonly used, although any other suture material is also acceptable). The suture type (interrupted, mattress, continuous) is not critical in our opinion; instead, what is critical is that the closure be tension-free. To achieve this, periosteal scoring under the flap may be required in some cases if closure is found to be difficult. When passing the needle through the tissue, the needle should enter the surface of the mucosa at a right angle, to make the smallest possible hole in the mucosal flap. If the needle passes through the tissue obliquely, the suture will tear through the surface layers of the flap when the suture knot is tied, which results in greater injury to the soft tissue. It is also important to ensure that adequate amount of tissue is taken when passing the needle through the flap, to prevent the needle or suture from pulling through the soft tissue flap. Once the sutures are passed through the mobile flap and immobile lingual tissue, they are tied with an instrument tie. Care must be taken not to excessively tighten the knots to avoid ischemia of flap margins. A reliable clinical indicator of flap ischemia is blanching of wound margins, which if it occurs should be dealt with immediately by reperforming the suture of the area.

Post-surgical considerations

Standard instructions that are used for minor oral surgical procedures are recommended. Oral antibiotics (7–10 days) and antimicrobial mouthwash (oral chlorhexidine for 1–3 weeks) should be routinely prescribed for all patients. Moderate-strength analgesics are generally required for the first 3–7 days, and then over-the-counter pain medications can be used. Rapid orthodontic treatment is then initiated within a few days (range 3–14 days) of surgery and continued until correction of malocclusion. It is imperative to remember that the goal is to complete as much orthodontic treatment as rapidly as possible while RAP peaks and exists. Thus, patients should be evaluated by their orthodontist weekly after surgery, and mechanics modified as and when required. All

patients undergo standard orthodontic retention treatment after treatment.

CLINICAL CASE PRESENTATIONS

Case 1

A 24-year-old female with convex facial profile, with significant upper and lower anterior dental crowding.

Primary problem: Significant dental crowding (8–9 mm)
Primary objective: Resolution of crowding without premolar extractions.
Secondary objective: Rapid orthodontics and shorten duration of treatment.

The patient was missing upper lateral incisors, had no lip incompetence, and showed 75% of her upper anterior teeth when smiling. Nasolabial angle was within normal limits. Dental model analysis revealed a full cusps class II molars and canines relationship with 4–5 mm overjet and 2 mm overbite; maxillary arch was mildly crowded (4 mm) and mandibular arch was severely crowded (8–9 mm) with the right lateral incisor lingually crowded. Upper dental midline was deviated to the right by 2 mm and lower midline was deviated 4 mm to the right when compared with the skeletal and facial midlines.

Traditional treatment would be approximately 2 years of orthodontic therapy, including lower premolar extractions to relieve the crowding, align the lower arch, and control possible bite opening during treatment (likely due to the hyperdivergent mandibular plane angle). The patient declined this option as she showed a genuine interest to have the orthodontic treatment completed as soon as possible and she preferred not extracting any teeth to relieve the crowding. The treatment plan involved the following comprehensive orthodontic treatment with fixed appliances to align the upper and lower teeth and correct the crowding and corticotomy procedure in both arches to accelerate the tooth movement. Owing to the congenitally missing upper lateral incisors and lack of space, it was decided that the canine teeth would substitute the missing lateral incisors and that first premolars will substitute the canines and the case would be finished in a class II molar relationship.

The patient was banded with fixed orthodontic brackets 2 weeks prior to surgery, and decortication was accomplished in all four quadrants under intravenous sedation. Full-thickness flaps were reflected after sulcular incisions and a high-speed handpiece and carbide bur were used for decortication, which was performed both labially/buccally and palatally/lingually. Orthodontic treatment was then resumed at the fifth post-operative day and the patient was debanded and placed into standard retention. The total treatment period with the fixed appliance therapy was 7.5 months. Figure 3.5a–h demonstrates the course of this patient.

Case 2

A 22-year-old female presented for consultation for surgical management of a large anterior open-bite malocclusion.

Primary problems: Large anterior open bite, multiple plane occlusion.
Primary objective: Avoid major (orthognathic) surgery.
Secondary objective: Rapid correction of malocclusion.

Clinical examination revealed a severe anterior open bite, proclined upper anterior teeth and a midline diastema. Orthodontic appliances were placed 2 weeks prior to surgery and selective alveolar decortication performed in a manner similar to patient in Case 1. Orthodontic therapy was started at the ninth post-operative

day and clinical examination at the 12th post-operative week interval revealed significant progress, including retroclining of the upper anterior teeth and closure of the midline diastema. Orthodontic treatment was completed and the patient debanded at post-operative week 15. Figure 3.6a–g demonstrates the successful use of selective alveolar decortication in this patient.

Case 3

A 23-year-old female who presented with facial and dental asymmetry after undergoing a complex orthognathic surgery procedure.

Primary problem: Skeletal and dental malocclusion resulting due to a complication from an orthognathic surgery procedure.
Primary objective: Minimally invasive surgery to correct dental malocclusion.
Secondary objective: Avoid repeat orthognathic surgery.

Verbal questions and history taking revealed that the patient had undergone complex reconstructive surgery 3 months previously. This had included a left temporomandibular joint (TMJ) surgery for rheumatoid arthritis and a right-sided mandibular sagittal split osteotomy with concomitant maxillary Le Fort 1 osteotomy. Post-operatively, the patient was found to have a 6–8 mm posterior open bite on the left side. The orthodontist indicated that it was not possible to correct the post-surgery malocclusion by orthodontic mechanics alone. There were two options: (1) repeat orthognathic surgery and (2) trial of corticotomy-facilitated orthodontic therapy. The patient declined to have another major surgical procedure performed; she indicated that she was OK with the facial asymmetry and canting and agreed to undergo decortication and orthodontics with the understanding that, at best, only the

(a)

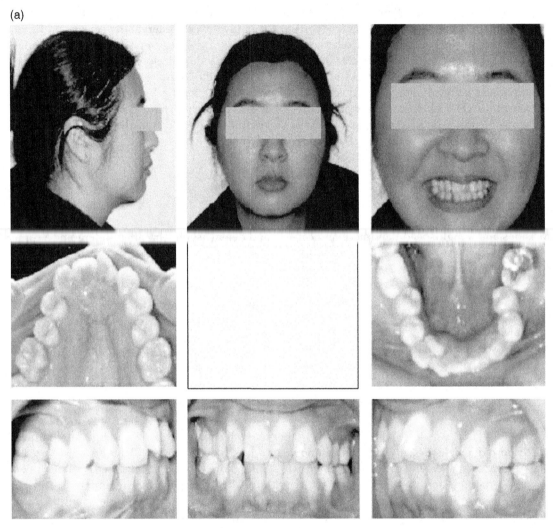

Figure 3.5 (a) Composite intraoral and extraoral photographs demonstrating patient with severe dental maloc-clusion and transverse maxillary hypoplasia and dental crowding. (b) Dental model analysis revealing skeletal and dental malocclusion, missing upper lateral incisors, and class II angle molar relationship. (c) Dental models demonstrating transverse maxillary hypoplasia and severe lower crowding. Note lingual positioning of right lower lateral incisor and severe lingual tipping of bilateral second premolars. (d) Exposure and decortication have been performed in bilateral maxillary as well as mandibular quadrants. Rotary surgical bur and handpiece were taken to perform decortication. (e) Pre-operative and 4-week post-operative views. Note increased transverse dimension, improvement and resolution of crowding in the maxillary anterior region and spacing in the lower right mandib-ular area, which would be subsequently used for bring the lateral incisors back into the alveolar arch form. (f) Pre-operative and 8-month post-operative views showing correction of severe dental crowding, dental malocclu-sion, and transverse maxillary hypoplasia with stable post-operative results. (g) Intraoral photographs revealing a retention phase and stable post-operative results with good arch form and resolution of crowding. (h) Pre-operative and post-operative extraoral photographs. Figure courtesy of Dr. Ruben Figueroa.

(b)

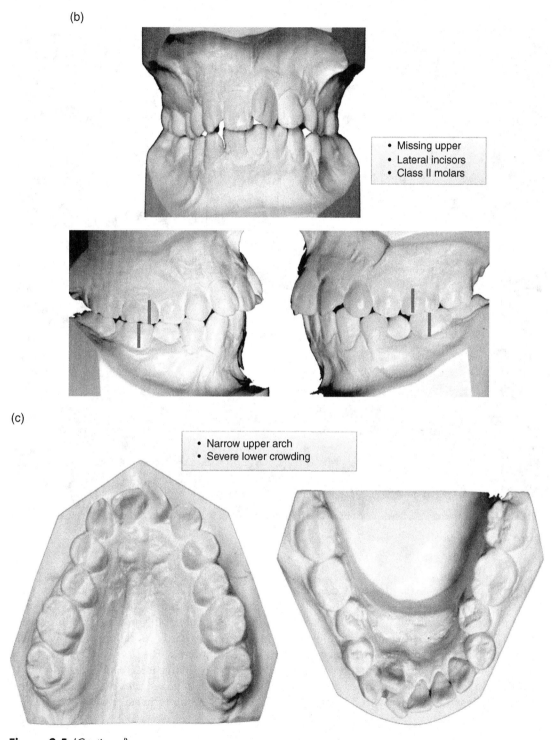

- Missing upper
- Lateral incisors
- Class II molars

(c)

- Narrow upper arch
- Severe lower crowding

Figure 3.5 (*Continued*)

(d)

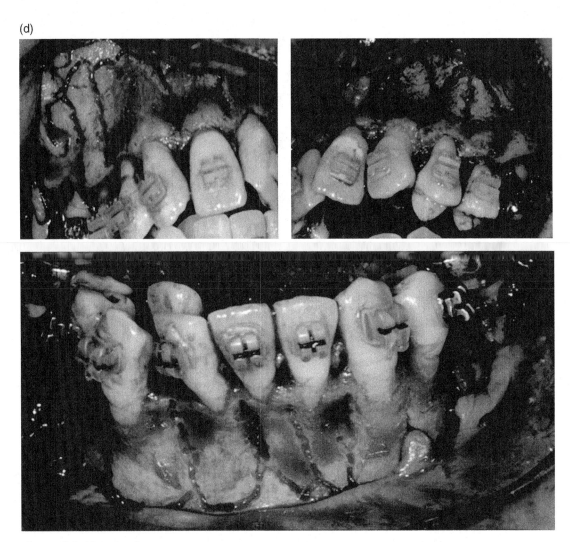

Figure 3.5 (Continued)

right-sided open-bite malocclusion would be corrected.

Full-thickness buccal and palatal flaps were reflected in the left maxillary and mandibular decortication accomplished under intravenous sedation using rotary instrumentation under irrigation. No grafting was performed and routine wound closure obtained with 3-0 chromic gut sutures. Post-surgical orthodontics was initiated on the ninth post-operative day and complete closure of the open bite accomplished in 3 weeks. No hard or soft tissue complications were encountered. Results were stable at the 1 year post-operative interval after decortication. Figure 3.7a–e demonstrates the effective use of SAD and the long-term successful outcome.

(e)

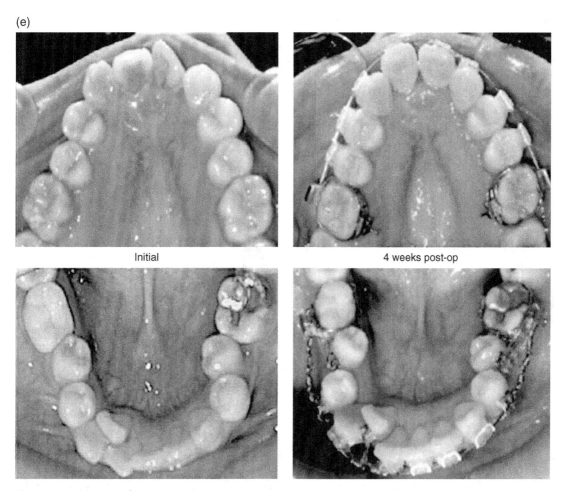

| Initial | 4 weeks post-op |

Figure 3.5 *(Continued)*

Case 4

A 26-year-old male who presented with a severe malocclusion after suffering from a malunion following surgical treatment for mandibular trauma (fracture).

Primary problem: Diagnostic workup showed that the malocclusion could not be corrected by orthodontics alone and/or segmental orthognathic surgery (this option would have required multiple single-tooth or two-teeth surgical segmentation of the mandible, risking inferior alveolar nerve injury and alveolar bone avascular necrosis besides damage to dental structures).

Primary objective: Modest improvement of dental relationships and occlusion.

Secondary objective: Level and align dentition in a manner so that, should the patient later desire, orthognathic surgery could be a viable alternative.

(f)

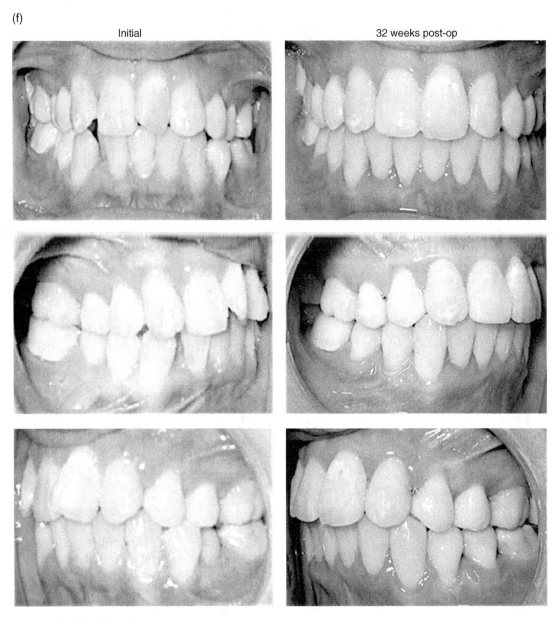

Figure 3.5 (*Continued*)

The patient presented with a severe malunion status post-correction of multiple mandibular fractures by another surgeon. Diagnostic study models were obtained and it was noted that it would be impossible to correct the dental malocclusion even with segmental mandibular surgery owing to the multiple planes of occlusion. The study models showed that complete intercuspation of teeth was not possible without long-term comprehensive orthodontic therapy,

(g)

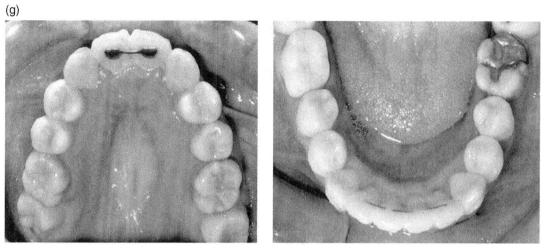

32 weeks post-op (8 months)

(h)   Initial   Final

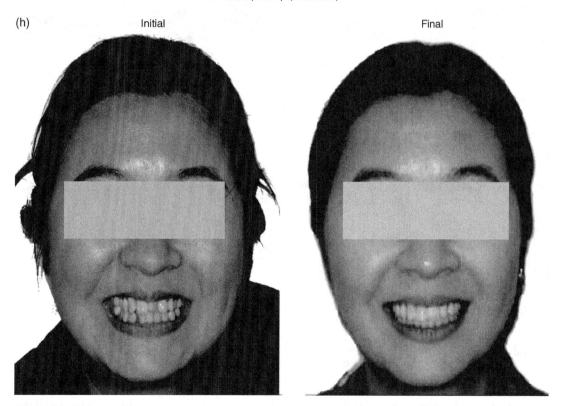

Figure 3.5 (*Continued*)

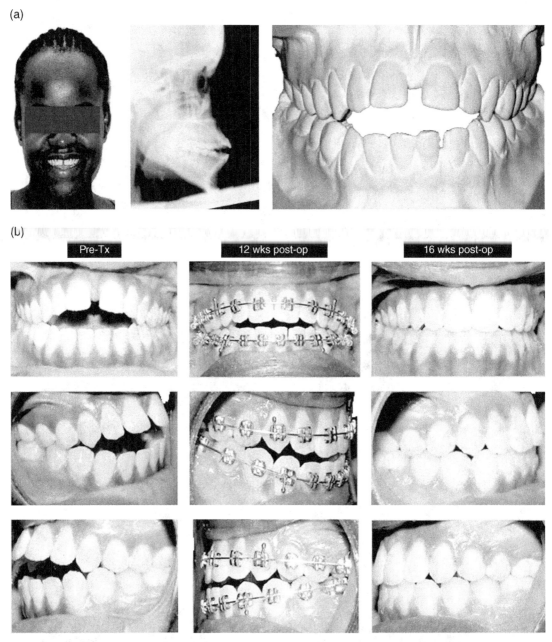

Figure 3.6 (a) Pre-operative photograph of a patient with large anterior open bite malocclusion, incisal diastema, and dentoskeletal deformity. (b) Composite pre-treatment, during treatment, and post-operative views demonstrating correction of anterior open-bite malocclusion in less than 4 months. (c) Dental models demonstrating effectiveness of technique and good intercuspation of dentition at the long-term follow-up stage. (d) Pre-operative and post-operative dental models showing effectiveness of results. (e) Pre-operative and post-operative cephalometric radiographs demonstrating successful treatment of combined skeletal and dental deformity in less than 4 months without orthognathic surgery. (f) Pre-operative and post-operative profile views. (g) Pre-operative and post-operative frontal views. Figure courtesy of Dr. Ruben Figueroa.

(c)

(d)

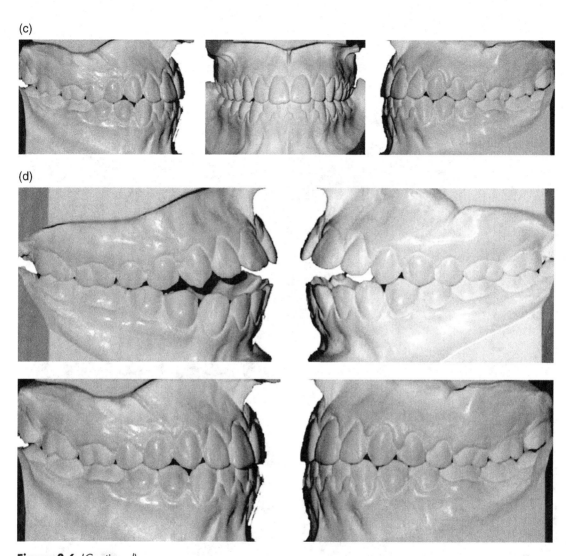

Figure 3.6 (*Continued*)

which the patient refused to undergo. Clinical examination also revealed poor periodontal status of much of the dentition on the right lower quadrant. The patient chose the option for corticotomy-facilitated orthodontic therapy with the understanding of all risks, including failure to correct malocclusion and loss of periodontally compromised teeth.

Orthodontic bands, brackets, and arch wires were placed 10 days prior to surgery and selective alveolar decortication was performed under local anesthesia on both the buccal and lingual aspects of the anterior and posterior portions of the right lower jaw. Buccal and lingual bone grafting were accomplished using particulate human freeze-dried bone. Post-operative orthodontic mechanics, including vertical elastics, were initiated on the eighth post-operative day. Significant improvement of the open bite was achieved within only

(e)

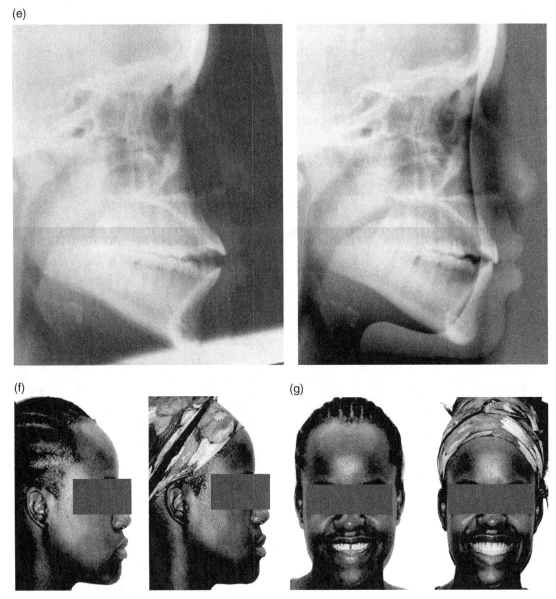

(f)

(g)

Figure 3.6 (*Continued*)

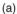

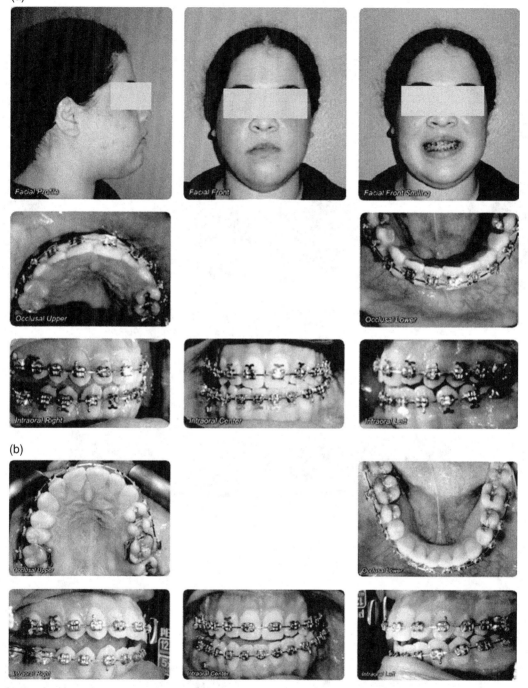

Figure 3.7 (a) Pre-operative photograph showing iatrogenic malocclusion on the right side with posterior open bite and canting following complex orthognathic and TMJ procedure. (b) Pre-operative radiograph at the time of banding approximately 7–10 days prior to selective alveolar decortication. (c) Pre-operative radiograph demonstrating orthognathic surgical procedure on both the maxilla and mandible. (d) Four-week post-operative results after selective alveolar decortication. Note that the right-sided open bite has completely been closed using a combination of selective alveolar decortication and orthodontic mechanics with vertical elastics in a rapid fashion. (e) Long-term retention results showing stability at the 6-month post-operative stage.

(c)

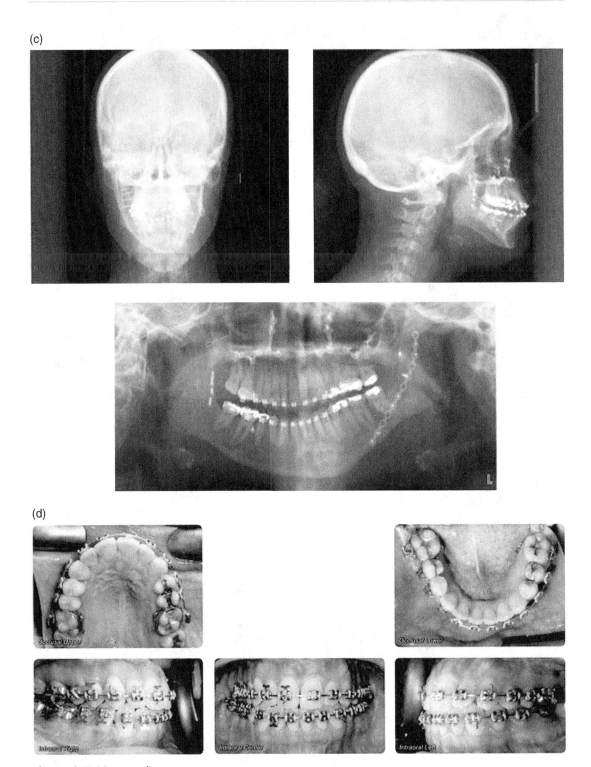

(d)

Figure 3.7 (*Continued*)

(e)

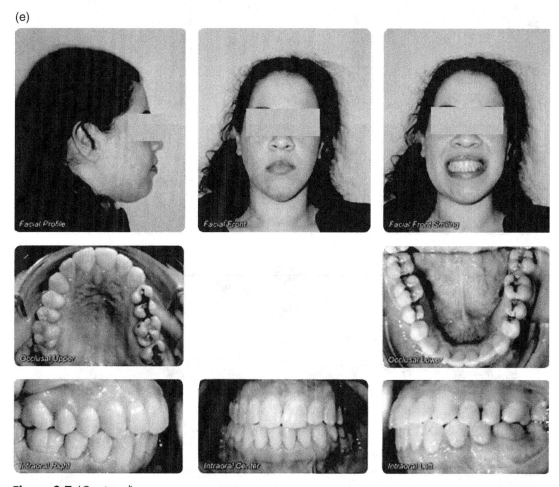

Figure 3.7 (*Continued*)

4 weeks post-surgery. Long-term results were found to be stable. Figure 3.8a–d shows the initial presentation, clinical progress, and final results.

Case 5

A 27-year-old male with severe maxillary transverse deficiency planned for a SARPE procedure.

Primary problem: Constricted maxilla in a skeletally mature patient.
Primary objective: Avoid hospital-based SARPE and thereby have decreased surgical and

anesthetic risk, shorter treatment, less invasive surgery and reduced costs.

Buccal and palatal flaps were made to expose all bony structures of the maxilla from tooth nos. 2 to 15. Selective decortication was next performed under sedation in an office setting using a rotary handpiece and carbide burs in a standard manner in all areas. The labial and buccal alveolar plates were then grafted with particulate human freeze-dried bone graft. Orthodontic therapy started on post-operative day 7 and the entire treatment, including transverse expansion (12 mm), completed in

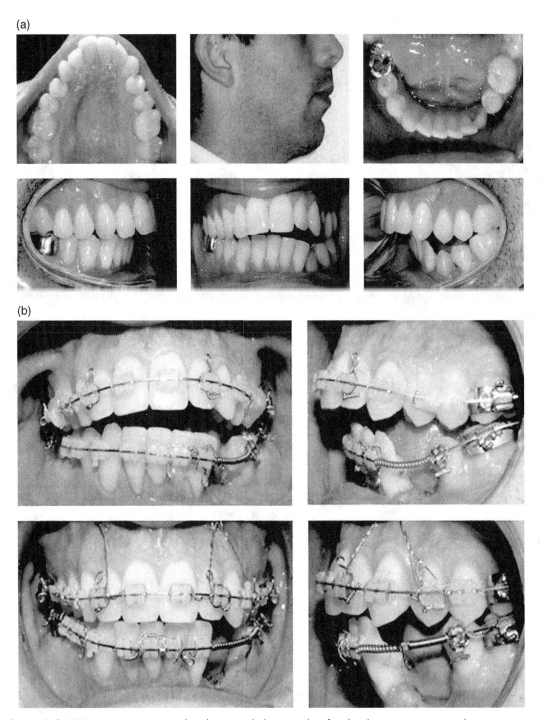

Figure 3.8 (a) Pre-operative intraoral and extraoral photographs of malocclusion status post-malunion treatment of fractures. The patient had multiple planes of occlusion in the maxilla and the anterior and left posterior mandible with a class II relationship. (b) Orthodontic hardware is in place on the maxillary and mandibular arches. A coil spring has been placed in the left mandible area and teeth extracted in preparation for selective alveolar decortication and correction of malocclusion. (c) Initial and 4-month post-operative views showing rapid correction of the severe skeletal and dental malocclusion. Implants have been placed for anchorage in the bilateral anterior maxilla (arrows). In this case, it was determined that orthognathic surgery was not a viable alternative owing to significant morbidity and complications. (d) Post-operative view of the same patient showing completion of results.

(c)

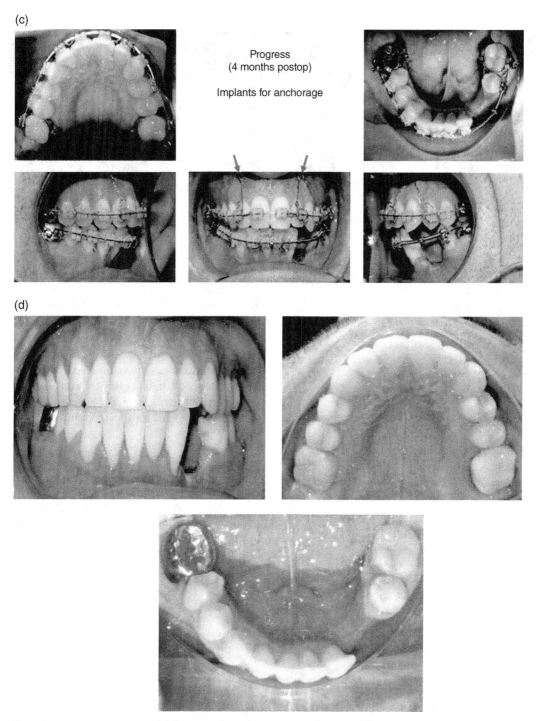

Progress
(4 months postop)

Implants for anchorage

(d)

Figure 3.8 (*Continued*)

(a)

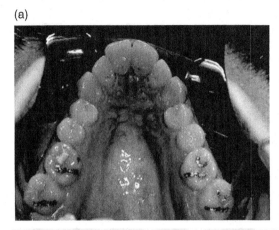

(b)

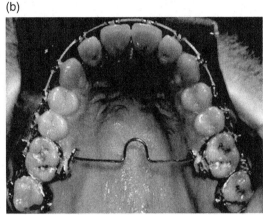

Figure 3.9 (a) Pre-operative radiograph of a patient with severe transverse maxillary hypoplasia. (b) Post-operative results showing correction of transverse maxillary hypoplasia with selective alveolar decortication without use of a maxillary expansion appliance or SARPE procedure.

16 weeks. Figure 3.9a and b shows the clinical course and final results.

RESEARCH EXPERIENCE

Statement of the problem

Hospital-based major orthognathic surgical procedures have been traditionally used for predictable surgical management of skeletal malocclusions. Recently, SAD has been proposed as an alternative option. However, no previous reports exist in the oral and maxillofacial surgery literature regarding long-term stability and/or limitations of this technique for correction of dentofacial deformities. We aimed to define specific indications, and present data showing failure and stability of treatment results with the use of SAD.

Materials and methods

The study involved a total of 48 patients with malocclusions who were surgically treated by combined SAD and orthodontic treatments. All surgical procedures were performed as outpatient surgery in an office setting under intravenous sedation. Buccal and lingual/palatal

decortication was performed using rotary high-speed instrumentation under irrigation. Alveolar augmentation was performed with particulate allograft, when indicated. Rapid orthodontic treatment was initiated within a few days (range 3–14 days) of surgery and continued until correction of malocclusion. All patients then underwent standard orthodontic retention.

Methods of data analysis

For study purposes, patients were divided into subgroups based on the presenting malocclusion: maxillary transverse deficiency ($n = 8$), dental crowding ($n = 8$), anterior open bite ($n = 8$), deep bite ($n = 8$), skeletal class II ($n = 8$), and skeletal class III ($n = 8$). Data were assessed for: (1) type of skeletal malocclusion corrected, (2) soft and hard tissue response, (3) surgical, orthodontic, and total treatment times, (4) cost of surgical treatment, and (5) long-term stability.

Results of investigation

The technique was extremely successful for correction of certain specific malocclusions, including dental crowding, transverse maxillary

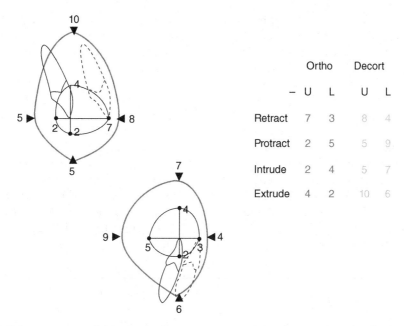

	Ortho		Decort	
–	U	L	U	L
Retract	7	3	8	4
Protract	2	5	5	9
Intrude	2	4	5	7
Extrude	4	2	10	6

Figure 3.10 Schematic view of the scope of treatment compared with conventional orthodontics. Note that decortication was effective in increasing the scope of treatment in most areas, excepting incisor retraction.

constriction, and some open-bite malocclusions. Scope of nonsurgical orthodontic treatment increased two to three times when compared with conventional treatment. Long-term results were extremely stable secondary to high tissue turnover and thicker cortical bone resulting from the augmentation grafting. The technique was not successful in treating skeletal anteroposterior (class II/III) discrepancies greater than 2 mm. Figure 3.10 shows preliminary results that were obtained during multiple research projects conducted by Dr Donald Ferguson in the early 2000s. These corroborate the increased scope of treatment via SAD compared with conventional orthodontics alone.

Although a relatively new technique, SAD has the potential to provide a solid platform for improvement in the efficiency and effectiveness of current-day orthodontic therapy. It significantly increases the scope of nonextraction

orthodontic treatment and has the potential to be an alternative to traditional orthognathic surgery when its use is limited to the management of certain specific types of minor dentoskeletal deformities. RAP occurs following purposeful SAD, thereby resulting in increased bone turnover and decreased bone density; these biological effects lead to accelerated tooth movement and reduced treatment duration, without adverse effects on the periodontium.

Besides increasing the scope of nonextraction orthodontic treatment, it hastens the results of conventional nonsurgical orthodontic therapy. It also has the potential to correct certain specific dentoskeletal malocclusions with minimally invasive, office-based surgery.

Even for patients requiring routine orthognathic surgery, SAD may be indicated as it decreases the pre-operative orthodontic treatment time by more than 50% (e.g., leveling and aligning of dental arches, relief of dental crowding, canine retraction). In the senior author's experience, rapid orthodontic tooth movement can be achieved in a third to a quarter of the time required for traditional orthodontics and without the need for dental extractions in many cases. Advantages of SAD include minimally invasive surgery, decreased treatment time, decreased health-care costs, and the ability to perform surgery in an office setting. SAD is excellent for vertical and transverse dental discrepancies. It is also very effective for relief of crowding by tipping and/or uprighting of the dentition. However, it must be remembered that it does not replace orthognathic surgery and should not be regarded as a standard treatment for moderate to severe skeletal class II or class III cases.

ACKNOWLEDGMENTS

The authors would like to acknowledge Dr. Ruben Figueroa and Dr. Donald Ferguson, both of whom actively participated with the senior author in the combined surgical and orthodontic management of the clinical cases presented in this chapter.

References

Frost HM (1983) The regional acceleratory phenomena: a review. *Henry Ford Hospital Medical Journal*, **31** (1), 3–9.

Frost HM (1989a) The biology of fracture healing: an overview for clinicians. Part 1. *Clinical Orthopedics and Related Research*, **248**, 283–293.

Frost HM (1989b) The biology of fracture healing: an overview for clinicians. Part II. *Clinical Orthopedics and Related Research*, **248**, 294–309.

Köle H (1959) Surgical operations on the alveolar ridge to correct occlusal abnormalities. *Oral Surgery Oral Medicine Oral Pathology*, **12**, 515–529.

Rusanen J, Lahti S, Tolvanen M *et al.* (2010) Quality of life in patients with severe malocclusion before treatment. *European Journal of Orthodontics*, **32** (1), 43–48.

Sebaoun JD, Kantarci A, Turner JW *et al.* (2008) Modeling of trabecular bone and lamina dura following selective alveolar decortication in rats. *Journal of Periodontology*, **79** (9), 1679–1688.

Shih MS, Norrdin RW (1985) Regional acceleration of remodeling during healing of bone defects in beagles of various ages. *Bone*, **5**, 377–379.

Suya H (1991) Corticotomy in orthodontics, in *Mechanical and Biological Basis in Orthodontic Therapy* (eds E Hosl, A Baldauf), HuthigBuchVerlag, Heidelberg, pp. 207–226.

Vig PS, Orth D, Weintraub JA *et al.* (1990) The duration of orthodontic treatment with and without extractions: a pilot study of five selected practices. *American Journal of Orthodontics Dentofacial Orthopedics*, **97** (1), 45–51.

Wilcko MW, Wilcko MT, Bouquot JE *et al.* (2001). Rapid orthodontics with alveolar reshaping: two case reports of decrowding. *International Journal of Periodontics and Restorative Dentistry*, **21**, 9–19.

Wilcko WM, Ferguson DJ, Bouquot JE *et al.* (2003) Rapid orthodontic decrowding with alveolar augmentation: case report. *World Journal of Orthodontics*, **4**, 197–205.

Yaffe A, Fine N, Binderman I (1994) Regional accelerated phenomenon the mandible following mucoperiosteal flap surgery. *Journal of Periodontology*, **65**, 79–83.

Orthodontic applications of alveolus decortication

Neal C. Murphy

Department of Orthodontics, Case Western Reserve University, School of Dental Medicine,
Cleveland, OH, USA
Department of Periodontics, Case Western Reserve University, School of Dental Medicine,
Cleveland, OH, USA

INTRODUCTION

The last half of the 20th century witnessed countless improvements in the orthodontic specialty, and those of the last 10–15 years have been particularly profound. Improvements of appliance aesthetics, self-ligating bracket systems, clear aligners, computerized imaging systems, implant-like anchorage screws, and many other developments have elevated the expectations of clinicians and patients alike. These recent advances offer convenience and esthetic advantages that make orthodontic therapy more acceptable, especially to adults. Despite all these innovative changes, the length of the orthodontic treatment still haunts the specialty as a major deterrent for many patients. So, in the last two decades, enterprising periodontists have resurrected and refined century-old methods of accelerating orthodontic therapy.

The procedures in general are referred to as "surgically facilitated orthodontic therapy" (SFOT). Originally, two basic procedures were performed, but these are now generally eschewed by periodontists because of their excessive morbidity. These traditional surgeries included crude segmental osteotomies luxated with chisels and mallets and rudimentary corticotomies that were undisciplined in their applications. Popularized largely by the intrepid studies of one clinical professor of periodontology,[1] the rudimentary methods have been refined to discrete and minor outpatient procedures using selective alveolar decortication (SAD). Today, a growing consortium of visionary clinicians worldwide is refining and developing new incarnations (Figure 4.1) of SAD and continuing this global renaissance for a new generation of periodontists and orthodontic specialists.

Orthodontically Driven Corticotomy: Tissue Engineering to Enhance Orthodontic and Multidisciplinary Treatment,
First Edition. Edited by Federico Brugnami and Alfonso Caiazzo.
© 2015 John Wiley & Sons, Inc. Published 2015 by John Wiley & Sons, Inc.
Companion Website: www.wiley.com/go/Brugnami/Corticotomy

(a)   (b)

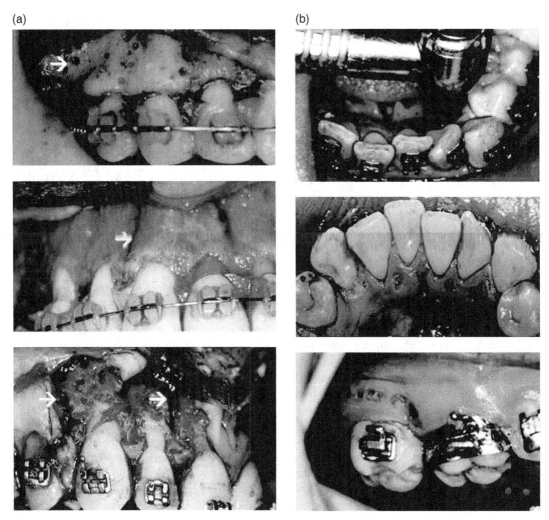

Figure 4.1 This demonstrates a series of selective alveolar decortication techniques to engineer accelerated tooth movement. The decortication quantitatively can be minimal, moderate, or aggressive. Qualitatively, they may be punctate or linear. Combinations vary by doctor preference and degree of osteopenia needed for a given amount of orthodontic tooth movement (OTM). (a) SAD induces a therapeutic, reversible regional osteopenia to facilitated accelerated OTM. The osteopenic state is extended by the strain of OTM or indefinitely by trans-mucosal perturbation (perforation) (TMP). The pattern of decortication is irrelevant, but the degree of decortication is commensurate with the degree of required therapeutic osteopenia. Here, we see three styles of decortication: top – a conservative punctate (arrow); middle – a moderate linear (arrow), and bottom – an aggressive combination (arrows). (b) TMP. This is an epigenetic perturbation of healing morphogenesis by perforation of the alveolus with a high-speed, surgical-length irrigated dental round bur. Top: TMP technique; middle: TMP to induce therapeutic transient osteopenia for mandibular incisor labial tipping; bottom: TMP to accelerate OTM of maxillary second molar. (*Source*: UniversityExperts.com used with permission.)

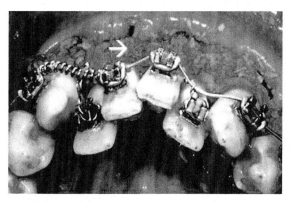 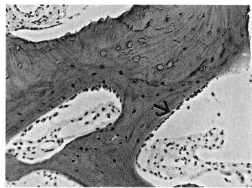

Figure 4.2 Refinements of SAD engineered to augment the mass of the alveolus bone. Left: PAOO is SAD with a demineralized bone matrix (DBM), so called "dead bone" at white arrow. DBM is also referred to as demineralized freeze-dried bone allograft (DFDBA). Right: H&E specimen of sample taken from alveolus after augmentation with PSCT, PAOO with a viable Mesenchimal Stem Cell (MSC) allograft, so-called "live bone," at black arrow. (*Source*: UniversityExperts.com used with permission.)

Most recently, even these manipulations have been enhanced with sophisticated grafting. Interestingly, these innovations – (Periodontally) Accelerated Osteogenic Orthodontics™ ((P) AOO™)[2] and periodontal stem cell therapy (PSCT) (Figure 4.2) – have been enthusiastically received by patients. But they are attracted to them neither for scientific reasons nor the minimal morbidity they enjoy. Rather, patients prefer them because they reduce total treatment time.

However, the surprisingly high degree of patient acceptance of such tissue engineering – singularly reducing treatment times by 200–400% – should not eclipse other professional advantages. These include but are not limited to, less infection, fewer caries, and less gingival damage (Waldrop, 2008), or attachment loss (Zachrisson and Alnaes, 1974). Traditional side effects, such as root resorption and decalcifications (Levander and Malmgren, 1988; Geiger *et al.*, 1992; Segal *et al.*, 2004; Fox, 2005; Bishara and Ostby, 2008; Pandis *et al.*, 2008) and compromised patient compliance (Royko *et al.*, 1999), also may be a thing of the past when SAD and its regenerative variants are employed.

In our fast-paced world there have been many other attempts to shorten the orthodontic treatment time, such as rapid distraction of the canines (Liou and Huang, 1998), local application of prostaglandin (Spielmann *et al.*, 1989), pulsed electromagnetic fields (Showkatbakhsh *et al.*, 2010), mechanical vibration (Nishimura *et al.*, 2008), low-intensity laser (Cruz *et al.*, 2004; Yamaguchi *et al.*, 2010), minor perforation (perturbation) of the adjacent alveolus bone (Murphy, 2006; Murphy *et al.*, 2012), and the derivatives, corticision (Kim *et al.*, 2009), Piezocision (Dibart *et al.*, 2009), and piezopuncture (Kim *et al.*, 2013).

However, these pale in comparison to the profound structural changes that are evoked by the salient incarnations of decortication-facilitated orthodontics (Bell and Levy, 1972; Anholm *et al.*, 1986; Gantes *et al.*, 1990; Suya, 1991; Wilcko *et al.*, 2001, 2003), PAOO and PSCT in particular. In a very recent study, Long *et al.* (2013) conducted a systematic review of interventions for accelerating tooth movement. They compared low-level laser therapy, corticotomy, electrical current, pulsed electromagnetic fields, and dentoalveolar or periodontal distraction. They concluded that, among these five interventions, the decortication procedure was safest and clearly able to accelerate orthodontic tooth movement.

THE BASIC CONCEPTS

SAD,[3] as it has evolved into the 21st century, employs an intentional, but minor, superficial "injury" to the cortical bone. Its origin lies in less discrete procedures first described in the late 19th century as an expedient way of surgically treating malocclusion and found its way into the American literature in the mid 20th century (Köle, 1959). At the cell level, mechanical microfractures of the osteon will induce remodeling that adapts the bone to novel mechanical stimuli, and SAD is the macroscopic, clinic-level analogue. At the turn of the 21st century, Wilcko et al. (2001) added the alveolar augmentation (bone grafting) to the SAD protocol and termed the innovation PAOO (Wilcko et al., 2001, 2003). This technique, combining alveolar decortication with bone grafting with DFDBA or MSCs to expand alveolar volume, exploits both the SAD-induced opportunity for rapid tooth movement and the enlargement of alveolus bone volume to accommodate dental arch expansion.

To explain the startling results of this pioneering work the designers called upon established histophysiologic mechanisms of decalcification and recalcification of the alveolus bone that is commonly encountered after periodontal osseous surgery. This posited mechanism is supported by the medical orthopedic literature (Bogoch et al., 1993; Frost, 1989) wherever it is applied to SAD. Therefore, a decalcification–recalcification description of the alveolus bone response is a direct and legitimate extrapolation of histophysiology seen in long bone fractures. The concept was extended further into 21st century tissue engineering with the addition of MSCs (Murphy et al., 2012).

Since the validity of SAD procedures has been scientifically validated by independent replication and the scientific justification is sound, the next developmental challenge is determining how predictable and realistic goals may be achieved with this nascent science: *oral tissue engineering*. Thus, the aim of this chapter

is to explain how various alveolar decortication procedures can play a significant role in orthodontic treatment.

ORTHODONTIC IMPLICATIONS OF BONE INJURY: THE REGIONAL ACCELERATORY PHENOMENON

When bone is traumatized in any way, a very specific and dynamic healing process occurs at the site of the bone "injury" that is proportional to the extent of the insult. This is best described by Frost in the orthopedic literature as a regional acceleratory phenomenon (RAP) (Shin and Norrdin, 1985; Frost, 1989a,b). The term "regional" refers to the demineralization of both the trauma site and histological reaction in the adjacent bone. The term "acceleratory" refers to an exaggerated or intensified metabolic response nearby that extends slightly into the marrow (spongiosa). This metabolic burst is a manifestation of normal remodeling that speeds up healing.

For SAD, the demineralization is later followed by subperiosteal appositional osteogenesis. There is a localized surge of coordinated osteoclastic and osteoblastic activity that, in the early phases, manifests a decrease in bone density with an increased bone turnover. The RAP begins within a few days of the surgery and becomes amenable to practical orthodontic tooth movement after 14 days. Then, depending on the degree of decortication, the demineralization peaks after 2–4 months – in the absence of orthodontically induced strain – and diminishes as remineralization sets in.

As alveolar decortication became popular, various animal experiments were conducted to explain its effects on the alveolar bone and orthodontic tooth movement potential. Sebaoun et al. (2008) evaluated the effects of decortication *per se* in the absence tooth movement in a split-mouth rat model. They found that at 3 weeks the catabolic activity (osteoclast count) and anabolic activity (apposition rate) were threefold greater in decortication sites. Calcified spongiosa decreased by twofold. Surgical injury to the alveolus that induced a significant increase in tissue turnover by week 3 dissipated to a steady state by postoperative week 11, and the impact of the injury was localized to the area immediately adjacent to the decortication. These data confirmed that alveolar decortication induced a RAP response in the alveolus like that in long bones, but Sebaoun *et al.* did not integrate the study with actual tooth movement.

Lee *et al.* (2008) investigated the effects of corticotomy-facilitated orthodontic therapy with micro-computed tomography (CT). Later, Baloul *et al.* (2011) compared the effects of alveolar decortication with and without tooth movement. In an award-winning[4] experiment, the researchers studied three groups: decortication only, tooth movement only, and a "combined group" (tooth movement and decortication). They used morphologic analysis, quantitative micro-CT for structural analysis, and quantitative polymerase chain reaction to analyze messenger RNA gene expression associated with both osteoclasts and osteoblasts. Their data conclusively established that alveolar decortication enhances the rate of tooth movement during the initial tooth displacement phase with a "coupled" mechanism of bone cell activation adding to the natural histologic phenomena of orthodontic treatment.

The term "coupling" refers to the fact that resorption and apposition are not strictly sequential or independent events; they are simultaneous and functionally connected with each other, overlapping in their effects (King and Keeling, 1995; Proff and Romer, 2009), and vary by location, intensity, and duration.

PRACTICAL APPLICATIONS

These findings are directly applicable to any clinical setting, because they suggest accelerating the rate of tooth movement treatment and engineering RAP can impact orthodontic treatment planning in two major ways. First, manipulating the consequent osteopenia with SAD enhances the relative degree of orthodontic anchorage. Second, to increase the mass of the alveolus and expand the envelope of possible tooth movement, treatment necessitates a kind of concentrated or focused biomechanical protocol during an osteopenic "window of opportunity."

ENHANCING RELATIVE ANCHORAGE

The practice of orthodontics is largely dependent on the availability of anchorage. Anchorage, by definition, is a body's resistance to displacement. Newton's third law suggests that for every force there is an equal and opposite reactive force. This explains differential rates of movement of two opposing objects which, practically speaking, is inversely related to the mass of the moved objects or resistance the force encounters. Thus, orthodontic treatments are designed with this law in mind, the goal being to resist unwanted tooth movement. According to Proffit (2000), in treatment planning,

> ...it is simply not possible to consider only the teeth whose movement is desired. Reciprocal effects throughout the dental arches must be carefully analyzed, evaluated, and controlled. An important aspect of treatment is maximizing the tooth movement that is desired, while minimizing undesirable side effects.

In orthodontic movement, segments of teeth that resist movement are often ligated together,

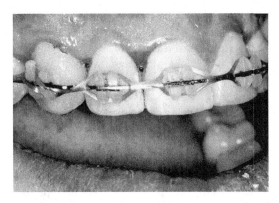

Figure 4.3 Orthodontic anchorage may consist of any combination of dental or tissue borne appliances. Usually, posterior teeth are ligated together for anchorage, but here, following SAD surgery, an elastic chain forms "anchor value" in the maxillary anterior sextant. (*Source*: UniversityExperts.com used with permission.)

with thin stainless steel wire or elastic chain (Figure 4.3), to serve as "anchors" and used to pull or push against other segments to be moved. Usually, the anchor segment will contain more teeth or teeth with greater "root enface"[5] (Murphy *et al.*, 1982) than the segment of teeth that are to be moved. This concept of differential anchorage is important in most orthodontic treatment, especially in cases of severe arch length deficiency (ALD); that is, "crowding" or skeletal dysplasias. In fact, treatment of certain malocclusions is often defined by the available anchorage; for example, "a maximum anchorage case."

There are numerous ways in which orthodontics has tried to augment anchorage, including auxiliary devices such as headgear, transpalatal arches, palatal acrylic pads (Nance appliances), and mini-implants of various designs. Many of these appliances are uncomfortable for patients or lead to "anchorage loss (slippage)," an untoward movement of dental anchorage units. Also, lower levels of patient compliance are common where extraoral traction or intraoral elastics interfere with patients' psycho-social imperatives. Thus, treatment outcomes can become compromised.

When movement of anchor teeth is not important the term "minimal anchorage" is employed. For example, if an extraction space needs closing by the mesial movement of posterior teeth in addition to the posterior movement of anterior teeth, the term "minimal anchorage" is appropriate. Where very little posterior tooth movement is desired as anterior teeth are pulled against them, the term "maximum anchorage" is used. However, maximum anchorage is often more of a wish than a reality because even in this ideal scheme some posterior tooth movement may occur.

Recently, titanium screws used as temporary anchorage devices (TADs) have been shown to provide excellent *absolute* anchorage where no posterior anchor movement whatsoever can be demonstrated. Because titanium screws do not have a reactive periodontal ligament the titanium anchors are as perfectly stable as ankylosed teeth. So TADs have, over the last two decades, emerged as very acceptable anchorage adjuncts to orthodontic treatment. However, owing to a number of limitations, such as patient disdain and premature exfoliation, they may be as unreliable as extraoral traction.

Tissue resistance to tooth movement must also be considered in assessing anchorage potential by estimating volume and density of the alveolar bone in addition to the cross-sectional area of the roots perpendicular to tooth movement vector sum. This osseous tissue that must be resorbed for a tooth to move thus contributes greater or lesser "anchorage value" (Roberts, 2005). That is, where there is less bone and less dense bone in the trajectory, there is less anchorage value. So, rendering a given volume of bone less dense through SAD increases the relative resistance of the opposing biomechanical anchorage units. This is why SAD, PAOO, PSCT, or TMP should not be used within 4–6 mm of ligated molars or TADs.

In addition to these histological assets, the shrewd use of "relative anchorage" provided by SAD allows orthodontists to avoid notoriously unpredictable anchorage paraphernalia, such as intraoral elastics and extraoral traction (headgear) that rely on capricious adolescent compliance.

MAXIMIZING THE WINDOW OF OPPORTUNITY

Following the reactive demineralization after SAD, there is a 3–4 month clinical "window of opportunity" to move teeth rapidly through demineralized bone before it remineralizes. But this can be extended to 4–6 months in orthodontically strained bone or indefinitely with transmucosal perforation (TMP) of the bone with an irrigated high-speed round bur (Murphy, 2006; Murphy *et al.*, 2012). Thus, the criticism (Mathews and Kokich, 2013) that RAP is too effete or transient for clinical use may be legitimately dismissed as spurious, naive, or premature.

If applying orthodontic force has the intention of lengthening the duration of the RAP effect, orthodontic activations must be made every 2 weeks after the decortication. The orthodontic force presumably delays the maturation of immature woven bone to mature lamellar bone around the decortication the way a mobile fracture fails to recalcify (malunion). This may occur by creating microfractures to the osteon and delays remineralization.

Since the effect of the decortication can diminish with time, the major tooth movements should be completed in the first few months of the treatment. So, the clinician should plan the mechanics to take advantage of this time frame. If possible, one should combine procedures using longer appointment times, if necessary to finish the major tooth movements. *Caveat:* undesirable delays caused by inefficient biomechanics, not an uncommon fate for unschooled neophytes, should not be unfairly attributed to SAD procedures *per se*. But fallacious critiques do indeed occur and, indeed, are inevitable with any clinical innovation.

A BRIEF HISTORY OF REDUCED TREATMENT TIME

Early scientific literature discussing SAD contains mostly clinical case analyses. For example, after the seminal article by Köle (1959) Gantes *et al.* (1990) reported a safe but undeniable reduction of orthodontic treatment time by approximately 50%. Later, Wilcko *et al.* (2001, 2003) presented cases safely treated in approximately 6 months with PAOO. Then more sophisticated research studied the efficacy of the SAD and PAOO technique with master's theses quality at St Louis and Boston universities under the astute and able tutelage of Professor DJ Ferguson. (See Chapter 1.)

Among these, Hajii (2000) studied decrowding of the mandibular anterior segment with conventional non-extraction and extraction treatment and then compared the outcomes with corticotomy-facilitated non-extraction therapies. This university-level research validated the hypothesis that PAOO significantly decreased the orthodontic treatment times in cases of mandibular Arch Length Deficiency (ALD). The average treatment times were 6.1 months for non-extraction PAOO in contrast to 18.7 months and 26.6 months for conventional non-extraction and extraction treatments respectively. Fulk (2001) reported similar results in mandibular crowding cases, demonstrating that average treatment times could be as short as 6.6 months for PAOO instead of 20.7 months for the conventional treatment group. Similar results were reported for maxillary ALD cases in replication studies by Skountrianos (2003).

MINIMAL EFFECTS

Fischer (2007) evaluated the effects of SAD (corticotomy) in patients with bilaterally impacted canines. In a split-mouth design, impacted canines were treated conventionally on one side and the other side had corticotomy-assisted exposure of the impacted canine. Fischer concluded that SAD could reduce treatment time by merely 30%, but a close analysis demonstrates major experimental design flaws that biased the results. So this has to be taken into account when analyzing Fischer's data. Had the bone volume on each side been equal then the accelerated rate would have been much greater than 30%. Yet Fischer's study shows that even when applied somewhat inappropriately, which may be the reality in private practice, SAD and PAOO can make a clinically significant contribution to the orthodontic treatment plan.

Another split-mouth design to evaluate the effects of corticotomy-facilitated orthodontics was done by Aboul-Ela et al. (2011), where canines were retracted following first premolar extractions in class II, division I cases. They found that during the first 2 months the average monthly rate of canine retraction was two times faster on the side subjected to decortication. These data suggest that PAOO outcomes can claim a treatment time almost universally faster than traditional methods.

It is important to note that the total "hands-on" treatment adjustment time – namely, time spent with the patient receiving specific personalized care ("chair time" or "doctor time") – is the same as conventional therapy. However, with SAD derivatives the time intervals *between adjustments* are compressed to reduce *total treatment time*, the time from bonding to debonding. This means that SAD-facilitated orthodontic therapy has earned a legitimate place in any informed consent where patients are concerned about notorious orthodontic time-related side effects like root resorption and infection-induced damage (Zachrisson and Alnaes, 1974; Wennstrom et al., 1993; Waldrop, 2008).

GRAFTING WITH DECORTICATION

Increased alveolus mass and increased distances through which teeth are moved may be greater gifts from PAOO than the mere acceleration of

tooth movement rate. The ultimate spatial limits of treatment prior to the introduction of the Wilcko research was dictated by perceptions that the "alveolar housing" of the dentition was *immutable*. This is not true. Alveolus bone by its very histological and ontological nature is *malleable*. However, this malleability, a kind of single-generation "phenotype plasticity," occurs only under specific conditions *in healthy tissue*. The functional matrix hypothesis of Moss (1997a–d; Moss-Salentijn and Moss, 1997) tells us that the roots are the supporting framework or *matrix* of alveolar bone. That is, the osteogenic framework and "container" of bone mass dictates the *functional* development of alveolar phenotype.

When the alveolus periosteum is supported further from a given point by more tooth eruption, a longer root, or periosteum elevated by a bone graft, a potential space is realized. Since bone is a reactive tissue, then, analogous to water, bone tends to "fill the container" in which it is placed. So the bone graft, besides providing bone morphogenetic protein or viable allografts to induce osteogenesis, also serves as a volumetric scaffold within which endogenous stem cells can replicate and differentiate into functional osteoblasts. This is the developmental basis of the alveolus form that justifies safe tooth movement and augmentation of periodontal–alveolus mass.

The limits of orthodontic tooth movement are thus defined by the "walls" of the alveolus; namely, the periosteum and the periodontal ligament. Wherever these "walls" are built, within a reasonable phenotypic range, the bone will develop within them. So orthodontist are wise to define "available space" not by a projection of an aligned and uprighted dentition, but rather by the labial limits of the marginal gingiva and bony walls of the alveolus.

Without PAOO, orthodontic treatment of teeth beyond the limits of the labial or lingual alveolar plate can lead to dehiscence formation (McComb, 1994; Wennstrom, 1996; Zachrisson, 1996; Melsen and Allais, 2005; Joss-Vassalli *et al.*, 2010) and predispose the patient to recession (Zachrisson, 1996; Melsen and Allais, 2005), especially where chronic infection inhibits adaptive fibroplasia (Aleo *et al.*, 1974). In a case where there is already alveolar dehiscence formation before the orthodontic treatment, tooth movement may be contraindicated. But in some cases the alternative – premolar extraction – can lead to a flattened profile, premature aging, arrested development and a generally unaesthetic, "dished-in" appearance to the lower face. PAOO and PSCT solve this dilemma by grafting the defective areas at the beginning of orthodontic treatment to help prevent further destruction and allow movement through a greater distance.

This saving grace was demonstrated by Ahn *et al.* (2012) and Kim *et al.* (2011) independently. They reported the use of alveolar decortication and bone augmentation in decompensation of the mandibular teeth in class III patients. Both reports concluded that alveolar decortication with bone augmentation reduced complications such as gingival recession, alveolar bone dehiscence, and bone loss in the mandibular anterior region in the treatment of class III patients undergoing orthognathic surgery.

Since bone grafting increases both the alveolar volume and the dimensions through which teeth can be moved, it follows that more severely crowded cases can now be treated without tooth extraction. Indeed, Ferguson *et al.* (2006) reported that the limits of orthodontic tooth movement, posited by Sarver and Profitt (2005) in adult patients can be expanded two- to threefold in all dimensions (except retraction) if PAOO is incorporated into orthodontic therapy.

Wilcko *et al.* (2001) reported non-extraction treatment of crowding with PAOO where maxillary intercanine distance was increased (by tipping) more than 7 mm using bone augmentation, and at the reentry 15 months later noted an increase in the post-treatment buccolingual thickness of the overlying buccal bone (Figure 4.4). It appears that this thickness is significant because it may relate to treatment stability. Rothe *et al.* (2006) evaluated mandibular incisor relapse and

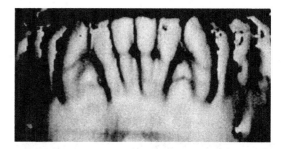
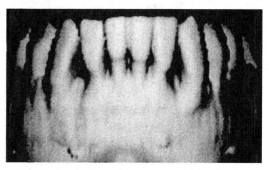
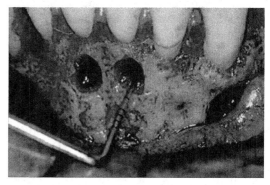

Figure 4.4 Significant augmentation of alveolus bone may be achieved by moving tooth roots into a bone graft. Top: Before PAOO, Middle: CT after PAOO, Bottom: Clinically healthy bone noted on surgical reentry for biopsy. (*Source:* Wiclkodontics, Inc. used with permission.)

found that patients with thinner mandibular cortices are at increased risk for dental relapse.

This observation suggests that bone augmentation during PAOO may increase stability of orthodontic outcomes due to the increased alveolar mass (Ferguson *et al.*, 2006). An incidentally positive effect of bone augmentation during alveolar decortication is that it improves the patient's

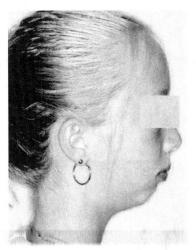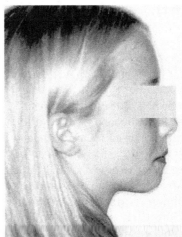

Figure 4.5 Lower facial profiles and labiomental folds may be profoundly improved with PAOO and PSCT. (*Source*: Wiclkodontics, Inc. used with permission.)

lower facial profile. By grafting the mandibular anterior region one may provide lip support, morph an unpleasing profile, and reduce an unaesthetic labiomental fold (Figure 4.5).

CONTRAINDICATIONS

SAD and PAOO, PSCT, and TMP are all limited by the same criteria that any oral surgery would suggest. These include, but are not limited to, bone pathoses that could reduce treatment quality, efficiency, or comfort. However, periodontal infection is not one of them. Indeed, periodontal surgery to eliminate infection and regenerate supporting alveolar bone has been combined with PSCT with impunity (Murphy *et al.*, 2012). However, where all infectious elements cannot be removed, then any bone graft is limited in its healing potential. That is axiomatic.

Despite these advances, publication of successful movement of implants or ankylosed teeth has not been available to date. Theoretically, a "bony block "movement could reposition such teeth, but these are SFOT procedures that reassemble bony parts and incur significantly more risk than a merely superficial re-engineering of the alveolus physiology to new forms.

Because of the inhibitory action of the immune system and osteoclastic potential, long-term use of immunosuppressants – such as corticosteroids and bisphosphonates respectively – may contraindicate decortication procedures categorically. There is no absolute age limit for decortication procedures because the physiologic mechanism of action is merely an acceleration of normal physiological bone healing. So, treatment in the mixed or deciduous dentitions is contraindicated only relative to other factors, such as compliance and the availability of less invasive alternatives.

APPLICATIONS

Segmental alveolar decortication

Alveolar decortication surgeries can be used in a generalized or localized manner, but an intelligent orthodontic effort suggests that the maxillary and mandibular arches should be treated simultaneously if possible. However, when the malocclusion is limited to a segment or only one arch, decortications may be used in a localized manner. An example would be using localized decortications where molars need to be distalized and uprighted in only one segment of the arch to open space for implant placement.

Where the malocclusion is localized to only one sextant of the dentition, SAD should also be limited to that area only. An anterior crowding case with a perfect posterior occlusion is an example of such a pattern. Other examples would be single tooth extrusions or intrusions for pre-prosthetic purposes.

Segmental decortications are particularly well utilized where miniscrews are used to intrude a few teeth. Combining miniscrews and decortication for relative anchorage enhancement now makes it possible to accomplish difficult orthodontic movements that required full mouth bracketing and complex biomechanical protocols in the past.

Decortication procedures with clear aligners

As long as a particular style of orthodontic tooth movement respects the basic physiology of decortication-enhanced orthodontic tooth movement then the particular brand or design of appliance is largely irrelevant. As the population is getting more esthetically conscious, the demand for clear orthodontic aligners and lingual braces has been increasing. Therefore, it is not surprising that the combination of decortication with clear aligner biomechanics would be attempted.

Such a combination was first reported by Owen (2001). After undergoing SAD he used Invisalign® to treat his own personal malocclusion. He reported very satisfactory results in correcting a class I ALD in about 8 weeks and provided unique first-person reportage. In such cases, decortication can be performed within 1 week of commencing treatment with aligners, which can be changed every 5 days instead of every 2 weeks. This protocol can be applied in cases where there are 30 aligners or less. If the number of aligners required to correct the malocclusion exceeds this number, a surgical revision or employment of TMP may be necessary to "reboot" (rejuvenate) the RAP.

Complications

It is important that the grafted material be resorbable (Figure 4.6). Synthetic nonresorbable grafts tend to give the misleading impression of regeneration when all that they achieve is a "long junctional epithelium." This collection of cells adheres to the root surface by

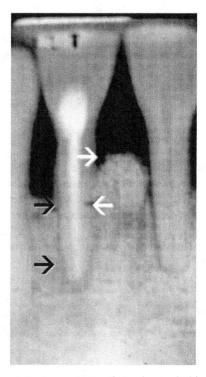

Figure 4.6 Demonstration that only resorbable bone should be use with PAOO. The non-resorbable bone between the incisor teeth that was placed in the central incisor extraction sockets prior to incisor space consolidation failed to integrate fully with native bone. The coronal–apical connection between the white arrows represents a long junctional epithelium, often *incorrectly* assumed to be regeneration of the periodontium, or so-called "new attachment." The junctional epithelium is attached to the root surface by a hemidesmosonal attachment and mucopolysaccharides, a bacterial nutrient. True regeneration of bone is considered a superior barrier to prevent apical migration ("unzipping") of the junctional epithelium when teeth are moved through an infected periodontal *milieu*. When teeth are moved in health, the attachment (bone) level remains stable between the black arrows. (*Source:* UniveristyExperts.com used with permission.)

means of mucopolysaccharide "glue," a bacterial nutrient, and an effete hemidesmosonal attachment. This friable attachment mechanism is considered less formidable than regenerated bone and connective tissue of a "new attachment (apparatus)" and can often rapidly detach ("unzip") from the root surface in the face of new infection. When this occurs, sudden "new," deep periodontal pockets form and acute, so-called "blow-out" abscesses can appear during orthodontic therapy. Such sudden abscesses can destroy bone very quickly and turn a seemingly controlled case into a major orthodontic complication (Ericsson *et al.*, 1978). However, when the periodontal disease is well controlled, simultaneous PAOO and periodontal pocket regeneration with bone grafting (Figure 4.7) can be executed in one surgery with impunity.

Complications and delays may arise from faulty or inefficient biomechanics or natural biodiversity. So it is better to speak in terms of *relative acceleration* instead of specific months or days anticipated. It is also wise to understate the anticipated success and slightly overstate the possible complications to winnow out

patients with skeptical attitudes, unrealistic expectations, or frank dentophobia.

Complications related to surgery include immediate post-operative edema, ecchymosis, and sub-periosteal hematomas, which are treated prophylactically or therapeutically in a conventional manner. One particularly odious occurrence is the exaggerated opening of labial embrasures upon leveling and alignment. The so-called "black triangle" appearance simulates the cosmetic compromise following reduced gingival inflammation in periodontal patients. This can be camouflaged with bonding, veneers, or interproximal enamel reduction with space consolidation. But without an explicit forewarning, patients often suspect that the occurrence is the result of clinical negligence.

Anterior teeth are often flared labially to eliminate the linguoversion ("pseudo-crowding") that can accompany a deep bite. The "decrowding" simultaneously treats excessive overbite/overjet relationships in the saggital plane. However, where a normal overbite/overjet relationship exists, a latent or occult

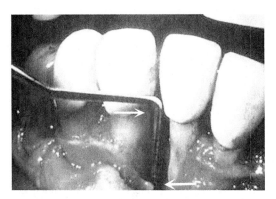 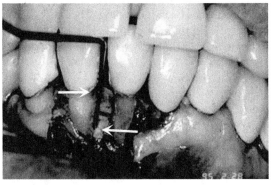

Figure 4.7 The left image demonstrates a 17 mm clinical periodontal pocket with a one-walled infrabony bony defect (arrows). The right image demonstrates the appearance of the defect 6 months later. Note periodontal regeneration (arrows), or so-called called "new attachment." The labial and lingual cortical bone adjacent to the pocket was untouched, while the infrabony defect itself was generously decorticated to liberate endogenous stem cells. Right image shows significant bone regeneration upon surgical reentry. The labial and lingual plates could have been simultaneously decorticated with impunity if the periodontal case required SFOT. (*Source*: UniveristyExperts. com used with permission.)

open bite is present in many case of severe ALD. In such cases, treatment may manifest an anterior open bite that can be mistaken as untoward.

Some orthodontic open bites are indeed iatrogenic, but not necessarily untoward or negligent. Iatrogenic changes are treatment-related empirical truths that may or may not be negligent acts according to a very specific set of constructive truths. As stated by Staggers (1990), most orthodontic mechanics are extrusive in nature, and this extrusion can sometimes increase the vertical dimension of occlusion, a phenomenon that may be useful or dysfunctional. The orthodontist should pay extra attention to the anterior vertical relationship during the initial leveling and alignment stage of the orthodontic treatment whenever alveolar decortication is planned for anterior sextants.

However, a significant cohort of orthodontists is overly mechanical in their orientation and unschooled in nuanced alveolus bone biology. Such nuances are the province of the periodontists and define their collegial obligation to support orthodontists' treatment plans. If necessary precautions are not taken as the bone is demineralized, the proclination effect of the initial archwires on the anterior segment combined with posterior tooth extrusion may create a precipitate iatrogenic anterior open bite of problematic proportions. When that occurs, a collaborative interdisciplinary effort can obviate the need for more morbid orthognathic surgery and produce a beautiful clinical outcome.

As mentioned above, a bite opening effect would be advantageous in deep bite cases; but in other cases, since ALD can mask an open bite tendency, patients may become alarmed at the appearance of a "new" pattern of the malocclusion. Treatment of such a complication may be especially problematic for patients with a tongue thrust habit. In such cases, using mechanics such as vertical elastics should be considered at the early stages of the treatment as soon as the complication arises. Moreover, patients should be warned before commencing treatment that the vexacious vertical elastics or uncomfortable vertical archwire bends may be necessary to reestablish normal incisor juxtapositions (Figure 4.8).

INTER-PROFESSIONAL COMMUNICATION

It is obvious that clear and unequivocal communication between the orthodontist and the periodontist is crucial during the treatment planning. However, owing to the insular development of specialty protocols, a body of jargon in each realm sometimes makes communication a Tower of Babel. And even ideal collaboration can be impaired by jargon or other semantic impediments. So each collaborator should understand universal terms of the others' databases. Moreover, the patient should be *explicitly informed*, in intelligible lay language where possible, about the specific location of treated anatomy, the specific treatment objectives, and contingency plans. Although the specific amount of the graft material may be indeterminate, the origins of the graft must be understood by the patient, philosophically accepted, and documented in a written informed consent to treat.

CASES PRESENTATION

Introductory note

The orthodontist employing PAOO must question what is changing in their treatment sequence, their so-called "biomechanics." The answer is: absolute nothing.

With PAOO, as Professor Wilcko has repeatedly pointed out, just the frequency of appointments changes; namely, the intervals between

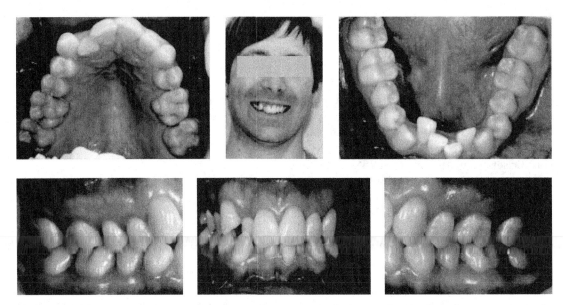

Figure 4.8 The patient presents a class I case of ALD, or so-called "crowding," which, by many standards, would be condemned to extraction therapy if the alveolus were considered immutable. Injudicious bicuspid extraction therapy is notorious for causing lower facial deformities, but prior to PAOO the only alternative to preserve facial esthetics was more risky orthognathic surgery. Here, the orthodontist decided to preserve facial esthetics by developing the dental alveolus bones. The patient also had anterior single-tooth cross bite in the upper right lateral incisor, deep bite, and an impacted upper left second premolar. It is helpful to note that all orthodontic treatment can be divided into three basic steps: (1) leveling (the curve of Spee) and aligning, (2) coordination of the dental arches with congruent archwires, (with or without extraction) and (3) finishing.

appointments must be no more than 2–3 weeks to sustain the osteopenic state.

If the orthodontists are dilatory in their biomechanical sequence then the above statement is not entirely true. It is categorically true for the orthodontist who is extremely efficient in their archwire adjustments and changes.

For example, many orthodontists start with the following "gentle" sequence of archwires:

0.012″ or 0.014″ braided (Wildcat) wire gradually progressing every 4 weeks to
0.016″ nickel–titanium,
0.016″ stainless steel,
0.018″ nickel–titanium,
0.018″ stainless steel,
0.016″ × 0.016″ stainless steel,

0.016″ × 0.022″ stainless steel, and finally
0.017″ × 0.018″ stainless steel, a "finishing" wire.

Eight archwire changes every 4 weeks means $8 \times 4 = 32$ weeks – nearly 7 months. This is done under the mistaken belief that such a sequence will be "appropriately gentle" to the periodontal tissue. This is a misleading shibboleth.

There is only a need for gradualism when one posits the potential irreversible damage by mechanical trauma per se and orthodontic force is seen as "controlled occlusal trauma." These are 1955 ways of thinking. The periodontium is quite resilient and, in the absence of those specific flora–host interactions known collectively as active periodontitis, there is little harm and great virtue in a bolder approach; for example:

0.018″ stainless steel wire,
0.016″ × 0.022″ stainless steel finishing wire.

With auxiliary use of coiled springs and elastic chain, many class I cases can be taken to completion in 3–6 months where prior protocols take 1–2 years.

So, in summary, there is a strong imperative to take advantage of the transient osteopenia by maximizing mechanical manipulations on each appointment and ensuring that each mechanical adjustment strains the bone to the presumptively osteogenic degree of at least 500–1000 microstrains.

Case 1

The patient presents a class I case of ALD, or so-called "crowding," which by many standards would be condemned to extraction therapy if the alveolus were considered immutable. Injudicious bicuspid extraction therapy is notorious for causing lower facial deformities, but prior to PAOO the only alternative to preserve facial esthetics was more risky orthognathic surgery. Here, the orthodontist decided to preserve facial esthetics by developing the dental alveolus bones. He also had anterior single-tooth cross bite in the upper right lateral incisor, deep bite and an impacted upper left second premolar (Figures 4.9–4.26).

Case 2

A young adult female presented with class I skeletal and dental relationship, severe ALD (crowding) in both maxillary and mandibular

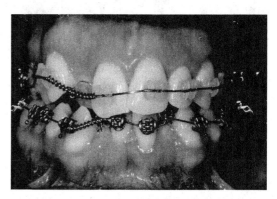

Figure 4.9 Here, at the first active orthodontic appointment, an initial leveling and aligning is demonstrated, displaying bonded brackets on the maxillary and mandibular dental arches and 0.016″ nickel–titanium alloy wires with a coiled spring. The process may involve a series of light archwires from 0.014″ nickel–titanium to 0.018″ stainless steel or a direct placement of 0.018″ stainless steel archwires. The general guideline is to insert, deeply into the bracket slot, the largest comfortable wire possible without permanent wire deformation. This preserves optimal load–deflection ratios, each of which is a function of Young's modulus of elasticity, a metallurgical parameter of flexibility. The coiled spring is used to open the arch space for an ectopic lateral incisor.

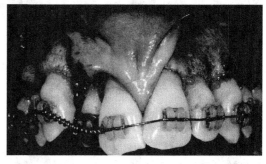

Figure 4.10 After the bonding and initial archwires are placed, surgery commences and linear decortications are made in the buccal and lingual alveolar cortices. Orthodontic appliance placement and activation may occur after the surgery, but no longer than 2–3 weeks if the RAP is to be sustained. Mucoperiosteal flaps are elevated with care to avoid compromising the esthetically sensitive incisal papilla.

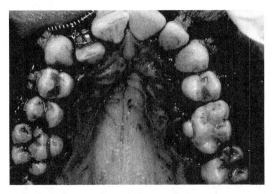

Figure 4.11 The palatal incision extends from tuberosity to tuberosity, a style that may not be entirely necessary where the dentition displays ideal interdigitation. The extent of the flap reflection is a province of the surgeon, but one must keep in mind that where flaps are elevated osteopenia ensues.

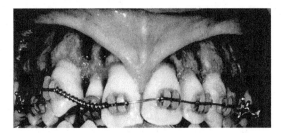

Figure 4.12 Alveolar decortication is achieved here with a surgical-length, high-speed round bur and copious irrigation.

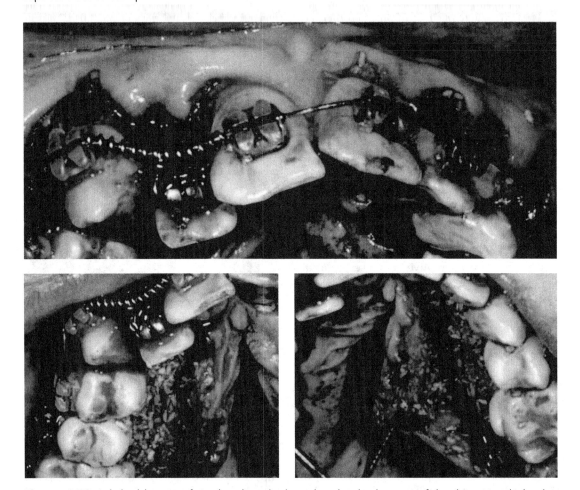

Figure 4.13 A hybrid bone graft is placed on the buccal and palatal aspect of the decorticated alveolus. Augmentation of the ridge is not strictly necessary where sufficient labial bone is present, but lies within the discretion of the treating professional team. The graft is a hybrid composed of DFDBA, with bovine-derived mineralized bone in a 2:1 ratio, prepared with a clindamycin phosphate lavage as a bacteriostatic precaution.

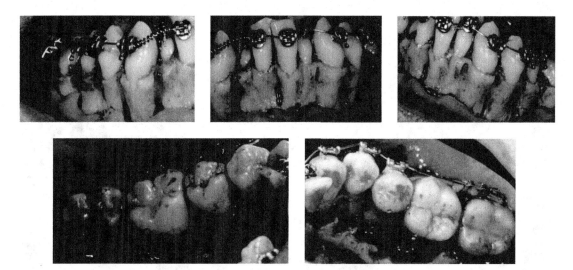

Figure 4.14 Alveolar decortication is performed on the lingual and buccal aspects of the mandibular alveolus bone.

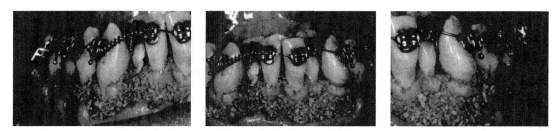

Figure 4.15 Bone grafting is demonstrated here for mandibular dental arch expansion.

(a) (b)

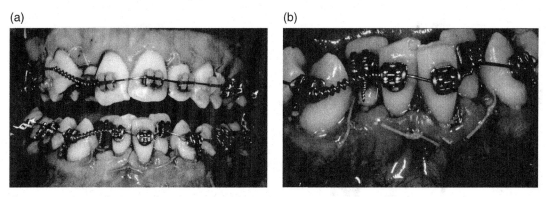

Figure 4.16 (a) The graft placement completely fills the space between the decorticated alveolus and the reflected mucoperiosteal flap, allowing the flap to be replaced to its original position as much as possible to protect the graft. (b) Note how the 0.016″ nickel–titanium archwire is nearly fully engaged into the bracket slots of the incisors and how normal uninfected granulation tissue is organizing into native tissue at the edge of the replaced flap. The alveolus morphotype, according to Professor Moss's revered functional matrix hypothesis, is determined by the position of the teeth. The load placed upon the periodontal ligament effects a novel, engineered alveolus phenotype consistent with that functional matrix. Applied force, internal strain, and surgical healing must all be choreographed harmoniously to ensure the best clinical outcome. But singularly conventional biomechanical thinking in the mind of the treatment team must surrender to a kind of 21st-century "NewThink," where emerging concepts of tissue engineering prevail for novel alveolus development to occur. This demonstrated state of healing is when the gingival tissue is most vulnerable to periodontal and gingival infection. So, the orthodontist must have at least a rudimentary understanding of bacteriology or acquiesce to the knowledge and skill of the periodontist.

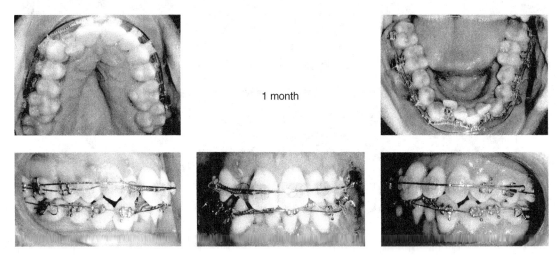

1 month

Figure 4.17 At 1 month, 0.016″ × 0.022″ a stainless steel overlay archwire is placed in the maxillary arch and 0.016″ stainless steel "stopped–advanced" mechanism is employed to expand the mandibular dental arch. Load is transferred to the osteogenic graft and stem cells in the healing wound and morphotype is being defined at the transcription stage of protein synthesis at the cell level. It is this coordination of clinic-level and cell/molecular-level biology that defines orthodontic "NewThink." Note how the osteogenic overlay archwire used for both dental expansion and alveolus development is coordinated with the dental archwires. This is synchronized with slot-inserted dental biomechanics that continues to align and level each dental arch, and the coiled spring opens space for an ectopic lateral incisor.

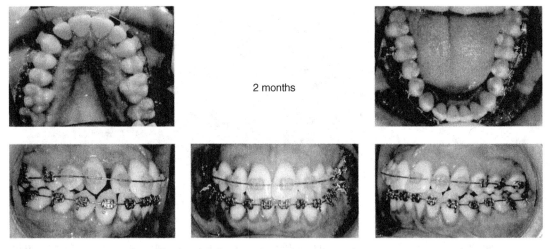

2 months

Figure 4.18 At 2 months, orthodontic follow-up shows that the overlay wire was removed on the previous appointment.

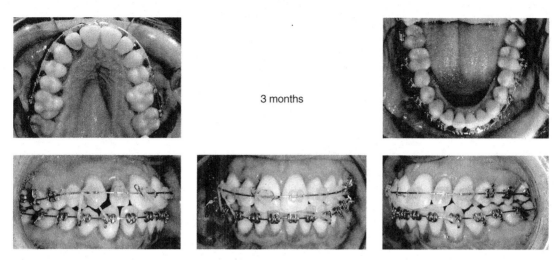

3 months

Figure 4.19 By 3 months the case demonstrates a 0.017″ × 0.025″ nickel-titanium archwire in the maxillary and mandibular arches, with intermaxillary elastics for closing a minor dental open bite. Skewed elastics are displayed on maxillary and mandibular arches.

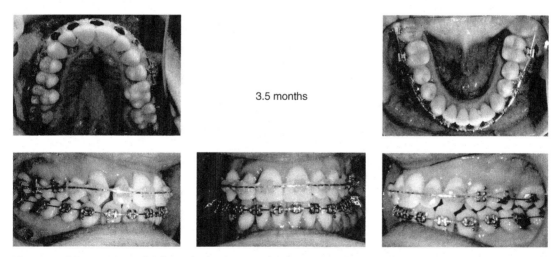

3.5 months

Figure 4.20 At 3.5 months the orthodontic care demonstrates 0.016″ × 0.022″ stainless steel wires in the maxillary and mandibular arches.

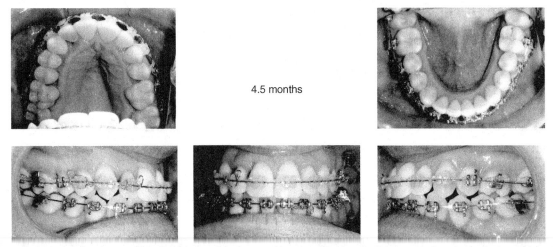

Figure 4.21 At 4.5 months the maxillary archwire was sectioned between the maxillary right lateral incisor and canine. Elastic chain was placed to connect the fist molars to hold interdental embrasures securely at a physiologic dimension and avoid opening protective contact points. A 0.016″ stainless steel archwire was placed in the maxillary arch with the power chain extended to the second molars and a box-elastic module was placed on the patient's right side to correct a dental midline discrepancy.

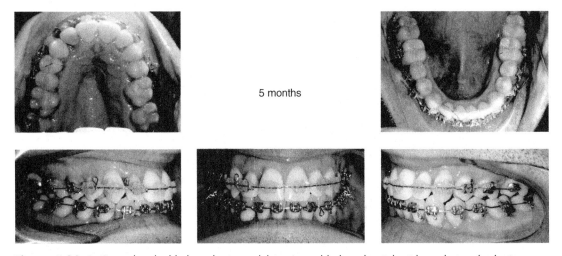

Figure 4.22 At 5 months, double box-elastic modules were added on the right side and triangle-elastics were worn at night on the left side.

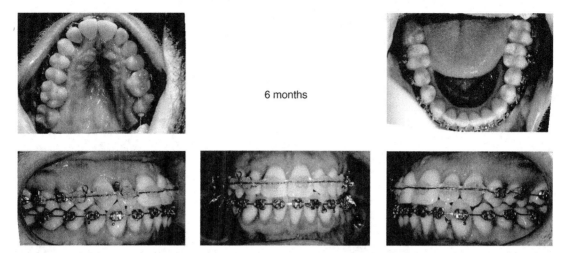

6 months

Figure 4.23 At 6 months, arch coordination is complete but inter-arch spaces and minor rotations remain to be corrected in the finishing stage. The maxillary archwire was sectioned at the maxillary canine and lateral incisor to allow for sextant movement, unimpeded by posterior occlusion. This allows an individualization of force application to as few as two or three teeth. Some orthodontists remove all brackets at this stage, hoping that normal settling of the dentition will eliminate the inter-arch "windows." Where this physiologic settling does not occur, teeth may need to be rebonded. Elastic chains are changed every 2 weeks to insure uninterrupted closure of interproximal spaces. The midlines are being adjusted with skewed elastic modules between the maxillary right lateral incisor and the mandibular left lateral incisor. The need to detail the posterior occlusion may have been obviated by maintaining the original occlusal pattern and rendering surgical correction only to the anterior sextant. Thus, this posterior malocclusion in this case may be iatrogenic, a common problem with rectangular archwires.

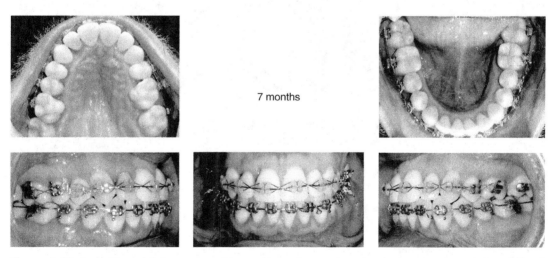

7 months

Figure 4.24 At the 7-month follow-up appointment the previous sectioned archwires are removed. A steel "lace" was placed between first molars and a "zig-zag patterned" inter-arch elastic was placed to facilitate tight interdigitation. This is commonly referred to as a "socked-in" occlusion in traditional orthodontic vernacular. However, this shibboleth is inconsistent with physiologic periodontal occlusion. Tight interdigitation between the dental arches can initiate both working and nonworking parafunctional interferences that are restrictive of mandibular movement tolerance. The overjet of the canines should always be less than the overjet of posterior teeth so that lateral excursions provide immediate disengagement ("lift-off") of contiguous posterior cuspal inclines. This ensures a mutually protected occlusion. Such oversight as rendered by "socked-in" occlusion is neither consistent with emerging biological principles nor with traditional gnathological data. A mechanical treatment devoid of biological sensibilities makes necessary a more intimate collaboration between periodontal and orthodontic clinicians.

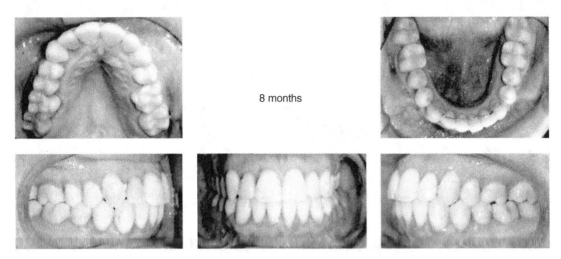

8 months

Figure 4.25 At 8 months the patient was debonded and fixed inter-canine retainer was delivered.

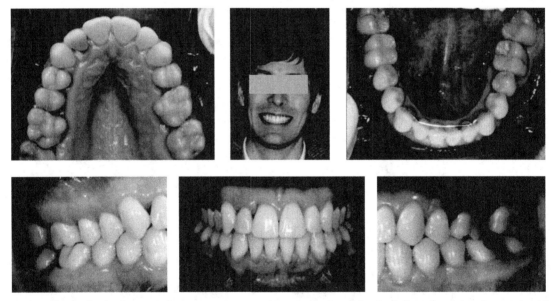

Figure 4.26 The final extraoral composite pictures demonstrate that a finished physiological occlusion should be adapted to the patient's unique needs by normal masticatory force vector sums. So, after 3–6 months, an occlusal equilibration should be rendered to eliminate any micro-malocclusion of aberrance occlusal morphology. This is often done by periodontists who are particularly aware of the pernicious effects of parafunction and lateral load vectors. Odontoplasty may also be employed for esthetic purposes. Here, the maxillary right canine should be recontoured to comport with universal principles of dental cosmesis.

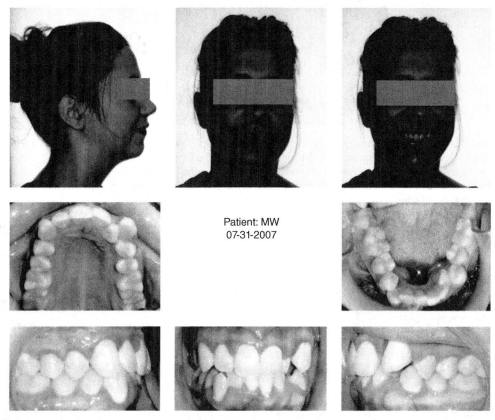

Patient: MW
07-31-2007

Figure 4.27 Here in case 2, a young adult female presented with class I skeletal and dental relationship, severe ALD (crowding) in both maxillary and mandibular dental arches, a deep anterior overbite, a maxillary midline discrepancy, inadequate oral hygiene standards, and impacted third molars.

dental arches, a deep anterior overbite, a maxillary midline discrepancy, inadequate oral hygiene standards, and impacted third molars (Figures 4.27–4.35).

CONCLUSION

Recent animal and clinical studies have helped us to understand the biology of tooth movement with alveolar decortication, and its effect on the teeth and bone. The journey of accelerated tooth movement that started in the 1890s has been continuing with constant and deliberative speed in the development of new techniques.

We are now understanding the underlying mechanisms and developing minimally invasive techniques to accelerate the treatment to satisfy both the patients' and the dental professionals' expectations. This achieves the best possible treatment, building on the clinical art of the past, to achieve outcomes that dentistry can be proud of and patients can safely count on, in a timely manner. That is a laudable goal for any doctor. We must collectively achieve it as a rational, scientific enterprise, unfettered by specious and unlettered criticism, progressively yet deliberatively.

Unfortunately, dentistry is surfeit with intemperate, ill-conceived criticism of SAD

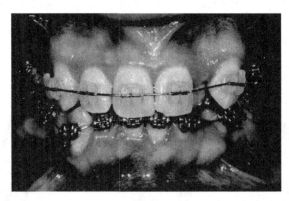

Figure 4.28 The patient was bonded with ideal orthodontic bracket positions 1 week prior to selective decortication (corticotomy). An initial 0.016″ nickel–titanium alloy archwire was placed in the maxillary and mandibular dental arches. At the second appointment 2 weeks later, 0.018″ nickel–titanium wire was secured in the slots of the maxillary arch and a stainless steel 0.016″ "stopped–advanced" archwire was placed in the mandibular arch. Coiled springs at the canines were also activated.

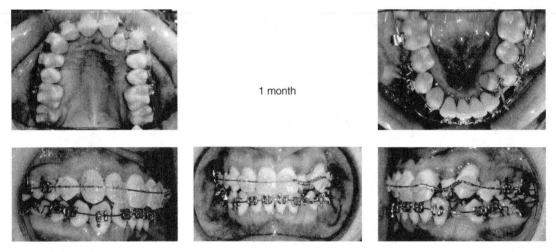

1 month

Figure 4.29 At the 1 month follow-up appointment an elastic chain was applied to the maxillary left canine to first molar and elastic thread was positioned between maxillary left lateral incisor and the lower left canine. A 0.016″ overlay arch was applied on the upper arch.

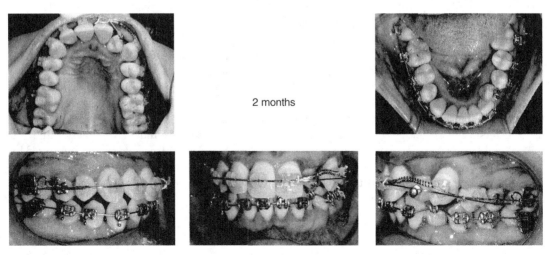

2 months

Figure 4.30 At 2 months an advancing maxillary overlay 0.0018″ wire is evident with a mandibular activated coiled spring and elastic thread.

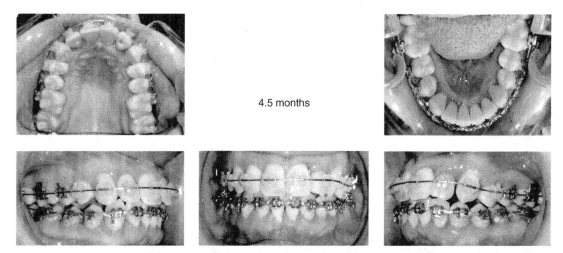

4.5 months

Figure 4.31 At 4.5 months one sees 0.017″×0.025″ nickel–titanium archwire, and in the mandibular arch an elastic chain module. Class II medium vertical elastics in a triangular pattern on the left and right side ensure closure of inter-arch spaces ("occlusal windows").

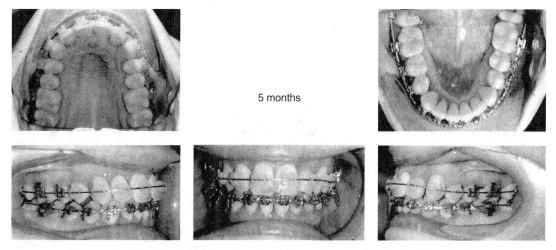

5 months

Figure 4.32 At 5 months 0.016″×0.022″ nickel–titanium archwires were placed in the mandibular arch.

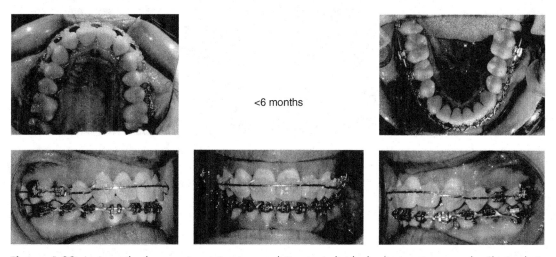

<6 months

Figure 4.33 At 6 months the case is coming to completion as individual adjustments are made. Elastic chain from maxillary and mandibular first molars sustains the orthodontic outcome and fortifies physiologic interdental contacts as the bone recalcifies out of its RAP.

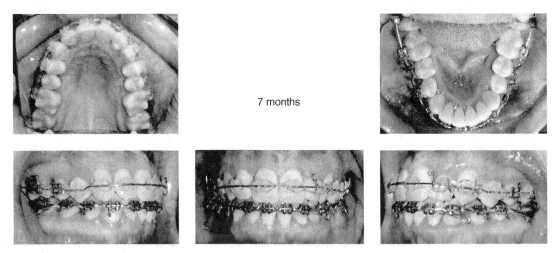

7 months

Figure 4.34 By the seventh month the maxillary left canine is disengaged. The protocol continues treatment with triangular elastic modules "full time" (24 h per day, 7 days per week) on the left side and during sleep on the right side.

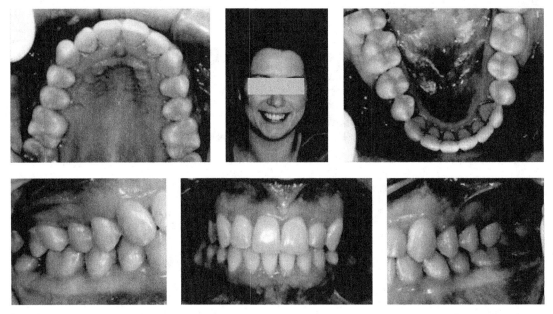

Figure 4.35 Case is completed in 8 months and 18 appointments, with no extractions; a bimaxillary protrusion ("full smile") consistent with contemporary standards of facial esthetics has been rendered with healthy periodontal support that satisfies the patient and is professionally gratifying to both the post-modern orthodontist and periodontist.

variants. This is to be expected with innovation and is not all bad. The specious claims are as common as the clinical variations of SAD and PAOO. Yet the science, the abiding and prolific epistemological tool of ultimate truth, is undeniable and, like the proverbial "genie out of the bottle," it tells us that SAD procedures, from crude corticotomy to PSCT, are here to stay.

Alas, so will the controversy, that inevitable cacophony of dialectical noise which gives birth to scientific innovation. Still, we live in a post-industrial, post-modern age that challenges the Enlightenment precepts of reason and scientific preeminence. So the clinicians employing enlightened perceptions must be the arbiters of truth as a fiduciary. He or she is charged with the directing of a final act on the stage of this manifest destiny – for better or worse.

The ultimate challenge is pernicious social forces which, manifest as inviolable artistic interpretations, can deconstruct the edifice of orthodontic science claiming it as irrelevant. This accounts for the disregard for scientific foundations that interfere with commercial exploitation of the specialty. Yet the scientific truths explicated by selective alveolar decortication and the nascent science of oral tissue engineering are difficult to exploit commercially. So the specialty can lie secure in the bosom of enlightened science and the absolute mathematical imperatives of the logical positivist. Whether one perspective – artistic, commercial, or scientific – will prevail over the others is an existential choice that each individual doctor and patient must make. Preferably, their choices will be concordant.

Carpe Diem!

DEDICATION

This chapter is dedicated to the visionary and intrepid leadership of Professors Mark Hans and Nabil F Bissada of Case Western Reserve University, Cleveland, OH, USA.

ACKNOWLEDGMENTS

We would like to thanks Dr Elif I. Keser for helping writing this chapter. Cases courtesy of periodontist Dr Nishant Joshi, Assistant Clinical Professor, Case Western Reserve University School of Dental, Medicine, Cleveland, OH, USA and orthodontist Dr Felix Gen, Private Practice, Twinsburg, OH, USA. Case commentary: Dr Neal C Murphy, Clinical Professor, Case Western Reserve University School of Dental, Medicine, Cleveland, OH, USA.

Notes

1 Professsor M. Thomas Wilcko at Case Western Reserve University in Cleveland, OH, USA, in collaboration with his orthodontist brother, Professor William M. Wilcko at the University of Pennsylvania.
2 (Periodontally) Accelerated Osteogenic Orthodontics™ ((P)AOO)™ are trademarks of Wilckodontics, Inc., Erie, Pennsylvania, USA.
3 For the purposes of this chapter, the terms "decortication" and "SAD" will replace the less discretely defined procedures collectively referred to as "corticotomy."
4 Baloul and her associates won the 2010 Milo Hellman Research Award presented by the American Association of Orthodontists.
5 Root surface area exposed to resistance.

References

Aboul-Ela SMBE, El-Beialy AR, El-Sayed KMF *et al.* (2011) Miniscrew implant supported maxillary canine retraction with and without corticotomy facilitated orthodontics. *American Journal of Orthodontics and Dentofacial Orthopedics*, **139**, 252–259.
Ahn HW, Lee DY, Park YG *et al.* (2012) Accelerated decompensation of mandibular incisors in surgical skeletal class III patients by using augmented corticotomy: a preliminary study. *American Journal of Orthodontics and Dentofacial Orthopedics*, **142**, 199–206.

Aleo JJ, De Renzis FA, Farber PA *et al.* (1974) The presence and biologic activity of cementum-bound endotoxin. *Journal of Periodontology*, **45** (9), 672–675.

Anholm JM, Crites DA, Hoff R *et al.* (1986) Corticotomy facilitated orthodontics. *California Dental Association Journal*, **14** (12), 7–11.

Baloul SS, Gerstenfeld LC, Morgan EF *et al.* (2011) Mechanism of action and morphologic changes in the alveolar bone in response to selective alveolar decortication-facilitated tooth movement. *American Journal of Orthodontics and Dentofacial Orthopedics*, **139**, S83–S101.

Bell W, Levy B (1972) Revascularization and bone healing after maxillary corticotomies. *Journal of Oral Surgery*, **30**, 640–648.

Bishara SE, Ostby AW (2008) White spot lesions: formation, prevention, and treatment. *Seminars in Orthodontics*, **14**, 174–182.

Bogoch E, Gschwend N, Rahn B *et al.* (1993) Healing of cancellous bone osteotomy in rabbits – Part I: regulation of bone volume and the regional acceleratory phenomenon in normal bone. *Journal of Orthopedic Research*, **11**, 285–291.

Cruz DR, Kohara EK, Ribeiro MS *et al.* (2004) Effects of low-intensity laser therapy on the orthodontic movement velocity of human teeth: a preliminary study. *Lasers in Surgery and Medicine*, **35**, 117–120.

Dibart S, Sebaoun JD, Surmenian J (2009) Piezocision: a minimally invasive, periodontally accelerated orthodontic tooth movement procedure. *Compendium of Continuing Education in Dentistry*, **30** (6), 342–350.

Ericsson B, Thilander B, Lindhe J (1978) Periodontal conditions after orthodontic tooth movements in the dog. *Angle Orthodontics*, **48** (3), 210–218.

Ferguson DJ, Wilcko WM, Wilcko MT (2006) Selective alveolar decortication for rapid surgical–orthodontic resolution of skeletal malocclusion, in *Distraction Osteogenesis of the Facial Skeleton* (eds WE Bell, C Guerrero), BC Decker, Hamilton, Ontario.

Fischer TJ (2007) Orthodontic treatment acceleration with corticotomy assisted exposure of palatally impacted canines. *Angle Orthodontics*, **77**, 417–420.

Fox N (2005) Longer orthodontic treatment may result in greater external apical root resorption. *Evidence Based Dentistry*, **6**, 21.

Frost MH (1989a) The biology of fracture healing: an overview for clinicians, part I. *Clinical Orthodontics*, **248**, 283–293.

Frost MH (1989b) The biology of fracture healing: an overview for clinicians, part II. *Clinical Orthodontics*, **248**, 294–309.

Fulk LA (2001) Lower arch decrowding comparing corticotomy facilitated, midline distraction and conventional orthodontic techniques. Thesis, St Louis University, St Louis, MO.

Gantes B, Rathbun E, Anholm M (1990) Effects on the periodontium following corticotomy facilitated orthodontics. Case reports. *Journal of Periodontology*, **61** (4), 234–238.

Geiger AM, Gorelick L, Gwinnett AJ *et al.* (1992) Reducing white spot lesions in orthodontic populations with fluoride rinsing. *American Journal of Orthodontics and Dentofacial Orthopedics*, **101**, 403–407.

Hajji SS (2000) The influence of accelerated osteogenic response on mandibular decrowding. Thesis, St Louis University, St Louis, MO.

Joss-Vassalli I, Grebenstein C, Topouzelis N *et al.* (2010) Orthodontic therapy and gingival recession: a systematic review. *Orthodontic and Craniofacial Research*, **13**, 127–141.

Kim SH, Kim I, Jeong DM (2011) Corticotomy assisted decompensation for augmentation of the mandibular anterior ridge. *American Journal of Orthodontics and Dentofacial Orthopedics*, **140**, 720–731.

Kim SJ, Park YG, Kang SG (2009) Effects of corticision on paradental remodeling in orthodontic tooth movement. *Angle Orthodontics*, **79**, 284–291.

Kim YS, Kim SJ, Yoon HJ *et al.* (2013) Effect of piezopuncture on tooth movement and bone remodeling in dogs. *American Journal of Orthodontics and Dentofacial Orthopedics*, **144** (1), 23–31.

King GJ, Keeling SD (1995) Orthodontic bone remodeling in relation to appliance decay. *Angle Orthodontics*, **65**, 129–140.

Köle H (1959) Surgical operations on the alveolar ridge to correct occlusal abnormalities. *Oral Surgery, Oral Medicine, Oral Pathology*, **12** (5), 515–529.

Lee W, Karapetyan G, Moats R *et al.* (2008) Corticotomy-/osteotomy-assisted tooth movement microCTs differ. *Journal of Dental Research*, **87** (9), 861–865.

Levander E, Malmgren O (1988) Evaluation of the risk of root resorption during orthodontic treatment: a study of upper incisors. *European Journal of Orthodontics*, **10**, 30–38.

Liou EJW, Huang CS (1998) Rapid canine retraction through distraction of the periodontal ligament. *American Journal of Orthodontics and Dentofacial Orthopedics*, **114**, 372–382.

Long H, Pyakurel U, Wang Y *et al.* (2013) Interventions for accelerating orthodontic tooth movement: a systematic review. *Angle Orthodontics*, **83** (1), 164–171.

Mathews D, Kokich VG (2013) Counterpoint: accelerating orthodontic tooth movement: the case against corticotomy-induced orthodontics. *American Journal of Orthodontics and Dentofacial Orthopedics*, **44** (1), 4–13.

McComb JL (1994) Orthodontic treatment and isolated gingival recession: a review. *British Journal of Orthodontics*, **21**, 151–159.

Melsen B, Allais D (2005) Factors of importance for the development of dehiscences during labial movement of mandibular incisors: a retrospective study of adult orthodontic patients. *American Journal of Orthodontics and Dentofacial Orthopedics*, **127**, 552–561.

Moss ML (1997a) The functional matrix hypothesis revisited. 1. The role of mechanotransduction. *American Journal of Ortho-* *dontics and Dentofacial Orthopedics*, **112** (4), 8–11.

Moss ML (1997b) The functional matrix hypothesis revisited. 2. The role of an osseous connected cellular network. *American Journal of Orthodontics and Dentofacial Orthopedics*, **112** (4), 221–226.

Moss ML (1997c) The functional matrix hypothesis revisited. 3. The genomic thesis. *American Journal of Orthodontics and Dentofacial Orthopedics*, **112** (4), 338–342.

Moss ML (1997d) The functional matrix hypothesis revisited. 4. The epigenetic antithesis and the resolving synthesis. *American Journal of Orthodontics and Dentofacial Orthopedics*, **112** (4), 410–417.

Moss-Salentijn L, Melvin L (1997) Moss and the functional matrix. *Journal of Dental Research*, **76** (12), 1814–1817.

Murphy NC (2006) *In vivo* tissue engineering for the orthodontist: a modest first step, in *Biologic Mechanisms of Tooth Eruption, Resorption and Movement* (eds Z Davidovitch, J Mah, S Suthanarak), Harvard Society for the Advancement of Orthodontics, Boston, MA (available under US free use doctrine at www.UniversityExperts.com).

Murphy NC, de Alba JA, Chaconas SJ *et al.* (1982) Experimental force analysis of the contraction utility arch wire. American Journal of Orthodontics, **82** (5), 411–417.

Murphy NC, Bissada, NF, Davidovitch, Z *et al.* (2012) Corticotomy and stem cell therapy for orthodontists and periodontists: rationale, hypotheses, and protocol, in *Integrated Clinical Orthodontics* (eds V Krishnan, Z Davidovitch), Elsevier, St Louis, MO, Chapter 21 (available under US free use doctrine at www. UniversityExperts.com).

Nishimura M, Chiba M, Ohashi T *et al.* (2008) Periodontal tissue activation by vibration: intermittent stimulation by resonance vibration accelerates experimental tooth movement hypothesis in rats. *American Journal of*

Orthodontics and Dentofacial Orthopedics, **133**, 572–583.

Owen AH (2001) Accelerated Invisalign treatment. *Journal of Clinical Orthodontics*, **35**, 381–385.

Pandis N, Nasika M, Polychronopoulou A *et al.* (2008) External apical root resorption in patients treated with conventional and self-ligating brackets. *American Journal of Orthodontics and Dentofacial Orthopedics*, **134**, 646–651.

Proff P, Romer P (2009) The molecular mechanism behind bone remodeling: a review. *Clinical Oral Investigations*, **13**, 355–362.

Proffit WR (2000) *Contemporary Orthodontics*, 3rd edition, Mosby, St Louis, MO.

Roberts WE (2005) Bone physiology, metabolism and biomechanics in orthodontic practice, in *Orthodontics: Current Principles and Techniques* (eds TM Graber, RL Vanarsdall Jr, KWL Vig), Elsevier, St Louis, MO, Chapter 6, p. 278.

Rothe LE, Bollen AM, Little RM *et al.* (2006) Trabecular and cortical bone as risk factors for orthodontic relapse. *American Journal of Orthodontics and Dentofacial Orthopedics*, **130**, 476–484.

Royko A, Denes Z, Razouk G (1999) The relationship between the length of orthodontic treatment and patient compliance. *Fogorvosi Szemle*, **92**, 79–86.

Sarver DM, Proffit WR (2005) Special considerations in diagnosis and treatment planning, in *Orthodontics: Current Principles and Techniques* (eds TM Graber, RL Vanarsdall, KWL Vig), Elsevier, St Louis, MO, p. 15.

Sebaoun JD, Kantarci A, Turner JW *et al.* (2008) Modeling of trabecular bone and lamina dura following selective alveolar decortication in rats. *Journal of Periodontology*, **79**, 1679–1688.

Segal GR, Schiffman PH, Tuncay OC (2004) Meta analysis of the treatment-related factors of external apical root resorption. *Orthodontic and Craniofacial Research*, **7**, 71–78.

Shin MS, Norrdin RW (1985) Regional acceleration of remodeling during healing of bone defect in beagles of various ages. *Bone*, **6**, 377–379.

Showkatbakhsh R, Jamilian A, Showkatbakhsh M (2010) The effect of pulsed electromagnetic fields on the acceleration of tooth movement. *World Journal of Orthodontics*, **11**, e52–e56.

Skountrianos HS (2003) Maxillary arch decrowding and stability with and without corticotomy facilitated orthodontics. Thesis, St Louis University, St Louis, MO.

Spielmann T, Wieslander L, Hefti AF (1989) Acceleration of orthodontically induced tooth movement through the local application of prostaglandin (PGE1). *Schweizer Monatsschrift für Zahnmedizin*, **99**, 162–165 (in German).

Staggers JA (1990) A comparison of results of second molar and first premolar extraction treatment. *American Journal of Orthodontics and Dentofacial Orthopedics*, **98**, 430–436.

Suya H (1991) Corticotomy in orthodontics, in *Mechanical and Biological Basics in Orthodontic Therapy* (eds E Hosl, A Baldauf), Huthig Buch Verlag, Heidelberg, pp. 207–226.

Waldrop T (2008) Gummy smiles: the challenge of gingival excess: prevalence and guidelines for clinical management. *Seminar in Orthodontics*, **14**, 260–271.

Wennstrom JL (1996) Mucogingival considerations in orthodontic treatment. *Seminars in Orthodontics*, **2**, 46–54.

Wennström JL, Stokland BL, Nyman S *et al.* (1993) Periodontal tissue response to orthodontic movement of teeth with infrabony pockets. *American Journal of Orthodontics and Dentofacial Orthopedics*, **103** (4), 313–319.

Wilcko WM, Wilcko MT, Bouquot JE *et al.* (2001) Rapid orthodontics with alveolar reshaping: two case reports of decrowding. *International Journal of Periodontics and Restorative Dentistry*, **21**, 9–19.

Wilcko WM, Ferguson DJ, Bouquot JE *et al.* (2003) Rapid orthodontic decrowding with alveolar augmentation: case report. *World Journal of Orthodontics*, **4**, 197–205.

Yamaguchi M, Hayashi M, Fujita S *et al.* (2010) Low energy laser irradiation facilitates the velocity of tooth movement and the expressions of matrix metalloproteinase-9, cathepsin K, and alpha(v) beta(3) integrin in rats. *European Journal of Orthodontics*, **32**, 131–139.

Zachrisson BU (1996) Clinical implications of recent orthodontic–periodontic research finding. *Seminars in Orthodontics*, **2**, 4–12.

Zachrisson BU, Alnaes L (1974) Periodontal condition in orthodontically treated and untreated individuals. *II*. Alveolar bone loss: radiographic findings. *Angle Orthodontics*, **44** (1), 48–55.

Piezocision™: Minimally invasive periodontally accelerated orthodontic tooth movement procedure

Serge Dibart[1,2] and Elif I. Keser[3,4]

[1] *Department of Periodontology and Oral Biology, Boston University Henry M. Goldman School of Dental Medicine, Boston, MA, USA*
[2] *Private Practice Limited to Periodontics and Implant Dentistry, Boston, MA, USA*
[3] *Department of Orthodontics, Boston University Henry M. Goldman School of Dental Medicine, Boston, MA, USA*
[4] *Private Practice, Istanbul, Turkey*

INTRODUCTION

As already seen in the previous chapters, surgical interventions on alveolar ridges aiming at facilitating orthodontic treatment are not a new concept (Köle, 1959a–c; Suya, 1991), but it was only in the late 1990s that the Wilcko brothers questioned the mechanical concept of bony block movement after reviewing radiographs and computed tomography scans of their patients who had undergone corticotomy-facilitated orthodontic therapy (Wilcko *et al.*, 2001). They hypothesized that rapid tooth movement resulted from a marked but transient decalcification–recalcification process of the alveolus. This concept is known in the orthopedic literature as the regional acceleratory phenomenon (RAP) described by Frost (1983). The Wilckos had understood and witnessed that in their own

patients. The elevation of buccal and lingual full-thickness flaps, with extensive decortications of the buccal and lingual alveolar bone, resulted in a physical injury that was responsible for the initiation of a temporary demineralization process coupled with an increased regional bone turnover that characterizes the RAP. They surmised that this transient osteopenia (diminished bone density, same bone volume) is responsible for the rapid tooth movement, as the teeth move in a more "pliable" environment (Wilcko WM *et al.*, 2003; Wilcko MT *et al.*, 2007). Their pioneering work, combining alveolar decortication concomitant with bone grafting to expand alveolar volume and allow for rapid tooth movement into the newly expanded sites, stands out as seminal. Then Vercelotti and Podesta (2007) introduced the use of piezosurgery in conjunction with the conventional flap elevations to create an

Orthodontically Driven Corticotomy: Tissue Engineering to Enhance Orthodontic and Multidisciplinary Treatment,
First Edition. Edited by Federico Brugnami and Alfonso Caiazzo.
© 2015 John Wiley & Sons, Inc. Published 2015 by John Wiley & Sons, Inc.
Companion Website: www.wiley.com/go/Brugnami/Corticotomy

environment conducive to rapid tooth movement. Although effective, these techniques require flap elevations. They have the potential to generate post-surgical discomfort as well as post-operative complications. Because of these shortcomings they have not been widely embraced by the patient or dental communities. Park *et al.* (2006) and Kim *et al.* (2009) introduced the corticision technique as a minimally invasive alternative to create surgical injury to the bone without flap reflection. In this technique, the authors use a reinforced scalpel and a mallet to go through the gingiva and cortical bone, without raising a flap bucally and lingually. The surgical injury created is enough to induce the RAP effect and move the teeth rapidly during orthodontic treatment. This technique, although innovative, has two drawbacks: the inability to graft soft or hard tissues during the procedure to correct inadequacies and reinforce the periodontium, and the repeated malleting, which may cause dizziness after surgery. We are describing here a new minimally invasive procedure that we called Piezocision™. This technique combines micro-incisions limited to the buccal side that will allow for the use of the piezoelectic knife and selective tunneling that allows for hard or soft tissue grafting (Dibart *et al.*, 2009).

PIEZOCISION™

Piezocision can be used to:

- Accelerate orthodontic treatment in a generalized, localized or sequential manner (including localized " boosters");
- Enhance the scope of tooth movement through grafting (i.e., posterior buccal expansion, decrowding without extractions due to the increased alveolar volume);
- Achieve differential tooth movement by altering anchorage value through changing the bone density at certain areas;
- Enhance the patient's profile in certain cases by altering the labiomental fold;

- Repair the alveolar cortical bone fenestrations and dehiscences, and improve the periodontium strength by adding hard or soft tissue grafting;
- Possibly enhance the stability of the orthodontic treatment through stronger alveolar cortices, when grafted.

Indications

- Class I malocclusions with moderate to severe crowding (extraction and nonextraction).
- Selected class II malocclusions (end-on).
- Selected class III malocclusions (dental).
- Correction of deep bite.
- Correction of open bite.
- Rapid adult orthodontic treatment.
- Orthodontic treatment with clear aligners (i.e., Invisalign®).
- Rapid intrusion and extrusion of teeth.
- Simultaneous correction of osseous and mucogingival defects.
- Prevention of mucogingival defects that may occur during or after orthodontic treatment.
- Multidisciplinary treatments.

Contra-indications

- Medically compromised patients.
- Patients taking drugs modifying normal bone physiology (i.e. biphosphanates, corticosteroids etc.).
- Any bone pathology.
- Ankylosed teeth.
- Noncompliant patients.
- Mixed dentition.
- Piezoelectric units must not be used if the patient and/or the operator has a pacemaker or any other active implant (e.g., a cochlear implant).

Armamentarium

1. Topical and local anesthetic.
2. Scalpel + blade no. 15C.

3. Periosteal elevator (24G, Hu-Friedy, Chicago, IL).
4. Piezotome (Satelec, Acteon group, Merignac France), insert BS1.
5. Bone allograft or xenograft.
6. 5-0 chromic gut suture.
7. Castroviejo needle holder.
8. Surgical scissors.
9. PeriAcryl®, cyanoacrylate glue.
10. Coe-pack if soft tissue grafting is needed.

Technique

Piezocision is performed 1 week after the placement of orthodontic appliances (Figure 5.1). The patient is anesthetized using Xylocaine 2% with 1/100000 epinephrine in infiltration. Once complete anesthesia is achieved, a small vertical incision is performed buccally and interproximally in the attached gingiva or mucosa. The incision into the attached gingiva is preferable as it will give less visible postoperative scarring. A mid-level incision between the roots of the teeth involved is made, keeping in mind that the soft tissues and the periosteum need to be cut to create an opening that will allow for the insertion of the piezoelectric knife.

At this point it is important to emphasize the following concept: Piezocision has a localized and selective effect on the teeth. Only the teeth or arch(es) to be moved need to be operated upon. The areas not surgerized have a higher anchorage value, since they are not affected by the demineralization process, and can be used as such in the global treatment plan. Once the vertical interproximal incisions are completed on the maxillary and mandibular arches or in localized segments, the tip of the Piezotome (BS1) is inserted in the openings previously made and a 3 mm piezoelectrical corticotomy is done (Figures 5.2–5.4).

The first mark on the BS1 insert can be used as the landmark for the decortication depth as it is located 3 mm from the tip (the decortication has to pass the cortical layer and reach the

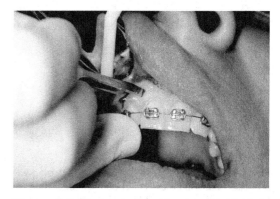

Figure 5.2 Interproximal incisions done with blade no. 15.

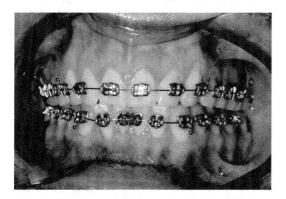

Figure 5.1 Class I malocclusion with moderate anterior crowding. Notice the mucogingival defect on tooth no. 11.

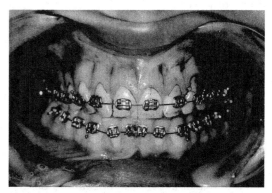

Figure 5.3 Interproximal incisions completed in the maxilla.

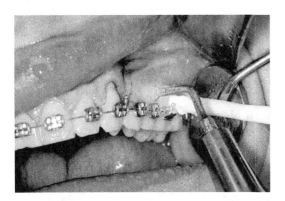

Figure 5.4 Piezoelectric corticotomy done with the Piezotome (tip BS1, Satelec, Acteon).

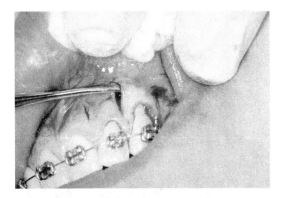

Figure 5.5 Tooth no. 11 presents with a gingival recession that will be corrected during Piezocision. A thin periosteal elevator (24 G, Hu-Friedy) is used to create a tunnel from one vertical incision to another. This tunnel will host the connective tissue graft needed to correct the recession.

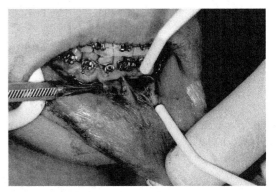

Figure 5.6 Tunneling is being done with the periosteal elevator from canine to canine to accommodate the bone graft needed to expand the mandibular alveolar bony envelope. This added bone will allow for the safe movement of the lower incisors forward.

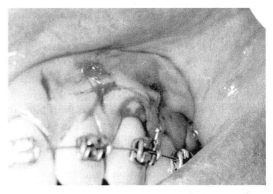

Figure 5.7 A subepithelial connective tissue graft has been harvested from the palate and placed into the tunnel and secured with 5-0 chromic gut sutures.

medullary bone to get the full effect of the RAP). One has to be very careful not to be too close to the interproximal papilla or to the roots, as irremediable damage may occur. In the areas with thin or little gingiva (recessions) or with thin or no cortical buccal bone (dehiscences, fenestrations), hard and soft tissue grafts can be added via a tunneling procedure (Figures 5.5 and 5.6).

From one of the vertical openings a periosteal elevator (24G, Hu-Friedy, Chicago, IL) is inserted between the periosteum and the bone and a blunt dissection is carried forward. This will create a tunnel that will host a soft tissue or a bone graft. Once the tunnel has been created, the piezoelectric corticotomy is done in between the roots of the teeth, and a bone graft or soft tissue graft is then added (Figures 5.7 and 5.8).

In the anterior mandible, this can be a little tricky, as only three vertical incisions in the soft tissue are made: between canines and laterals and between the two lower central incisors. This allows for a longer pouch, helping with the retention of the bone graft. Once the procedure is finished, only the areas that have

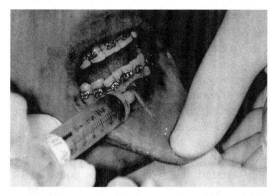

Figure 5.8 A bone allograft is being syringed into the prepared tunnel. This will enhance the bone volume and allow for anterior tooth movement with minimal risk.

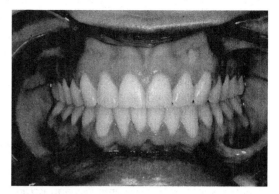

Figure 5.10 Case completed after 12 months.

Piezocision and allow for faster tooth movement and early completion of treatment (Figures 5.9 and 5.10).

DIFFERENCES BETWEEN CONVENTIONAL ORTHODONTICS AND PIEZOCISION ORTHODONTICS

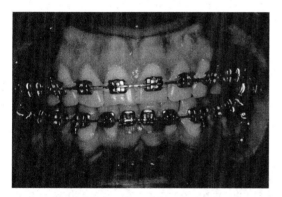

Figure 5.9 At 3 months into treatment, notice the correction of the recession on tooth no. 11 and the appearance of tooth no. 26.

been tunneled will require suturing with a 5-0 chromic gut interrupted sutures. A few drops of cyanoacrylate glue (PeriAcryl) can also be useful to protect these sutures.

The remaining areas (verticals with corticotomy that have not been tunneled) do not need suturing or gluing. The patient is seen a week after the surgery for a follow-up visit and 2 weeks post surgery to start the active phase of the orthodontic treatment. It is very critical for the patient to be seen every 2 weeks thereafter by the orthodontist in order to benefit from the temporary demineralization phase created by

Piezocision was designed to accelerate orthodontic treatment and at the same time improve the periodontium by hard and/or soft tissue grafting. As mentioned above, this procedure combines micro-incisions limited to the buccal gingiva that allow for the use of the piezoelectric knife to decorticate the alveolar bone without flap elevations and initiate RAP. It also has the advantage of allowing for hard and/or soft tissue grafting via selective tunneling when needed. Virtually all aspects of the accelerated orthodontic treatment utilizing Periodontally Accelerated Osteogenic Orthodontics™ (PAOO) discussed in Chapter 4 also apply to the Piezocision procedure, and therefore the orthodontic considerations in relation to both procedures are very similar. While we will not repeat that discussion here, certain considerations will be briefly reviewed in order to give the Piezocision procedure its proper context.

When the bone is injured, a very dynamic healing process occurs at the site of the bone injury that is proportional to the extent of the surgical insult (Frost, 1989a,b). There is a localized surge in osteoclastic and osteoblastic activity that results, in the early phases, in a decrease in bone density with an increased bone turnover. The RAP begins within a few days of the surgery and usually peaks in 1–2 months and then slows down and disappears as remineralization sets in.

Various animal experiments (Sebaoun et al. 2008, Baloul et al. 2011) have confirmed that alveolar decortication induced a RAP response, and these were discussed in Chapter 4.

More recently, similar research has been done to show the effects of Piezocision on the alveolar bone and tooth movement (Dibart et al., 2013). It has been shown that a similar RAP effect is produced when decortications are done by the piezoelectric knife. In a preliminary study on animals we have found that, although more conservative as a surgical procedure, Piezocision and the use of the piezoelectric knife appear to induce a more extensive and diffuse demineralization effect on the bone than the bur.

When these findings are applied to the clinical setting, it can be suggested that, in addition to accelerating the treatment, the RAP changes the orthodontic treatment planning in two major ways: (1) in anchorage planning, by creating a more "pliable" bone due to the transient osteopenia, and (2) the treatment timing and progress during the "window of opportunity," where the teeth move faster.

ANCHORAGE

The practice of orthodontics is largely dependent on the availability of anchorage.

The density of the alveolar bone and the cross-sectional area of the roots in the plan perpendicular to the direction of tooth movement are the primary considerations for assessing anchorage potential. The volume of osseous tissue that must be resorbed for a tooth to move a given distance is its anchorage value (Roberts, 2005).

Piezocision can now be defined as another tool for creating differential anchorage. Since it has been shown that the density of the bone around the Piezocision cut is less, the anchorage values of the teeth at the decortication site would be different. Piezocision can be done only around the teeth that are going to be moved, and the anchorage values of these teeth can be decreased. Therefore, the need for additional anchorage devices can be eliminated by designing the alveolar decortication according to the desired tooth movements.

WINDOW OF OPPORTUNITY

The theory behind accelerated tooth movement is that injury to the alveolar cortex induces a bimodal response in the alveolar bone (RAP) that can demineralize the bone around the dental roots. Looking at the literature, once the bone has demineralized following bur corticotomy, there is a 3–4 month window of opportunity to move teeth rapidly through the demineralized bone matrix before the alveolar bone remineralizes (Lee et al., 2008). The effect of Piezocision on the length of this window of opportunity is being investigated. Preliminary results indicate that owing to the more extensive nature of the demineralization engendered by the piezoelectric knife this RAP could last up to 6 months.

This concept is best observed by the patients treated with Invisalign. When Piezocision is done in combination with the Invisalign treatment, the patient changes the aligners every 5 days instead of every 2 weeks. In our practice, Piezocision-assisted Invisalign cases reported that after the fifth or sixth month in treatment, the pressure felt by the aligner decreases much more slowly compared with the earlier months in treatment. This would seem to indicate that the tooth movement starts to slow down back to the normal speed 5–6 months after the Piezocision.

REDUCED TREATMENT TIME

A split-mouth study was done by Gun and Cakirer (2013), to evaluate the effects of Piezocision on the canine distalization rate and rotation, in first premolar extraction cases. When the movement was studied at 10 weeks the canine distalization was two times more on the Piezocision side than the control side, and the canine rotation was similar on both sides. The study concluded that Piezocision is a minimally invasive alternative to corticotomies, significantly shortening the orthodontic treatment time.

GRAFTING: INCREASING THE SCOPE OF TOOTH MOVEMENT AND IMPROVEMENT OF THE PERIODONTIUM

The orthodontic treatment of teeth beyond the limits of the labial or lingual alveolar plate can lead to dehiscence formation (McComb, 1994; Wennstrom, 1996; Joss-Vassalli *et al.*, 2010) and predispose the patient to recession (Zachrisson, 1996; Melsen and Allais, 2005).

Bone grafting increases alveolar volume, thereby increasing the scope of orthodontic tooth movement. Crowding cases can be treated without extraction by the expansion of the alveolus with bone augmentation (Ferguson *et al.*, 2006).

When Piezocision is used, the graft can be placed without the need of a flap elevation. The area where bone graft is needed can be tunneled, the graft material can be placed with a syringe and sutured, and the alveolus of that area can be expanded.

Another positive effect of bone augmentation during alveolar decortication is that it improves the patient's profile. By grafting the mandibular anterior region, a deep labiomental fold can be corrected and the profile can be enhanced (Figure 5.11).

APPLICATIONS

Piezocision can be used in a generalized, localized, or sequential manner.

If the correction of the malocclusion requires the movement of all the teeth in both the maxilla and mandible at the same time, the decortications should be done in both arches in a single step, and in a generalized manner. Certain cases can benefit from a sequential approach, where the RAP effect is induced at certain areas of the arch at a specific time. And once the desired tooth movement is achieved at these specific locations, the other areas are decorticated to induce the RAP. Since a sequential approach requires decortications at different time points throughout the treatment (meaning multiple surgeries), Piezocision is the preferred option. Piezocision is a minor surgical intervention and does not require flap elevations; therefore, a sequential approach can be clinically applicable by using this minimally invasive method.

When the malocclusion is limited to a segment or only one arch, Piezocision can be used in a localized manner. An example of this would be using localized Piezocision where molars needed to be distalized and uprighted in one segment of the arch to open space for implant placement.

Anchorage requirements are the key factor and should be well planned before deciding what type of Piezocision should be performed.

LOCALIZED PIEZOCISION

In many cases, the malocclusion or the misalignment can be localized to only one part of the dentition. In such cases, the tooth movement

(a)

(b)

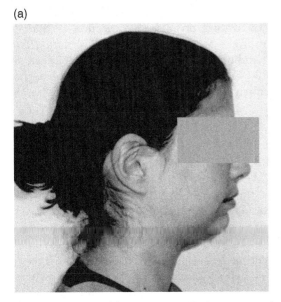
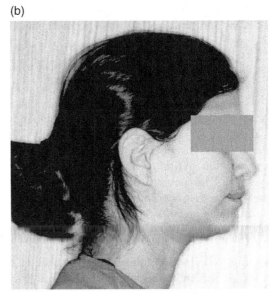

Figure 5.11 (a) Deep labiomental fold. Courtesy of Dr Eleni Kanasi. (b) Improvement of the labiomental fold after grafting. Courtesy of Dr Eleni Kanasi.

that needs to be done is also localized to that part of the dentition. An anterior crowding case with a perfect posterior occlusion is an example of such cases. Other examples would be single tooth extrusions–intrusions, molar distalization to open adequate space for implant placement, and other malocclusions that require localized tooth movement. The most important advantage of Piezocision in correction of localized problems is the differential anchorage. Piezocision should be done only around the teeth that need to be moved, creating a more pliable bone at these sites and therefore minimizing the undesired tooth movement at the other sites.

Localized piezocision is primarily used to facilitate interdisciplinary treatment. It could be used for one arch or one segment of the arch (segmental Piezocision).

A 26-year-old female was seen in consultation complaining about her smile. She had lost no. 8 to trauma and was not happy with the fixed partial denture she had (Figure 5.12). After

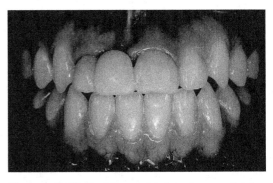

Figure 5.12 A 26-year-old female complaining about her smile. She had lost no. 8 to trauma and was not happy with the fixed partial denture she had.

removal of the existing partial denture and doing a chairside composite mockup to assess space and volume needs it became apparent that there was not enough space to replace no. 8 with a better esthetic outcome. The decision was made to distalize nos. 7 and 9 to create the space needed for a more harmonious restoration (Figure 5.13). Segmental Piezocision-assisted

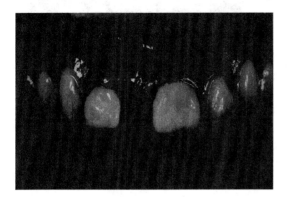

Figure 5.13 After composite mock up, it becomes apparent that the space for no. 8 is insufficient for a satisfactory restoration. Courtesy of Dr. Galip Gurel.

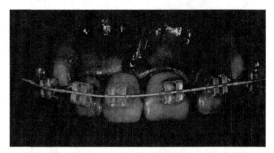

Figure 5.14 One week after bracketing, Piezocision is done distal of no. 7 and no. 9. Courtesy of Dr Elif Keser.

orthodontics was used to open that space in a timely fashion that would be acceptable to the patient. The patient was bracketed a week prior to the surgery. After local anesthesia was achieved, two Piezocision cuts were done (distal of no. 7 and distal of no. 9) to locally demineralize the areas around these teeth and allow for faster tooth movement (Figure 5.14). The surgery was performed in less than 10 min. The patient was dismissed and reported no discomfort or adverse events in the following days. The wires were activated and the patient saw the orthodontist every 2 weeks until completion of the treatment. After 7 weeks the space had opened and the patient was sent to the restorative dentist for further treatment (Figure 5.15). The space gain was 2.5 mm; this was achieved in 7 weeks as opposed to 3 months with conventional orthodontics.

SEQUENTIAL PIEZOCISION

In recent years, the Piezocision technique has evolved from being used throughout the whole mouth in one surgical setting (Dibart *et al.* 2009, 2010; Keser and Dibart, 2011), to a more "staged" approach, where demineralization of selected areas or segments of the arch are being demineralized at different times during

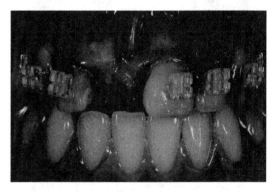

Figure 5.15 After 7 weeks the space gain was 2.5 mm; the patient now can start the restorative phase of the treatment. Courtesy of Dr Elif Keser.

orthodontic treatment to help achieve specific results (Keser and Dibart, 2013). The case presented in Figure 5.16 illustrates the sequential Piezocision approach.

The patient had a severe maxillary crowding that required more tooth movement to correct the malocclusion, compared with the mandible. She also exhibited multiple crossbites due to the skeletal discrepancy. Bonding both arches at the same time would have created some buccal movement of the lower incisors, making it hard to control the overbite and correct the crossbite. Since Piezocision creates a more pliable bone, the effects of a nickel–titanium wire become exaggerated. Subsequently, the decreased resistance now created by the Piezocision effect allows for a

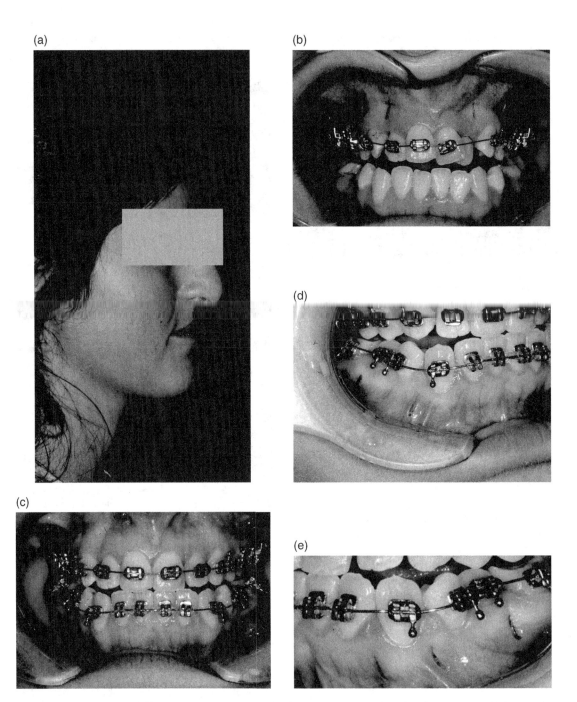

Figure 5.16 (a) Initial profile view. *Source:* Keser and Dibart (2013). Reproduced with permission of Elsevier. (b) Piezocision was initially done only on the maxilla to correct the crossbite and expand the upper arch at first. *Source:* Keser and Dibart (2013). Reproduced with permission of Elsevier. (c) The mandibular teeth were bonded after the maxillary crowding was resolved. *Source:* Keser and Dibart (2013). Reproduced with permission of Elsevier. (d) Piezocision was done on the mandible 2 weeks after mandibular arch was bonded (sequential Piezocision). *Source:* Keser and Dibart (2013). Reproduced with permission of Elsevier. (e) Piezocision was done on the mandible 2 weeks after mandibular arch was bonded (sequential Piezocision). *Source:* Keser and Dibart (2013). Reproduced with permission of Elsevier. (f) Profile view at the end of the treatment. Notice the improvement of the patient's profile. *Source:* Keser and Dibart (2013). Reproduced with permission of Elsevier. (g) Completion of the orthodontic treatment, day of debanding.

(f)

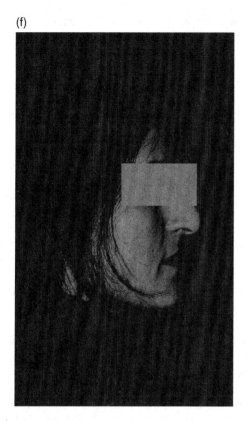

(g)

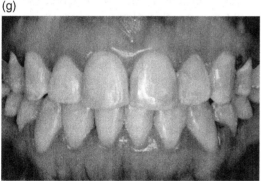

Figure 5.16 (*Continued*)

faster buccal movement of the lower incisors, which compromises the control on the overbite, especially in the anterior crossbite cases. For this reason, initially the maxillary teeth were bonded and Piezocision was done on the upper arch, the crowding was resolved, and the crossbites were

corrected. A rectangular stainless steel wire was placed on the maxilla with simultaneous bonding of the lower arch. Piezocision cuts on the mandible were done 2 weeks following the lower bracket placement. Six vertical interproximal incisions were made in the same manner as described for the maxilla. Mandibular bracket placement was done 2.5 months after the maxillary Piezocision cuts, when the RAP effect was at its peak, enhancing and complementing the effects of class III elastics on the maxilla. The total treatment time was 8 months in this case.

The RAP in the adult patient lasts approximately 6 months, and then tooth movement starts to slow down as bone remineralization sets in (data not shown). It is sometimes necessary, in the finishing phase of the orthodontic treatment, to go back and "reactivate" the RAP around a couple of teeth in order to give a "booster" to the final phase of the orthodontic treatment.

Piezocision with clear orthodontic aligners

Piezocision can be combined with clear orthodontic aligners such as Invisalign (Keser and Dibart, 2011). The patient should be wearing the first aligner and the Piezocision can be performed 1 week after the patient starts to wear the first aligner. After Piezocision the aligners are changed every 5 days instead of 2 weeks. This protocol can be applied in cases where there are 30 aligners or less. If the number of aligners required to correct the malocclusion exceeds this number, redoing the Piezocision should be considered or the subsequent aligners should be changed every 10–14 days instead of 5 days.

"ClinCheck" as a planning tool for Piezocision

When combining Piezocision with Invisalign, Align Technology's software "ClinCheck" is a very helpful tool. The superimposition feature

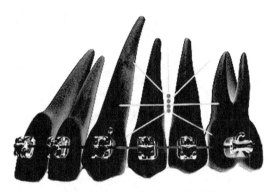

Figure 5.17 The demineralization effect of Piezocision is more extensive and diffuse on the bone than the bur.

gives the clinician a very accurate picture of the tooth movement planned. Since the idea with alveolar bur decortication/Piezocision is to demineralize the bone around the teeth that are going to be moved, the location of the cuts can be planned according to the tooth movement predicted on the superpositions. The effect of Piezocision has been shown to extend to 1.5 teeth from each side of the surgical cut (Figure 5.17). Therefore, in certain cases, decorticating every other tooth can be a viable option.

It should be kept in mind that patient compliance is crucial in Piezocision treatment, especially combined with a removable appliance like Invisalign.

Having combined Invisalign and Piezocision in many cases, it was observed that changing the aligners quickly and seeing the results faster improves the compliance and had been very well accepted by the adult patients.

An interdisciplinary case treated with Invisalign and Piezocision is illustrated in Figures 5.18–5.20.

The case involves an adult male whose chief complaint is an unaesthetic smile. He had a class I canine and molar relationship with maxillary diastemas and mandibular crowding. His anterior overbite was decreased, especially on the left segment. The gingival margins were not leveled and the incisor edges of the anterior teeth were chipped. His upper right second

premolar was missing and the space for tooth no. 4 was decreased (Figure 5.18).

As the patient's chief complaint was to achieve a pleasing smile, he needed extensive restorations on the upper arch to restore the worn dentition and altered tooth proportions, as well as the decreased overbite.

Lately, one of the most important considerations in restorative dentistry is being minimally invasive. It has been shown that when the preparations of porcelain laminate veneers were limited to the enamel, the failure rate resulting from debonding and microleakage decreased to 0% and minimal preparations significantly increased the performance of the restorations (Gurel *et al.*, 2012). Therefore, in most of the restorative cases an interdisciplinary approach increases the success rate of the treatment. The case illustrated here is an example of an interdisciplinary case where the orthodontic treatment was a crucial part of the overall treatment needed to achieve the best possible result. The goal of the orthodontic treatment was to achieve a positive overbite and to retract the upper incisors to create space for the porcelain laminate veneers, so that the amount of tooth preparation would be minimal, or almost none.

Correction of the lower crowding and lower incisor retraction was also planned in order to have space to retract the upper incisors and achieve an ideal overbite. Another goal was to create the ideal space for the implant placement for tooth no. 4.

Orthodontic tooth movement was planned to be achieved by Invisalign and Piezocision, since the patient was concerned about the look and the length of the treatment.

His ClinCheck analysis revealed that he needed 10 aligners in the maxilla and in the mandible to achieve the desired result. Interproximal reduction (IPR) of 3.5 mm was needed to correct the lower crowding and retract the lower incisors. After careful evaluation and discussion of the ClinCheck results with the team members and the patient, the treatment plan was accepted. The ClinCheck superimpositions of the initial

(a)

(b)

(c)

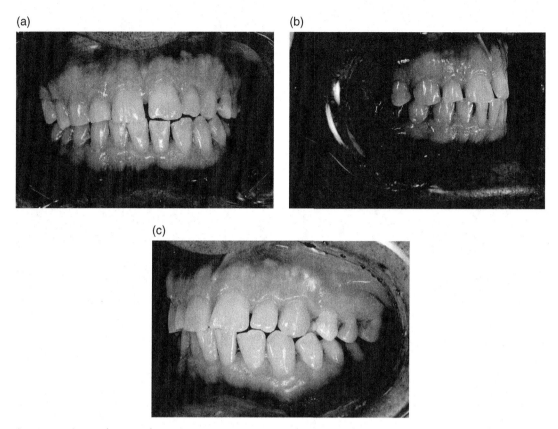

Figure 5.18 Initial intraoral views.

and planned final views showed the amount of tooth movement that was planned, and these superimpositions were used as an important tool to determine the location of the Piezocision cuts (Figure 5.19a–f). There was no movement planned distal to the upper right first premolar; therefore, no Piezocision cuts were made there. However, on the upper left segment, a Piezocision cut was planned on the mesial of the first molar to accelerate the movement of the molar. Similarly, cuts were planned mesial and distal of the canines to accelerate the anterior and canine movement on both jaws, and two cuts mesial to the first mandibular molars to help the movement of the lower posterior teeth. Piezocision was performed 1 week following placement of the first set of aligners (Figure 5.19g–i). Local anesthesia was given; vertical interproxi-

mal incisions were made, below the interdental papilla, on the buccal aspect of the maxilla using a blade. These incisions were kept minimal, just to give access to the piezo surgical knife, which was then used to create the alveolar decortication through the gingival opening and to a depth of approximately 3 mm.

Because of the rapid and temporary demineralization that occurs after Piezocision, as a result of the RAP effect, the patient was asked to change his aligners every 5 days instead of 14 days. His maxillary teeth were aligned, retracted, and extruded in 7 weeks with 10 aligners. His mandibular teeth were aligned and retracted in 7 weeks with 10 aligners. Upper and lower fixed lingual retainers were placed and the patient was sent to complete the restorative treatment (Figure 5.20).

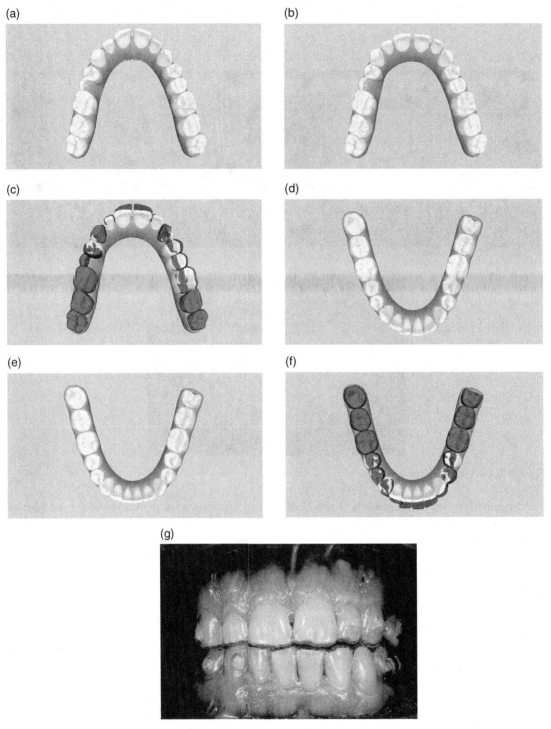

Figure 5.19 ClinCheck views of: (a) the initial malocclusion, maxilla; (b) the simulated result of the invisalign treatment, maxilla; (c) the superimposition of the initial and simulated result of the invisalign treatment, maxilla; (d) the initial malocclusion, mandible; (e) the simulated result of the invisalign treatment, mandible; (f) the superimposition of the initial and simulated result of the invisalign treatment, mandible. Piezocision cuts were done (g) 1 week after insertion of the first aligners and (h,i) with aligner in place.

(h)

(i)

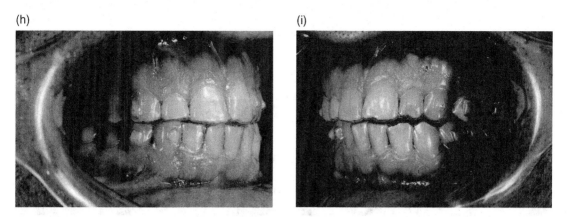

Figure 5.19 (Continued)

(a)

(b)

(c)

(d)

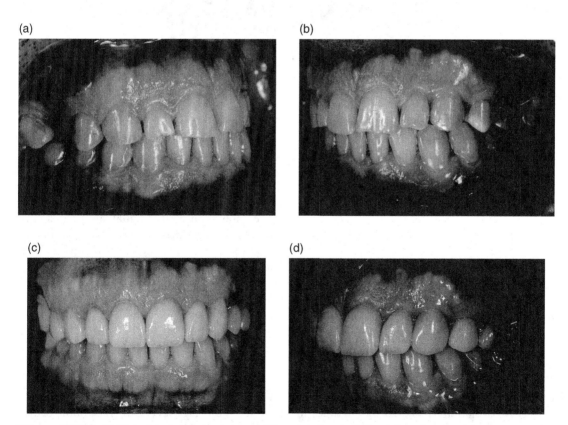

Figure 5.20 (a,b) End of orthodontic treatment (7 weeks' duration). (c–e) Porcelain laminate veneers were placed after orthodontic treatment. Restorative work by Dr Galip Gurel, Ceramist Adriano Schayder. (f) Initial smile. (g) Final smile.

(e)

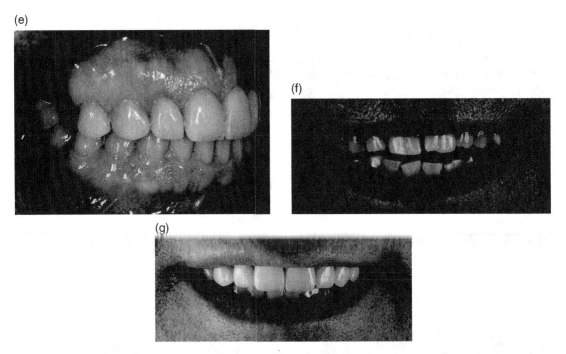

(f)

(g)

Figure 5.20 (*Continued*)

Reducing the orthodontic treatment time positively affects the patient's acceptance of the "ideal" treatment in interdisciplinary cases and makes it possible to achieve a better esthetic result by correctly positioning the teeth. Thus, accelerating the orthodontic treatment helps the dental team.

Piezocision with lingual appliances

Lingual appliances were not the most popular treatment modality for many years, mainly for reasons such as the higher rate of bracket loss, the complex and imprecise indirect rebonding technique, the difficult and time-consuming finishing process, and the average quality being not as good as that of labial cases (Rummel *et al.*, 1999; Stamm *et al.*, 2000). Significant improvements have been made in the manufacturing of the lingual appliances with the help of technological advances. Custom-made lingual brackets and wires are overcoming most of the previously experienced shortcomings, and lingual orthodontic appliances are becoming more popular everyday.

Piezocision can be used in combination with these systems as well. When Piezocision is used in combination with lingual appliances, the incisions and the decortications are done on the buccal side only and there will be no need for decortication on the lingual side. The orthodontic adjustments should be done every 2 weeks and the wires should be advanced as fast as possible.

POSSIBLE COMPLICATIONS

Anterior bite control

As stated by Staggers (1990), most of the orthodontic mechanics are extrusive in nature, and this extrusion appears to maintain or even increase the vertical dimension. The orthodontist should pay extra attention to the anterior vertical relationship during the initial leveling and alignment stage of the orthodontic treatment when alveolar decortication is done at

the anterior segment. If necessary precautions are not taken, as the bone is demineralized at the decorticated areas, the proclination effect of the initial archwires on the anterior segment would be exaggerated and the bite will open. A

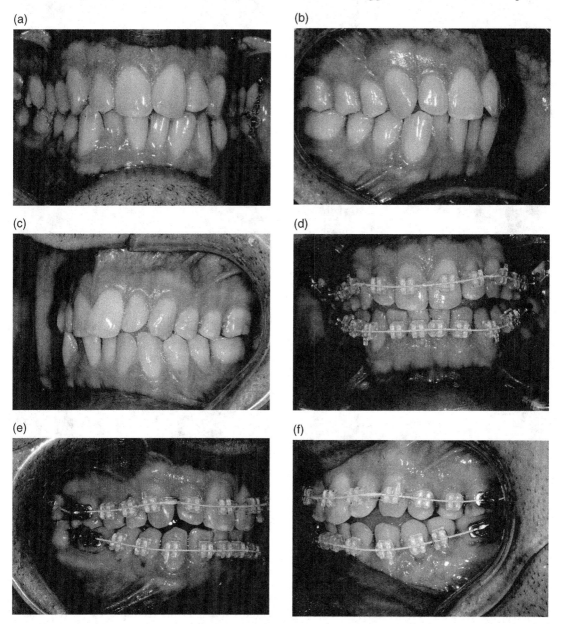

Figure 5.21 (a–c) Initial intraoral views. (d–f) At 5 months in treatment; notice the developing open bite. (g–i) Completion of orthodontic treatment (9 months' duration). (j–l) At 2 years in retention; the case looks stable.

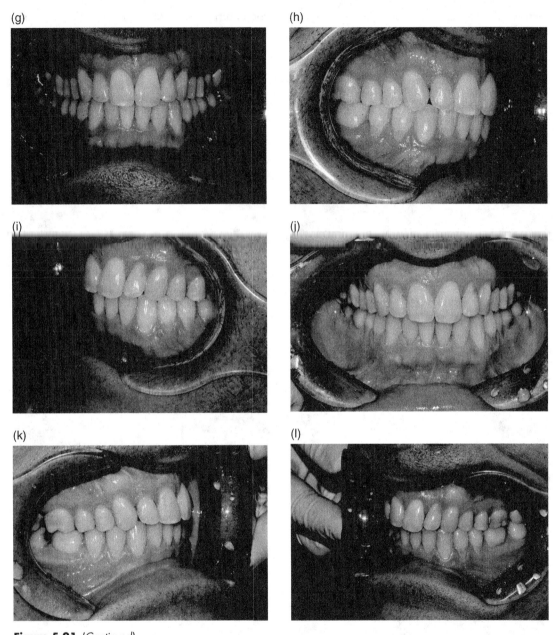

Figure 5.21 (Continued)

bite opening effect would be advantageous in deepbite cases, but in other cases, if it is not controlled from the beginning, anterior openbites will develop, especially in patients with a tongue thrust habit. The patient illustrated (Figure 5.21) is an example of such a case. He had a class I malocclusion with anterior crowding.

(a)

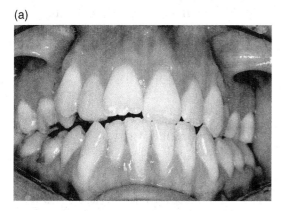

(b)

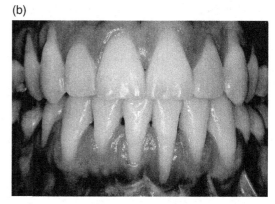

Figure 5.22 (a) Initial intraoral view. (b) Completion of the orthodontic treatment. Severe periodontal problems due to the lack of communication and proper treatment planning by the orthodontist and the periodontist. A soft and hard tissue graft should have been planned in conjunction with the orthodontic treatment.

His treatment was started with bracketing the upper and lower arch. Piezocision cuts were done on both jaws 2 weeks after bracketing. As the treatment progressed and the crowding was being resolved, the bite started to open. As the necessary precautions were not taken at the beginning of the treatment, at 5 months, around the time the treatment should have been finished, mechanics had to be started to control the bite. The total treatment time was 9 months for this case, much longer than anticipated. However, the results were stable 2 years after the completion of the treatment. If the vertical control had been started at the beginning of the treatment then the goal of accelerating the treatment time would have been accomplished.

Perio–ortho miscommunication

Communication between the orthodontist and the periodontist is crucial during the treatment planning. Figure 5.22 is an example of a case where necessary grafting procedures were not planned and the arch was expanded, creating major periodontal defects at the end of the orthodontic treatment.

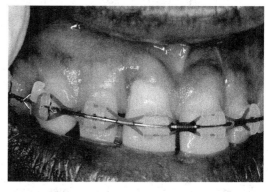

Figure 5.23 Piezocision done too close to interproximal papilla resulting in gingival recession in tooth no. 8. The defect has been there for 2 months.

Complications related to surgery

Possible complications are:

1. Loss of the interdental papilla (Figure 5.23). This may happen if the incision and Piezocision are done too close to the interdental papilla. It is of paramount importance to stay away from the papilla and do the incisions at mid root level.
2. Damage to the roots. This may happen when not using the proper tip or not evaluating properly

the underlying anatomy. In the case of close root proximity, it is best, if unsure, to skip that site.

ADVANTAGES OF PIEZOCISION COMPARED WITH OTHER ALVEOLAR DECORTICATION TECHNIQUES

Flapless versus flap

Piezocision is a flapless technique, only requiring minimal incisions on the buccal aspect. This minimally invasive approach dramatically shortens the surgical time and, therefore, minimizes the postoperative discomfort, pain, and swelling. This technique also makes it possible to apply it at different time points throughout the orthodontic treatment, making a sequential application possible. Although it would still be possible to apply PAOO or alveolar decortication with raising flaps, it would not be clinically easy to have the patient go through the same invasive procedure many times.

From an orthodontic standpoint, the sequential approach by Piezocision makes a positive modification in the orthodontic mechanics in selected cases. Although it is a flapless technique, hard and soft tissue grafting can still be done through tunneling.

Piezoelectric knife versus bur decortication

When alveolar decortications are performed using burs, some damage could be done to the teeth and to the bone due to the excessive heat generated and could produce marginal osteonecrosis (Vercellotti and Podesta, 2007). On the other hand, piezoelectric incisions have been reported to be safe and effective in osseous surgeries and lead to precise osteotomies without any osteonecrotic damage (Robiony *et al.*, 2004; Kotrikova *et al.*, 2006).

The effect of the piezoelectric cut on the bone is not only safe, but also appears, at least in the animal model, to be more extensive in terms of demineralization than the bur is.

Some important points

- Patient compliance is crucial in accelerated orthodontic treatment.
- Orthodontic activations every 2 weeks are needed with fixed appliances. When aligners are used they should be changed every 5 days.
- Wires should be advanced as fast as possible.
- Vertical control is important, starting from the beginning of the treatment.
- Regular retention protocol is used after the treatment.
- The surgical piezoelectrical cut should pass the alveolar cortex to reach the medullary bone. This is very important to get the most RAP effect.

Summarizing, the advantages of Piezocision are as follows:

1. Minimally invasive, innovative procedure.
2. Minimal post-operative discomfort.
3. Short surgical time.
4. Allows concomitant soft and/or hard tissue augmentation.
5. Very versatile. It can be used in orthodontic therapy or can be included as part of a comprehensive interdisciplinary treatment approach (large perio-prosthetic-implant rehabilitations).
6. Challenging orthodontic movements (i.e., lingual or palatal tipping of roots, etc.).
7. High patient acceptance.
8. Can be repeated several times during the course of treatment to reactivate the RAP if necessary.

DISCUSSION

Various surgical techniques have been proposed and will continue to be developed to shorten the orthodontic treatment time; they all make use of the RAP effect to various degrees following cortical bone injury. Surgical burs, blades, and bone chisels have been used to decorticate the bone and initiate the RAP. In recent years the use of the piezoelectric knife for osseous surgery has gained popularity. Vercellotti *et al.* (2005) investigated the use of a piezoelectric instrument vibrating in the ultrasonic frequency range for its potential use in periodontal resective therapy. They compared the rate of postoperative wound healing in a dog model following surgical ostectomy and osteoplasty done with the piezoelectric knife, a carbide bur, or a diamond bur. They reported that the surgical sites treated by the carbide or diamond burs lost bone, while the surgical sites treated by the piezoelectric knife revealed a gain in the bone level. They concluded that the use of the piezoelectric knife provided more favorable osseous repair and remodeling than the bur when surgical ostectomy and osteoplasty procedures were performed. This has prompted the use of the piezoelectric knife to do our decortications during Piezocision surgery. The piezoelectric knife we used (Piezotome, Satelec, Acteongroup, Merignac) has proven to achieve bone demineralization that would extend to a tooth and a half of each side of the Piezocision cut in the animal model as well as achieve profound demineralization corono-apically (Figures 5.24, 5.25, and 5.26).

Hence, there is a necessity to place the Piezocision cut at mid root level in the adult patient to get this "3D" demineralization effect. At this stage, this low mineral bone matrix milieu offers little resistance to tooth movement and the teeth are carried into place quickly using orthodontic mechanics. The bone surrounding these teeth (which have been now moved orthodontically to their desired position) gets mineralized as the anabolic phase of the RAP takes over.

Furthermore, it is important to remember that this is an orthodontically guided surgical procedure, designed by the orthodontist and performed by the periodontist/oral surgeon. After thorough data collection and analysis, the

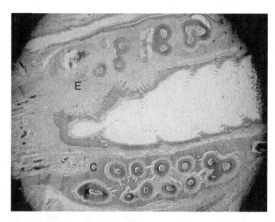

Figure 5.24 Horizontal cross-section of the rat's maxilla 2 weeks after Piezocision. Coronal level cut. E: experimental side, where piezocision was done; C: control side (untouched; notice the bone is intact).

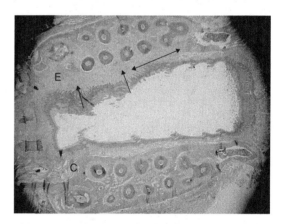

Figure 5.25 Horizontal cross-section of the rat's maxilla two weeks after piezocision. Mid-level root cut. E: experimental side, where piezocision was done; C: control side. The arrow point at the site of the piezocision (mesial and distal of the first molar). Notice the amount of demineralization following Piezocision mesio-distally. The effect reaches approximately 1.5 teeth away from the last site of piezocision (double-ended arrow).

orthodontist and the surgeon sit together and discuss the surgical treatment planning of the case. At this point the orthodontist has made their diagnosis and treatment plan. They will tell the surgeon which teeth or segments are going to move and where, and the areas that

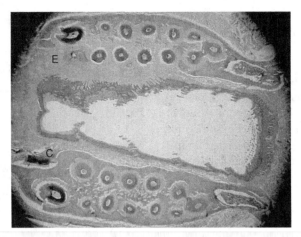

Figure 5.26 Horizontal cross section of the rat's maxilla 2 weeks after Piezocision. Apical level root cut. E: experimental side, where piezocision was done; C: control side. Notice the amount of demineralization following piezocision mesio-distally and apico-coronally (when you look at the three cuts).

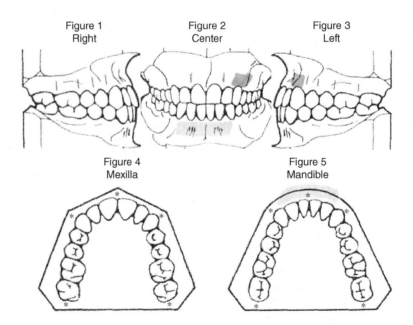

Figure 5.27 Surgical sheet ("road map") indicating where the cuts are going to take place (red), the bone graft (blue) and the soft tissue graft (dark red).

will need hard or soft tissue augmentation. The surgeon will then offer their input regarding the feasibility of the procedure, the incision design, place of incision, type of graft, and so on. The outcome of this meeting is the creation of a surgical "road map" that the surgeon will bring in the operating room and will follow (Figure 5.27).

The technique is extremely versatile as it allows for soft tissue as well as hard tissue grafting in the areas of need; as a cause of concern for the orthodontist is the possibility of creating or aggravating an existing mucogingival problem after orthodontic treatment. These areas are determined after thorough clinical and radiographic examination by the treating team (Figure 5.28) This can be addressed by grafting bone or connective tissue at the time of

(a)

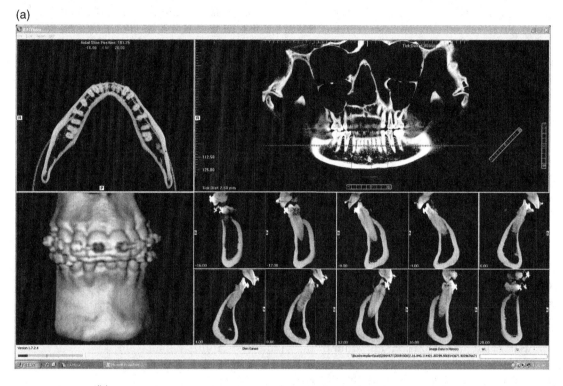

(b)

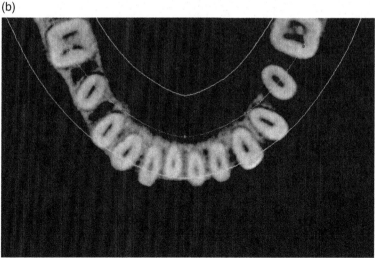

Figure 5.28 Vertical (a) and horizontal (b) cross-sections of mandible shown in Figure 5.13, confirming the need for bone graft in the lower anterior region prior to orthodontic tooth movement.

Piezocision surgery. This is done via tunneling and only after the decortication of the alveolar bone has taken place. Frost (1983, 1989a,1989b) and others demonstrated that regional noxious stimuli of sufficient magnitude result in accelerated reorganizing activity in the osseous and soft tissues. This is characterized by a burst of the localized remodeling process, which accelerates healing, particularly following the surgical wounding of cortical bone. Grafting bone or connective tissue at the time of Piezocision would take advantage of this phenomenon and greatly improve the outcome of such grafts as they are "incorporated" during the healing phase. This may create a stronger periodontium and prevent fenestrations or dehiscence from occurring during or after orthodontic therapy.

CONCLUSIONS

The novelty of Piezocision resides in the "one-sided" flapless buccal approach, where there is no need to operate palatally or lingually. This combination of buccal interproximal micro-incisions and localized piezoelectric corticotomies is able to create a significant amount of demineralization all around the teeth in the areas of tooth movement, making this a very attractive alternative to the conventional and more aggressive techniques. Unlike conventional orthodontics and during the course of treatment, a sharp increase in tooth mobility is observed resulting from the transient osteopenia induced by the surgery. This is normal and expected. Also important is the fact that orthodontic forces are applied to the teeth in order to maintain mechanical stimulation of the alveolar bone and the transient osteopenic state allowing for rapid treatment. Finally, it is of paramount importance for the orthodontist and surgeon to understand that the surgically induced high tissue turnover is restricted to the surgical areas, creating what might be referred to as a localized spatio-temporal window of opportunity. Attention must be given to

perform the bony incisions only around the teeth where tooth movement is planned. As such, the relative anchorage value of the teeth away from the surgical site remains high and the anchorage value of teeth adjacent to the surgical site is low. RAP is transient, but the continuous mechanical stimulation of the teeth would prolong the osteopenic effect induced by the procedure. Hence, there is a need to see the patient and adjust the orthodontic appliance every 2 weeks during treatment.

Piezocision is an innovative, minimally invasive technique that allows rapid orthodontic tooth movement without the downside of the extensive and traumatic classical surgical approach. Because of its minimal morbidity it can be repeated several times during the same treatment to reactivate the RAP when specific movements are required (i.e., distalization of molars, intrusion and lingual torque of roots, etc.). Piezocision proves to be efficient from the patients' and clinicians' standpoints and offers advantages that should lead to greater acceptance in the dental and patient communities.

This new treatment approach that combines minimally invasive surgery and orthodontics can be a powerful tool in the armamentarium of the 21st-century dental team.

References

Baloul SS, Gerstenfeld LC, Morgan EF *et al.* (2011) Mechanism of action and morphologic changes in the alveolar bone in response to selective alveolar decortication-facilitated tooth movement. *American Journal of Orthodontics and Dentofacial Orthopedics*, **139**, S83–S101.

Dibart S, Sebaoun JD, Surmenian J (2009) Piezocision: a minimally invasive, periodontally accelerated orthodontic tooth movement procedure. *Compendium of Continuing Education in Dentistry*, **30**, 342–350.

Dibart S, Surmenian J, Sebaoun JD *et al.* (2010) Rapid treatment of class II malocclusion with piezocision: two case reports. *International*

Journal of Periodontics and Restorative Dentistry, **30** (5), 487–493.

Dibart S, Yee C, Surmenian J *et al.* (2013) Tissue response during Piezocision-assisted tooth movement: a histological study in rats. *European Journal of Orthodontics* [Epub ahead of print]. doi: 10.1093/ejo/cjt079.

Ferguson DJ, Wilcko WM, Wilcko MT (2006) Selective alveolar decortication for rapid surgical– orthodontic resolution of skeletal malocclusion, in *Distraction Osteogenesis of the Facial Skeleton* (eds WE Bell, C Guerrero), BC Decker, Hamilton, Ontario.

Frost HA (1983) The regional acceleratory phenomena: a review. *Henry Ford Hospital Medical Journal*, **31**, 3–9.

Frost HM (1989a) The biology of fracture healing. An overview for clinicians. Part I. *Clinical Orthopaedics and Related Research*, **248**, 283–293.

Frost HM (1989b) The biology of fracture healing. An overview for clinicians. Part II. *Clinical Orthopaedics and Related Research*, **248**, 294–309.

Gun I, Cakirer B (2013) Canine distalization with Piezocision. Pilot study. Part of PhD thesis, Marmara University, Istanbul.

Gurel G, Morimoto S, Calamita MA *et al.* (2012) Clinical performance of porcelain laminate veneers: outcomes of the aesthetic pre-evaluative temporary (APT) technique. *International Journal of Periodontics and Restorative Dentistry*, **32** (6), 625–635.

Joss-Vassalli I, Grebenstein C, Topouzelis N *et al.* (2010) Orthodontic therapy and gingival recession: a systematic review. *Orthodontics and Craniofacial Research*, **13**, 127–141.

Keser EI, Dibart S (2011) Piezocision assisted Invisalign treatment. *Compendium of Continuing Education in Dentistry*, **32** (2), 46–51.

Keser EI, Dibart S (2013) Sequential Piezocision: a novel approach to accelerated orthodontic treatment. *American Journal of Orthodontics & Dentofacial Orthopedics*, **144**, 879–889.

Kim SJ, Park YG, Kang SG (2009) Effects of corticision on paradental remodeling in orthodontic tooth movement. *The Angle Orthodontist*, **79** (2), 284–291.

Kotrikova B, Wirtz R, Krempien R *et al.* (2006) Piezosurgery – a new safe technique in cranial osteoplasty? *International Journal of Oral and Maxillofacial Surgery*, **35** (5), 461–465.

Köle H. (1959a) Surgical operations on the alveolar ridge to correct occlusal abnormalities. *Oral Surgery, Oral Medicine, Oral Pathology*, **12**, 515-529.

Köle H. (1959b) Surgical operations on the alveolar ridge to correct occlusal abnormalities. *Oral Surgery, Oral Medicine, Oral Pathology*, **12**, 413–420.

Köle H. (1959c) Surgical operations on the alveolar ridge to correct occlusal abnormalities. *Oral Surgery, Oral Medicine, Oral Pathology*, **12**, 277–288.

Lee W, Karapetyan G, Moats R *et al.* (2008) Corticotomy-/osteotomy-assisted tooth movement microCTs differ. *Journal of Dental Research*, **87** (9), 861–865.

McComb JL (1994) Orthodontic treatment and isolated gingival recession: a review. *British Journal of Orthodontics*, **21**, 151–159.

Melsen B, Allais D (2005) Factors of importance for the development of dehiscences during labial movement of mandibular incisors: a retrospective study of adult orthodontic patients. *American Journal of Orthodontics and Dentofacial Orthopedics*, **127**, 552–561.

Park YG, Kang SG, Kin SJ (2006) Accelerated tooth movement by corticision as an osseous orthodontic paradigm. *Kinki Tokai Kyosei Shika Gakkai Gakujutsu Taikai, Sokai*, **28**, 6.

Roberts WE (2005) Bone physiology, metabolism and biomechanics in orthodontic practice, in *Orthodontics Current Principles and Techniques* (eds T Graber, R Vanarsdall, K Vig), Elsevier, St Louis, MO, Chapter 6, p. 278.

Robiony M, Polini F, Costa F *et al.* (2004) Piezoelectric bone cutting in multipiece maxillary osteotomies. *Journal of Oral and Maxillofacial Surgery*, **62** (6), 759–761.

Rummel V, Wiechmann D, Sachdeva R (1999) Precision finishing in lingual orthodontics. *Journal of Clinical Orthodontics*, **23**, 101–113.

Sebaoun JD, Kantarci A, Turner JW *et al.* (2008) Modeling of trabecular bone and lamina dura following selective alveolar decortication in rats. *Journal of Periodontology*, **79**, 1679–1688.

Staggers JA (1990) A comparison of results of second molar and first premolar extraction treatment. *American Journal of Orthodontics and Dentofacial Orthopedics*, **98**, 430–436.

Stamm T, Wiechmann D, Heinecken A *et al.* (2000) Relation between second and third order problems in lingual orthodontic treatment. *Journal of Lingual Orthodontics*, **3**, 5–11.

Suya H. (1991) Corticotomy in orthodontics, in *Mechanical and Biological Basics in Orthodontic Theraphy* (eds E Hosl, A Baldauf), Huthig Buch Verlag, Heidelberg, pp. 207–226.

Vercellotti T, Podesta A (2007) Orthodontic microsurgery: a new surgically guided technique for dental movement. *International Journal of Periodontics and Restorative Dentistry*, **27** (4), 325–331.

Vercellotti T, Nevins ML, Kim DM *et al.* (2005) Osseous response following resective therapy with piezosurgery. *International Journal of Periodontics and Restorative Dentistry*, **25** (6), 543–549.

Wennstrom JL (1996) Mucogingival considerations in orthodontic treatment. *Seminars in Orthodontics*, **2**, 46–54.

Wilcko MT, Wilcko WM, Marquez MG *et al.* (2007) The contribution of periodontics to orthodontic therapy, in *Practical Advanced Periodontal Surgery* (ed. S Dibart), Wiley–Blackwell, Ames, IA, pp. 23–50.

Wilcko WM, Wilcko T, Bouquot JE *et al.* (2001) Rapid orthodontics with alveolar reshaping: two case reports of decrowding. *International Journal of Periodontics and Restorative Dentistry*, **21**, 9–19.

Wilcko WM, Ferguson DJ, Bouguot JE *et al.* (2003) Rapid orthodontic decrowding with alveolar augmentation: case report. *World Journal of Orthodontics*, **4**, 197–205.

Zachrisson BU (1996) Clinical implications of recent orthodontic–periodontic research finding. *Seminars in Orthodontics*, **2**, 4–12.

Orthodontically driven corticotomy: Tissue engineering to enhance the treatment, guided by the orthodontist

Federico Brugnami[1] and Alfonso Caiazzo[2,3]

[1]*Private Practice Limited to Periodontics, Oral Implants and Adult Orthodontics, Piazza dei Prati degli Strozzi 21, Rome, Italy*
[2]*Department of Oral and Maxillofacial Surgery, Boston University Henry M. Goldman School of Dental Medicine, Boston, MA, USA*
[3]*Centro Odontoiatrico Salernitano, Via Bottiglieri 13, Salerno, Italy*

INTRODUCTION

"Corticotomy facilitated therapy does not create anatomical fragments or separate 'parts'. Corticotomies re-engineer physiology seek to re-engineer epigenetic potential in both the basic physiology of healing and ultimate morphogenesis at the molecular level of DNA and (endogenous and grafted) stem cells." Tissue engineering is the sum of: "Tissue – a collection of cells for a common purpose" and "Engineering – marshaling natural forces and manipulating them to a predetermined design" (Williams and Murphy, 2008).

In the oral surgery and orthodontic literature, the term "corticotomy" is often confused with "osteotomy." As described in Chapter 3, corticotomy is the cut of the cortices and osteotomy is the cut through the entire thicknesses, including the interposed medullary bone between the cortices, potentially creating a mobilized segment of bone and teeth. The confusion was mainly created because the earlier concept of rapid tooth movement was based on bony block movement in corticotomy techniques. Suya (1991) had proposed, in fact, that the tooth embedded within a block of medullary bone served as the handle by which the bands of less dense medullary bone surrounding the teeth were moved block by block. Unfortunately, this theory is still influencing surgeons in attempting to design a block of bone, therefore including buccal and lingual vertical and sub-apical full-thickness horizontal cuts circumscribing the roots of the teeth, as it would be done in osteo-distraction cases. The Wilckos were the first to demonstrate that the movement does not result from repositioning of tooth–bone blocks (Figure 6.1), but rather from a cascade of transient localized reactions in the

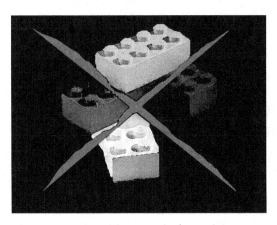

Figure 6.1 The Wilckos were the first to demonstrate that the movement does not result from repositioning of tooth–bone blocks.

bony alveolar housing leading to bone healing (Wilcko *et al.*, 2001).

The historical background and the development of the surgical technique is described in Chapter 1. For the purpose of this book we will consider the work of the Wilcko brothers as the renaissance of modern corticotomy. They started to work in the early 1990 on a combined surgical–orthodontic therapy with an innovative technique of combining corticotomy surgery with alveolar grafting. They initially termed their technique Accelerated Osteogenic Orthodontics® (AOO®) and more recently changed the terminology to Periodontally Accelerated Osteogenic Orthodontics® (PAOO®) (Wilcko *et al.*, 2001). In this chapter and mainly in the rest of the book the term corticotomy and PAOO® may be used synonymously.

SURGICAL TECHNIQUES: THE BEGINNING OF TISSUE ENGINEERING IN ORTHODONTICS

As described in previous chapters, corticotomy was originally planned as an in-office alternative to orthognathic surgery, which is quite invasive,

technical demanding, time consuming, and not so friendly for the patient (Köle, 1959). During the following years, and especially after Suya's (1991) publication, the surgery was modified to make it gradually less invasive and comparable to a full-mouth periodontal surgery (Wilcko *et al.*, 2001). More recently it has been modified to the point that it can be done in a flapless fashion (Dibart *et al.*, 2009). Regardless of the type of surgical approach that made the procedure more and more applicable and acceptable for the patient, the major shift has been made on the rationale of the technique. Thanks to the work of the Wilcko brothers and their PAOO® technique, corticotomy became a tool not only to speed up orthodontics, but also to enhance it. Adding a bone graft to the area of decortication allowed a profound modification of the alveolar basis and exceptionally boosted the treatment options (Wilcko *et al.*, 2001). It was the start of a concept that is leading toward bone engineering to modify and mold the alveolar basis, stretching the limits of orthodontic treatment. Corticotomy offers the following advantages: the possibility of solving crowding without the need for routine extraction of premolars; a more robust periodontium, and therefore a lesser risk of periodontal damage; less risk of root resorption; wider movements; less relapse; the possibility to correct transverse and mild sagittal discrepancy, modify differential anchorage of teeth, and the ability to modify the lower third of the face (Wilcko *et al.*, 2003). In other words, it exponentially expanded the scope of orthodontics and the limits of safe orthodontic treatment, and the speed merely became a marketing bonus to enhance patient acceptance. The treatment was, yes, much faster than the traditional one, but speed was overtaken by the other advantages.

Single-flap corticotomy

In the previous chapters, two major distinct surgical approaches have been described: the original one, described by the Wilcko brothers, namely, PAOO® (Wilcko *et al.*, 2001); and the most notable modifications described by Dibart *et al.* (2009), named Piezocision®. The Wilckos' approach is classically contemplating a full-mouth, full-thickness flap elevation, both in the vestibular and palatal/lingual side with or without bone graft, and it is generally involving the entire dentition in both jaws. In the Piezocision® approach, the regional acceleratory phenomenon (RAP) is started in a flapless fashion, with the surgical insult being carried out with a piezoelectric scalpel through incisions of the mucosa. (For a more comprehensive description of the techniques, please refer to Chapters 1, 3, and 5.)

We would like to introduce a third surgical approach that we routinely use in corticotomy treatment, which is a slight modification of the PAOO® protocol. This involves only a single full-thickness flap elevation in the anticipated direction of the orthodontic movement. This is, normally, a vestibular flap, and we term it single-flap corticotomy (SFC). For example, for decrowding, which is one of the most common types of orthodontic problems where corticotomy is used (Brugnami *et al.*, 2010), only the vestibular flap is elevated. For arch expansion, the same approach would be utilized. On the other hand, if a lingualization is planned, a single flap on the lingual side can be performed (Figure 6.2).

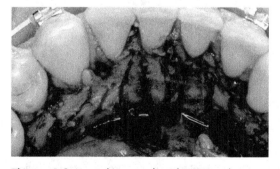

Figure 6.2 Lingual approach in the SFC technique.

Surgical technique

Since the surgical technique used is very similar to the one described in Chapter 3, only the small differences will be outlined here. Cone-beam computed tomography (CBCT) scans become critical, depending on the type and entity of movement and the periodontal biotype, in evaluating three-dimensional (3D) alveolar bone morphology and the indications for corticotomy and bone grafting. If the anticipated movement is beyond the alveolar bone surrounding the tooth (i.e., expansion or proclination) and/or the bone is <1 mm, the combination of corticotomy and bone graft is strongly suggested.

Incision design. In SFC, only one flap is elevated by definition. In most cases it is also segmental and performed only in the area where the anticipated movements will take place. It is comparable to periodontal surgery, where rarely one arch is treated simultaneously, but rather in quadrants or sextants fashion. The incision will be influenced accordingly. In most cases we may need to place vertical releasing incisions to avoid periodontal involvement of teeth in the area where corticotomy would not be performed and to increase flap mobility. The vertical incisions may be placed at least one tooth and a half away for the most mesial and the most distal area where corticotomy is going to be performed. Intra-sulcular incision is carried out with a no. 15 Bard-Parker surgical blade. In adult patients with thin periodontium, a papilla preservation approach may be used so that the base of the papilla will not be elevated. Therefore, the horizontal incision will run at the base of the papilla, from the mesial line angle at the cemento-enamel junction of one tooth to the distal line angle of the contiguous one. Vertical incisions and periosteal undermining at the base of the flap are also useful for mobilization, positioning of the graft, and tension-free closure of the flap, as recommended in Chapter 3.

Flap reflection and exposure. Same as Chapter 3.

Corticotomy/surgical decortication. Authors suggest a combination of rear-vented high-speed, rotary surgical instrumentation under copious irrigation for speed and outlining of corticotomy (Figure 6.3) and a piezoelectric scalpel for refinement and small interproximal corticotomies, especially in the presence of root proximities (Figure 6.4). Some authors suggest that the piezoelectric scalpel may be superior to burs in terms of postoperative swelling (Sivolella *et al.*, 2011). On the other hand, others have shown a higher increase in temperature and increase in surgical length compared with rotative instruments (Maurer *et al.*, 2008). Thus, to date, there

(a)   (b)

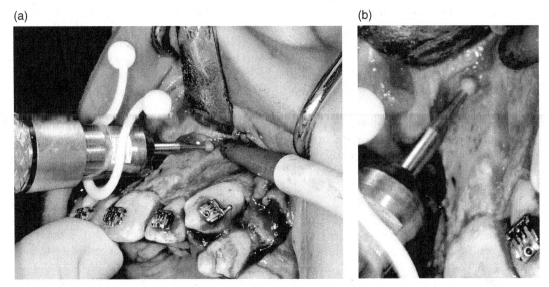

Figure 6.3 Use of rotatory instrument under copious irrigation in corticotomy: (a) for initial and faster corticotomy design; (b) close-up of a rotatory instrument used for initial corticotomy.

(a)   (b)

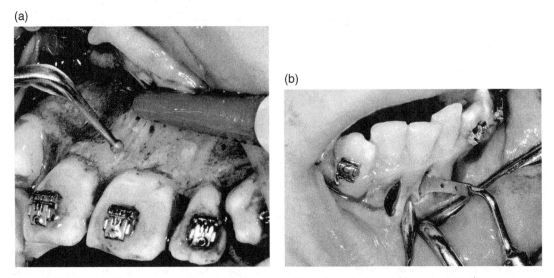

Figure 6.4 Use of piezoelectric scalpel: (a) refinement of initial corticotomy; (b) interproximal corticotomies, especially in the presence of root proximities.

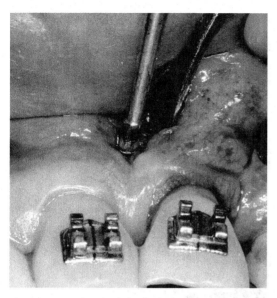

Figure 6.5 The use of rotatory instruments is less indicated than a piezoelectric scalpel in a flapless approach because the risk of soft tissue's tearing.

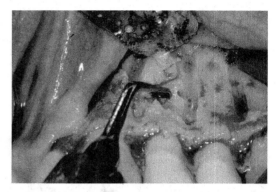

Figure 6.6 Thinning of the alveolar bone surrounding the tooth in the anticipated direction of movement.

is no definitive evidence that piezoelectric scalpels are comparable or superior to classical rotary instruments (Cassetta *et al.*, 2012), merely becoming a choice of the surgeon. In the flapless approach, a piezoelectric scalpel, for example, becomes much more practical and safe for the surgeon compared with a rotating bur (Figure 6.5).

The design of decortication is not relevant, but we try to overcome the fact that we do not elevate both flaps by deepening the interproximal cuts of at least 3 mm in the bucco-lingual direction and being at least 3 mm from the level of bone crest in the apico-coronal direction. We also perform a thinning of the alveolar bone surrounding the tooth in the anticipated direction of movement (Figure 6.6). This is an important part of the corticotomy, often ignored and difficult to perform in a flapless fashion (Piezocision®).

Bone grafting and membrane. The use of bone grafting has already been widely discussed in Chapter 3. In grafting selection, slow resorp- tion bovine xenograft or freeze-dried allograft are preferred (Figure 6.7). Autogenous and demineralized freeze-dried bone graft, which are more rapidly resorbed, should be avoided, unless utilized with a membrane and/or in layers with slow resorbing grafting material acting as a membrane (see Chapter 7). Calcium sulfate and other quick resorbing material should also be avoided, since they have shown a limited stability even in a short period of time (Figure 6.8).

The volume of the graft material used is dictated by the direction and amount of tooth movement predicted, the pretreatment thickness of the alveolar bone, and the need for labial support by the alveolar bone.

Lingual and buccal plates are very thin close to the margin. An inclination of the tooth will produce a stress and a potential resorption at the marginal cervical level in the direction of the rotation and at the opposite apical side. It is important, therefore, to try to deliver the bone graft where the bone is thinner and where the anticipated movement will produce the resorbing stress.

For these reasons, a tunnel approach to grafting is not suggested, since it is very difficult to place the graft under the attached gingiva and the graft has the tendency to be displaced too apically (Figures 6.9 and 6.10).

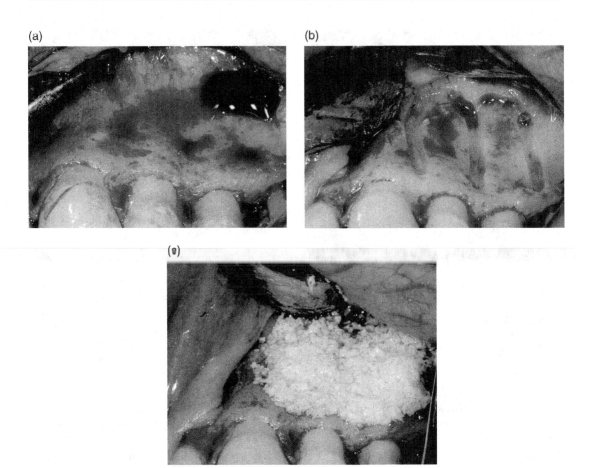

Figure 6.7 Application of a xenogeneic grafting material at the corticotomy site: (a) flap elevation and bone exposure on the corticotomy site; (b) corticotomy design; (c) application of a xenogeneic graft material on the site of corticotomy.

Since, as already described, most SFCs are done in sextants or quadrants, the mobility of the flap may be inferior compared with a full arch design, when elevation has been carried out as described in Chapter 3. This is somehow limiting the quantity of bone graft we can deliver (0.5 cm³ for approximately three or four teeth) and being still able to achieve a tension-free reapproximation of the flap. We often try to overcome the lesser volume of graft by following the principle of guided bone regeneration (GBR) and place a resorbable, collagen membrane over the graft (Figure 6.11).

Care should be taken to avoid fixation pins, which may interfere with orthodontic movements (Figure 6.12).

A membrane will also enhance the possibility of true bone regeneration, compared with a fibro-encapsulation of at least the most superficial layers of the graft.

Only in those rare cases where thickness of cortical plates in the direction of movements is more than 2 mm and the entity of anticipated movement is very limited can bone grafting be avoided.

Suture and postsurgical considerations. Resorbable sutures (4-0 or 5-0 vicryl) are recommended

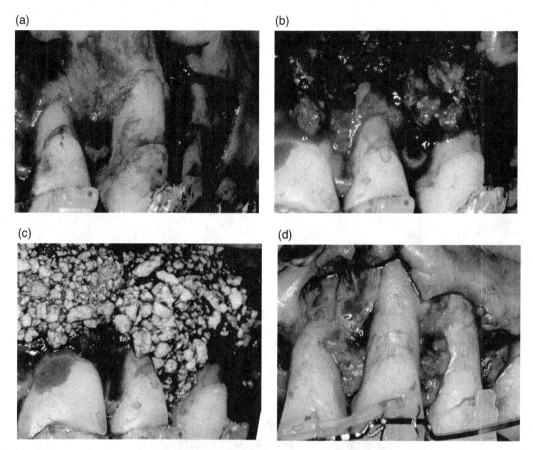

Figure 6.8 Fast resorbing grafting materials should be avoided in corticotomy: (a) flap elevation and bone exposure; (b) autologous bone graft in place; (c) application of calcium sulfate grafting material; (d) at 3 months post operation, a connective tissue graft was requested to correct a muco-gingival problem, created by persistent prolonged inflammation in the area of grafting. After elevation of the flap, no signs of grafting or regeneration were present; actually, the level of bone was worse than the pre-operative level.

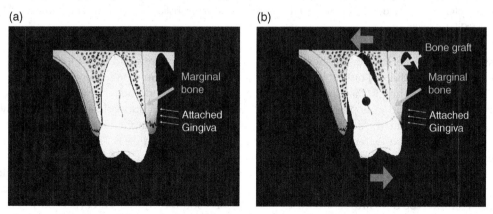

Figure 6.9 (a) The volume of the graft material used is dictated by the direction and amount of tooth movement predicted, the pre-treatment thickness of the alveolar bone, and the need for labial support by the alveolar bone. (b) In the case of tooth inclination, it would be useful to place the bone graft as close as possible to the cervical bone margin. A tunnel approach has a tendency to displace the graft too apically, far from the anticipated resorptive stress caused by the orthodontic movement, which in case of inclination would be at the marginal level in the direction of the inclination and at the apical level on the opposite side.

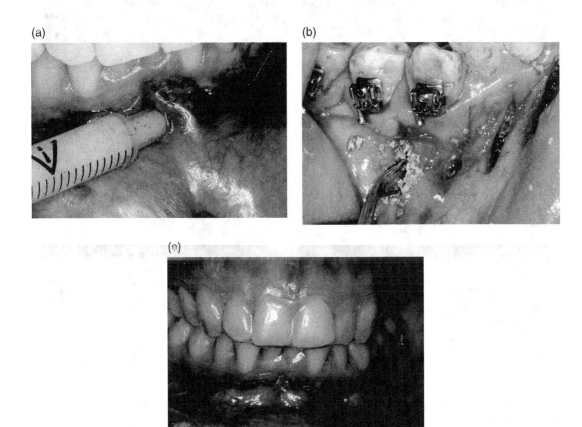

Figure 6.10 In some cases a tunnel approach to grafting is not suggested, since it is very difficult to place the graft under the attached gingiva and the graft has the tendency to be displaced too apically: (a) insertion of grafting material with a syringe into the tunnelized flap; (b) positioning of the grafting material by means of a thin periosteal elevator; (c) 10 days follow-up in a different case – note the bulk of the graft material, positioned below the muco-gingival line.

for suturing. Post-operative instructions include oral antibiotics (7–10 days) only if bone graft is used and chlorhexidine 0.2% b.i.d. rinsing for 2 weeks. Pain medication is prescribed twice a day and used as required. Although swelling is anticipated, it may be extremely variable and seems to be due to the extent of the surgery (i.e., full arch versus sextant) or the type of flap elevation (flapless versus one flap versus both flaps) rather than the type of instrument used to perform corticotomies (round burs versus piezo-electric scalpel). An in-office retrospective examination also indicates that most of the patients will stop the analgesic before the second post-operative day, and only a very minor

percentage continued for more than 4 days. Liquid diet should be followed for 1 week post-operatively and then a soft diet until suture removal, which normally takes place 1–2 weeks after surgery. Rapid orthodontic treatment is initiated immediately. The segmental and/or sequential approach to the surgery allows multiple surgery in sextants according to the orthodontic treatment plan (that is why we call it "orthodontically driven corticotomy" (ODC)). Contrary to the "classical" Wilcko technique and surgical design, it is, in fact, not mandatory to combine different mechanics to take as much advantage as possible of the RAP. It will be the RAP that will be initiated according to the

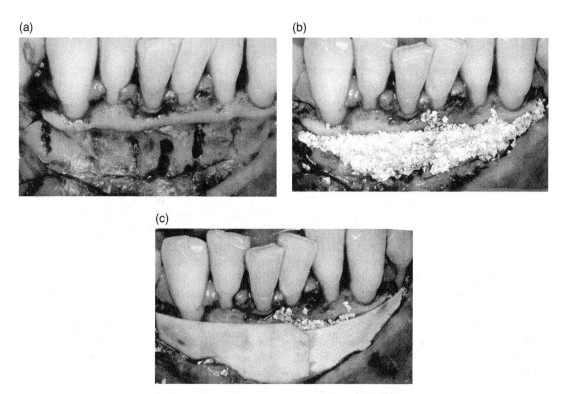

Figure 6.11 Since most SFCs are done in sextants or quadrants, the mobility of the flap may be inferior compared with a full arch design. This is somehow limiting the quantity of bone graft we can deliver (0.5 cm³ for approximately three or four teeth) and being still able to achieve a tension-free reapproximation of the flap. We often try to overcome the lesser volume of graft by following the principle of GBR and place a resorbable, collagen membrane over the graft. (a) Flap elevation and bone exposure. (b) Application of the grafting material. (c) Collagen membrane positioning.

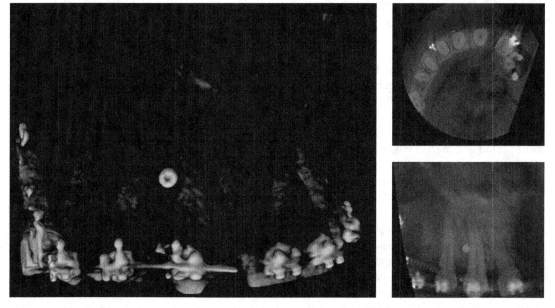

Figure 6.12 Fixation pins may interfere with tooth movement and should be avoided to fix the resorbable membrane.

orthodontic treatment plan. The segmental approach also amplifies the duration of the RAP. Being in fact performed when the actual orthodontic movements take place according to the orthodontic treatment plan and mechanics, the 4-month window of opportunity is not wasted while correcting other problems.

PAOO® versus Piezocision® versus single-flap corticotomy

Do we need another surgical approach? And how do we choose when to apply one technique over the others? We would like to answer that in this section, underlining the fact that most of the following considerations come from our clinical experiences and small retrospective analysis, and therefore they should not be taken as conclusive evidence. We would like to see some of our considerations validated or refused in an experimental model sooner or later, but for the time being this is what it is: not more than clinical experience and empirical observations and some retrospective analysis on a small pool of patients. The quest for the most minimally invasive technique that still does the job is not over yet. Although the concept of a very minimal surgical technique is somehow attractive, if this does not accomplish the goal then it becomes a useless tool. In our experience, the PAOO® approach is a long in-office procedure that may require up to 3 hours, and although generally well tolerated by the patients may be tedious. It also forces the orthodontist to make the majority of movements in a short period of time. As we know, the window of opportunity is, in fact, limited in time and may require the orthodontist to combine different mechanics in order to take advantage of the RAP. For example, in a treatment of a class II case, with anterior crowding and transverse discrepancy, it may be necessary to combine the wire mechanics to other appliances, such as a distalizer or a palatal expander. In other words, once the surgeon is done with a single-

shot surgery, the orthodontist is trying to keep up with the window of opportunity and modify the treatment planning accordingly.

On the other hand, a Piezocision® approach could be feasible for the decrowding phase, but can be less predictable in mesio-distal bodily movements or traverse expansion. Most of the time a thinning of the bone toward the direction of movement is required and a simple cut in the interproximal bone may not be sufficient. The large amount of demineralization and the superiority of the piezoelectric surgery is far from being widely accepted and demonstrated (Sivolella et al., 2011). The most salient advantages compared with conventional techniques are selective cutting of hard tissue and a gentle and precise cut without the need for excessive force. This device does not harm the surrounding soft tissues, which makes it especially suitable for surgery in areas adjacent to vulnerable structures, such as blood vessels, nerves, and the meninges. Still, it has to be used with caution, since damage may eventually occur in the hands of careless surgeons. A clear disadvantage in clinical routine use is the longer time required for osteotomies (Schaller et al., 2005).

Research experience

Statement of the problem

Recently, PAOO® or SFC and Piezocision® have been proposed as an effective tool to accelerate orthodontic treatment. However, no previous reports exist comparing the differences between PAOO®/SFC and Piezocision®. We aimed to define specific indications on when the use of one technique is indicated over the other.

Materials and methods

The study involved a retrospective analysis of 25 patients with moderate to severe crowding malocclusion or mesialization/distalization for opening/closing space treated by combining selective alveolus decortication and orthodontic treatments either with the PAOO®, SFC, or Piezocision® protocol. We also compared both procedures with a group of 20 patients randomly selected from a pool of patients with similar characteristics as age and type of malocclusion to the one in the study. All surgical procedures were performed in an office setting under local anesthesia. In the decrowding treatment ($n = 20$), SFC was compared with Piezocision®. Ten cases were treated according to SFC, with buccal decortication performed using a combination of rotary high-speed instrumentation under irrigation and piezoelectric scalpel. In the other 10 cases, surgical injury of bone was performed through vertical incisions of the mucosa, according to the protocol explained on Chapter 5. Alveolar augmentation was performed with particulate xenogeneic bovine bone, when indicated. Patients were bracketed at least 1 week before surgery. Rapid orthodontic treatment was initiated on the day of surgery and continued until correction of malocclusion. Nickel–titanium arches of increasing dimension were changed whenever possible; crowding was considered resolved, for the purpose of this investigation, when it was possible to engage a rectangular stainless steel arch.

In the mesialization/distalization cases ($n = 12$), PAOO® was compared with Piezocision® or SFC. Seven cases were treated according to the PAOO® protocol, raising both lingual and vestibular flaps and performing corticotomy on both sides; five cases were treated with a Piezocision®/SFC approach. The procedures were performed at the time of engagement of a rectangular stainless steel arch. Rapid orthodontics were started at the time of surgery. Application of forces included open and closed nickel–titanium coils of 150/200 g. One- to three-year follow-ups were also available for stability evaluation.

Methods of data analysis

For study purposes, 25 patients were divided into subgroups based on the presenting malocclusion: moderate to severe dental crowding ($n = 20$), opening or closing spaces ($n = 12$). Seven patients had both type of problems. Data were assessed for (1) soft and hard tissue response, (2) surgical, orthodontic, and total treatment times, (3) and (4) stability.

Results of investigation

In the decrowding treatment, both techniques were more efficient than traditional nonsurgical orthodontics (189.7 ± 35.4 days), although the treatment time in the SFC group was shorter (62.5 ± 13.4 days) than in the Piezocision® group (89.7 ± 16.7 days) (Figures 6.13–6.15).

In the mesialization/distalization groups, not only was the PAOO® quicker than the SFC/Piezocision® group (180.6 ± 33.2 days compared with 210.6 ± 43 days), but also more efficient in enhancing molar movement, with proper control of the roots and no tipping of the crown. SFC/Piezocision® failed to notably accelerate molar movement, and treatment mostly resulted in molar tipping. Stability also increased in PAOO®, since with no contention only one case out of seven slightly relapsed compared with five out of five in the SFC/Piezocision® group, where relapsing was also more pronounced (Figures 6.16–6.19).

Conclusions

Both procedures were effective in speeding treatment of decrowding, but SFC resulted in faster treatment than Piezocision® did. In the opening and closing spaces in the molar area, only PAOO® was effective in enhancing treatment and increasing stability, while the results in the Piezocision® group were less evident, and particularly negative on relapse.

Therefore, when a mesiodistal movement is desired, the design of choice is a dual-flap exposure with interproximal cuts and copious thinning of bone in the anticipated area of movement, as clearly represented by the PAOO® of the Wilcko brothers.

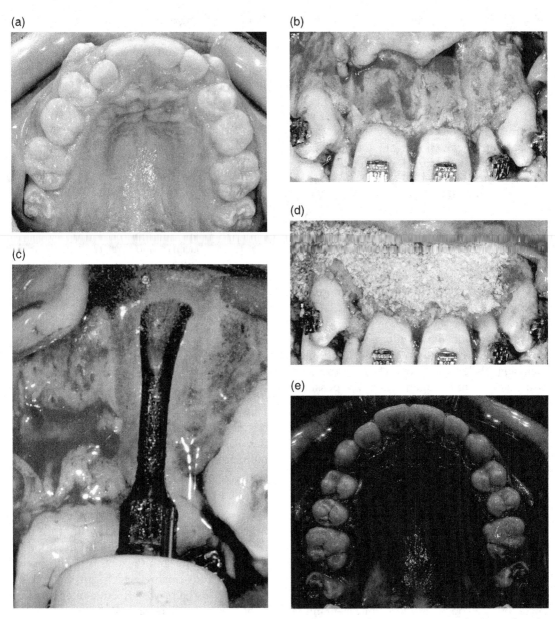

Figure 6.13 A case of palatal expansion in which an SFC was used with a Piezocision® scalpel to outline the corticotomy design and obtain a thinning of the cortical bone a xenogeneic graft material was then used: (a) initial occlusal view (upper arch); (b) corticotomy design from canine to canine only in the direction of the expected teeth movement; (c) use of piezoelectric scalpel for bone thinning; (d) application of a xenogeneic grafting material; (e) final occlusal view (upper arch). (Orthodontics by Dr F. Pedetta, Pisa, Italy.)

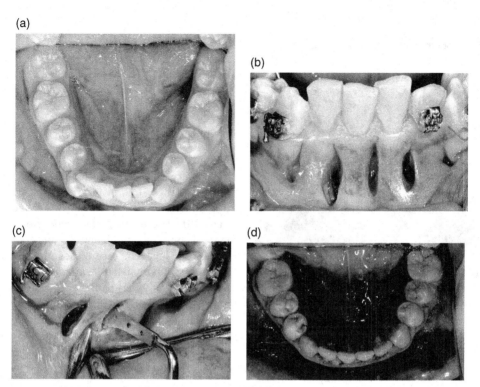

Figure 6.14 A case of moderate lower arch crowding in which the Piezocision® approach was used without flap elevation as described by Dibart *et al.*: (a) initial occlusal view; (b) small incisions to allow insertion of a piezoelectric scalpel; (c) use of a piezoelectric scalpel to create an interproximal bony insult; (d) final occlusal view. (Orthodontics by Dr F. Pedetta, Pisa, Italy.)

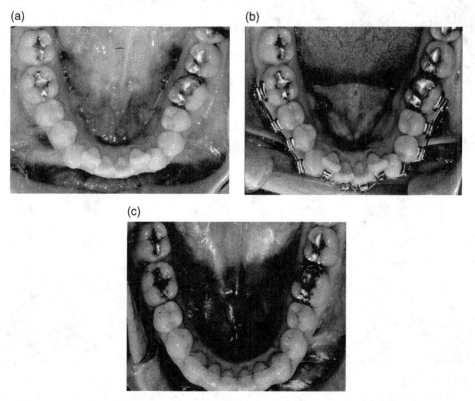

Figure 6.15 A case of moderate lower arch crowding treated without corticotomy: (a) initial occlusal view; (b) patient with brackets; (c) final occlusal view. (Orthodontics by Dr F. Pedetta, Pisa, Italy.)

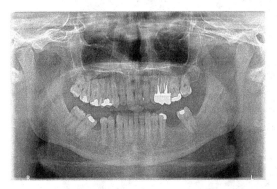

Figure 6.16 Pre-operative orthopantomography (OPT) of a patient with missing first lower right molar and first and second lower left molars. The treatment plan included closing the space in the right side and mesializing the wisdom tooth on the left and placing an implant to replace the missing first molar.

Clinical considerations: Single-flap corticotomy versus Piezocision®

In the Piezocision® technique, the grafting through a tunnel can be difficult to perform in a precise manner. It is, in fact, quite hard, if not impossible, to deliver the graft under the keratinized attached gingiva; therefore, the grafting material has the tendency to be displaced at mid-root level. In case of severe crowding, with minimal bony bases available, we feel that Piezocision® may be insufficient and still want to have an alternative to the Wilckos' full-mouth approach. That is why in certain clinical situations we rather perform an SFC, in segmental

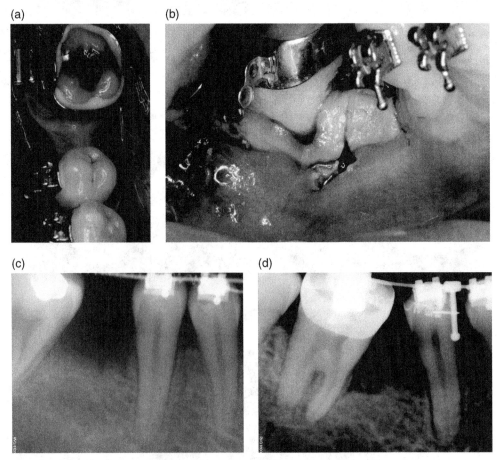

(a) (b) (c) (d)

Figure 6.17 The right side was treated with a Piezocision®: (a) pre-operative occlusal view; (b) design of the surgery; (c) pre-operative periapical radiograph; (d) periapical post-operative radiograph showing an almost complete closure of the space, with a tipping of the crown.

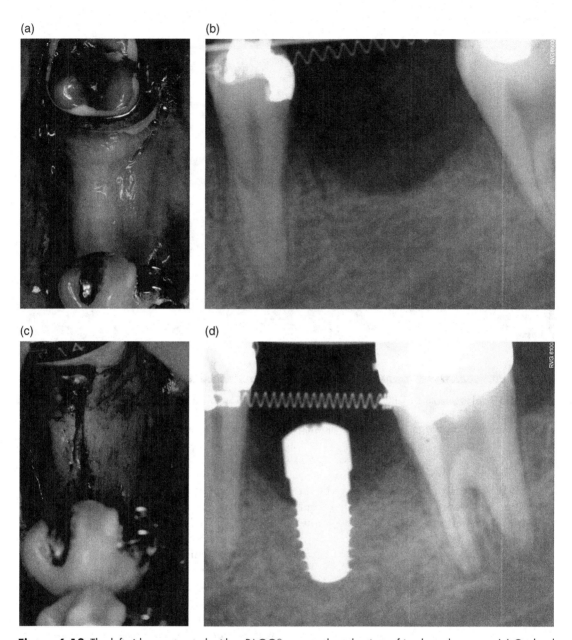

Figure 6.18 The left side was treated with a PAOO® approach at the time of implant placement. (a) Occlusal view at the surgery. Note the buccal and lingual flap elevation to perform corticotomies on both sides, and ridge expansion to allow implant placement. (b) Pre-operative periapical radiograph. (c) Surgery design. (d) Completion of anticipated movement with good control of crown tipping.

(a)

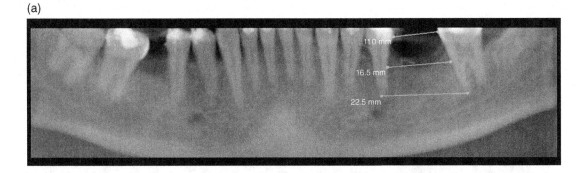

(b)

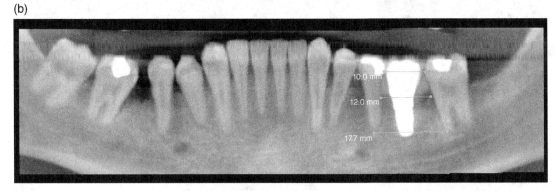

Figure 6.19 (a) Pre-treatment CBCT panorex showing the missing teeth and inclinations of molars at both sides. (b) The 1-year CBCT panorex showing good control of root uprighting of the left side treated with PAOO®, and no relapse, without contention. The right side showing less control root uprighting and some relapse.

fashion. We feel that this approach may be an interesting and less invasive alternative, but allowing one to perform the grafting and stimulate the RAP in a more adequate way.

Segmental, sequential, segmental and sequential

Segmental approach

In 1985, a segmental approach to corticotomy was introduced by Mostafa *et al.* (1985). In 2007, the segmental surgical approach for corticotomy was utilized (Spena *et al.*, 2007) to demonstrate how corticotomy was able to significantly modify the anchorage of teeth, and in fact a bodily

distalization of the upper molars was obtained without accessory anchorage (Figures 6.20–6.23).

This showed another important property of corticotomy: the modification of differential anchorage, which was the logical consequence of the RAP theory that the Wilckos introduced. More importantly, it opened up to a different concept: it was the surgery that was following the needs of the orthodontist and not the other way around. In case of decrowding, for example, regardless of the type of surgery (with or without flap elevation), we want to limit the surgery to the area where the decrowding is necessary. This opens up another important concept in the corticotomy's design and application: the segmental approach. We further developed the concept and named the

(a)
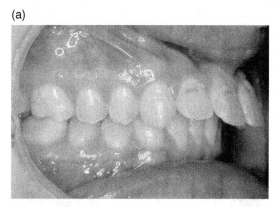

(b)
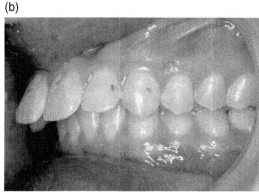

Figure 6.20 Lateral intraoral view of the patient with a class II malocclusion. (a) Right side. *Source:* Spena *et al.* (2007). Reproduced with permission from JCO, Inc. (b) Left side. *Source:* Spena *et al.* (2007). Reproduced with permission from JCO, Inc.

approach ODC, which is a surgical aid to orthodontic treatment performed by the surgeon according the treatment needs of the orthodontist, which is the real play-maker of ODC. In other words, the surgeon does the surgery, but it is the orthodontist that dictates when and where to do it.

Sequential approach

The concept is going to be developed during the entire chapter; but in order to be able to understand it, we also need to introduce the concept of sequential corticotomy. The sequential approach involves the application of corticotomy to one arch and then to the other. For example, in maxillary expansion it may be applied to the upper jaw and then, when enough expansion is achieved, it may be applied to the lower jaw if needed. The sequential approach can also be applied to a limited part of the arch, and in this case will be sequential and segmental: for example, in the case of upper expansion of an arch where rotated teeth are present, it can be designed to facilitate de-rotation only in the proximity of the rotated teeth when elastic nickel–titanium wires are used, and to the entire arch when

de-rotation is accomplished and expansion is required.

To summarize, we can have a segmental approach, where only a part of the arch is involved in corticotomy. We can also have a sequential approach, where an arch is treated before the other. And we can have a segmental and sequential approach in which a part of the arch is of interest first and another part (or the entire arch) in sequence (Table 6.1; see website for Videos 6.1 and 6.2).

WHAT IS ORTHODONTICALLY DRIVEN CORTICOTOMY?

As we already mentioned, in the ODC approach the design of the surgery is carefully projected in an attempt to follow the needs of the orthodontist. In this way, the orthodontist dictates when and where, and the surgeon decides how to do it. The advantages of this approach over the traditional Wilckos' approach is that the surgery is quicker and easier for the surgeon and more friendly for the patient. It also allows one to design the surgery in a segmental fashion according to the orthodontic treatment. For example, in the case of

(a) (b)

(c) (d)

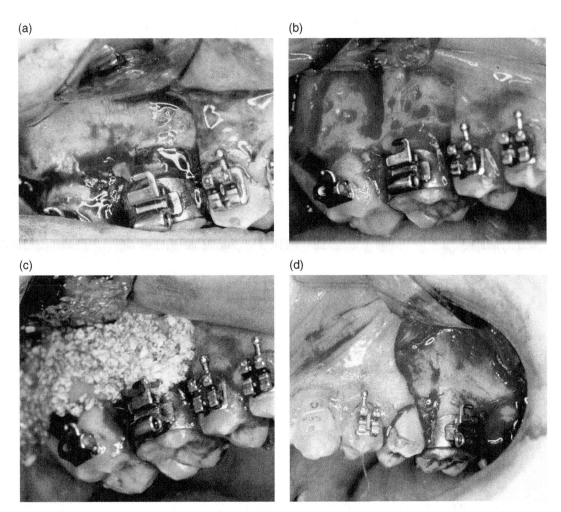

Figure 6.21 Corticotomy was performed on the upper arch bilaterally at the site of the first and second molars. Since a bodily movement into the bony bed was anticipated, the corticotomy was done at the lingual side as well. (a) Flap elevation and bone exposure on the right side revealing a fenestration on the second molar. *Source:* Spena *et al.* (2007). Reproduced with permission from JCO, Inc. (b) Corticotomy design (right side). *Source:* Spena *et al.* (2007). Reproduced with permission from JCO, Inc. (c) Application of a xenogeneic grafting material (right side). *Source:* Spena *et al.* (2007). Reproduced with permission from JCO, Inc. (d) Flap elevation and bone exposure on the left side revealing a fenestration on the mesial root of the first molar. *Source:* Spena *et al.* (2007). Reproduced with permission from JCO, Inc. (e) Corticotomy design (left side). *Source:* Spena *et al.* (2007). Reproduced with permission from JCO, Inc. (f) Application of a xenogeneic grafting material. *Source:* Spena *et al.* (2007). Reproduced with permission from JCO, Inc.

(e)

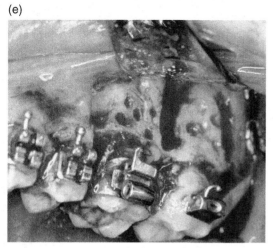

(f)

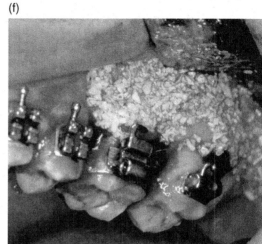

Figure 6.21 (*Continued*)

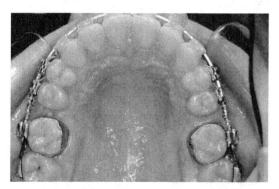

Figure 6.22 Occlusal view at 8 weeks after corticotomy*Source:* Spena *et al.* (2007). Reproduced with permission from JCO, Inc.

(a)

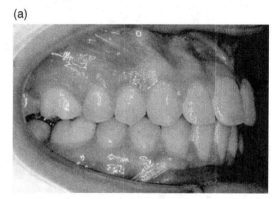

(b)

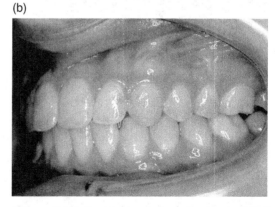

Figure 6.23 Final intraoral view after 11 months of treatment: (a) right side; (b) left side. *Source:* Spena *et al.* (2007). Reproduced with permission from JCO, Inc.

transverse discrepancy and anterior decrowding, the corticotomy can be designed in the anterior sextant when leveling and aligning is performed with elastic nickel–titanium wires. Then, when the orthodontist starts to use a more robust arch in stainless steel, the surgery can be performed in the lateral sextants. The advantages of vestibular-only flap over Piezocision®, in our hands, are a more precise control of grafting compared with a flapless blind technique, a visualization of the areas of fenestration and/or dehiscence, and, from our clinical experience, a faster resolution, especially in more severe cases.

Table 6.1

Type of procedure	Surgical approach	Surgical design	Surgical instrument	Indications	Bone graft
SFC	Single flap in the direction of movement	**Segmental** (one or more sextant or quadrants) **Sequential** (one arch at the time) **Segmental/sequential** (one or more sextant or quadrants, followed by another procedure according to orthodontic needs)	**Surgical burs** Outline corticotomy, Speed, Thinning of thick bone **Piezoelectric scalpel** refinement, Deepening of interproximal cuts, Small thinning, Limited surgical access and vicinity to vital structures **Bone scraper** Thinning and collection of autologous bone graft in case	Light decrowding Medium to severe decrowding, Arch expansion, Sagittal discrepancy (max 3 mm)	Very thin bone (<0.5 mm) Dehiscences and/or fenestrations Yes (with bone <2 mm) Yes+membrane Yes+membrane
Piezocision®	Flapless (through vertical cuts in the mucosa)	**Segmental** (one or more sextant or quadrants) **Sequential** (one arch at the time) **Segmental/Sequential** (one or more sextant or quadrants, followed by another procedure according to orthodontic needs)	Piezoelectric scalpel	Light to medium decrowding, Derotation of 1–2 teeth	
PAOO®	Lingual and buccal flaps	**Segmental** **Full arch** (classical Wilcko)	Surgical burs and piezolectric scalpel as above	Mesio-distal movements inside the alveolar boundaries, Intrusion, Extraction cases	Very thin bone Fenestrations and/or dehiscences

CASE PRESENTATION

Case 1

The patient is a 31-year-old female previously treated by another orthodontist who addressed only the upper arch with conventional orthodontics. She presented with class I occlusion and a bilateral mandibular scissor bite (Figure 6.24). The decision was made to treat her with clear aligners and inferior corticotomy to improve and augment the range of possible movements. Corticotomy was performed on the lower anterior arch with a vestibular-only flap 2 weeks from the beginning of treatment; surgical insult to the bone was carried out according to the Wilckos' technique. Following the bony cuts, a xenograft and a collagen membrane were used above the corticotomy sites (Figure 6.25).

To take advantage of the window of opportunity that will follow the surgery (RAP), aligners were changed every week instead of every 2 weeks for 4 months. The case was completed in 6 months with complete resolution of the malocclusion . The improvement of soft tissue should be noticed compared with the initial biotype (Figure 6.26).

At the end of treatment a CBCT was taken to show the presence of the graft (Figure 6.27).

Orthodontic treatment: Dr Giulia Vitale, private practice, Salerno, Italy.

Case 2

A 44-year-old business woman presented for orthodontic treatment, wishing to improve her smile. She had a skeletal and dental class I with moderate crowding in the upper and light crowding in the lower. Her chief complaint was related to the blocked out position of the upper right canine (Figures 6.28 and 6.29).

She had a connective tissue graft several years before in the upper left lateral and canine

to correct a periodontal recession and was quite sensitive to health/appearance of the gums.

She was informed about the possibility to accelerate the treatment and minimizing the risk of side effect on the periodontium to orthodontic treatment and accepted to combine a classical orthodontic treatment with corticotomy.

At the first appointment she was bracketed with indirect bonding in the upper and lower jaws (Figure 6.30). Being very busy, she also requested to have the surgical procedure combined at the same appointment. Since the crowding was mainly concentrated in the upper sextant, the corticotomy was designed in a segmental fashion (Figure 6.31).

A scraping instrument was utilized to refine corticotomy and perform thinning over the roots, combining triggering of the RAP and collection of autologous graft. In the lower jaw it was used through a tunnel approach. The graft collected was used in the upper jaw (Figure 6.32).

The Patient was orthodontically activated at the end of surgery and seen every 2 weeks, for the first 3 months and once a month for the following 3 months, for a total of nine appointments and 22 weeks of treatment. The arch sequence was as follows: nickel–titanium 0.016″ and 0.018″, stainless steel 0.16″ and 0.020″, 0.019″ × 0.25″ nickel–titanium and 0.019″ × 0.025″ stainless steel (Figures 6.33 and 6.34).

Case 3

A 42-year-old female with sagittal and transverse maxillary discrepancy presented for dental and orthodontic comprehensive treatment. She had congenitally missing upper lateral incisors, the upper second right and left, lower first right and left molars missing for extractions caused by decay. Overjet and overbite were 0 mm. She also had a 90° rotation of the lower left second premolars and 45° rotation of both upper right premolars (Figures 6.35–6.37).

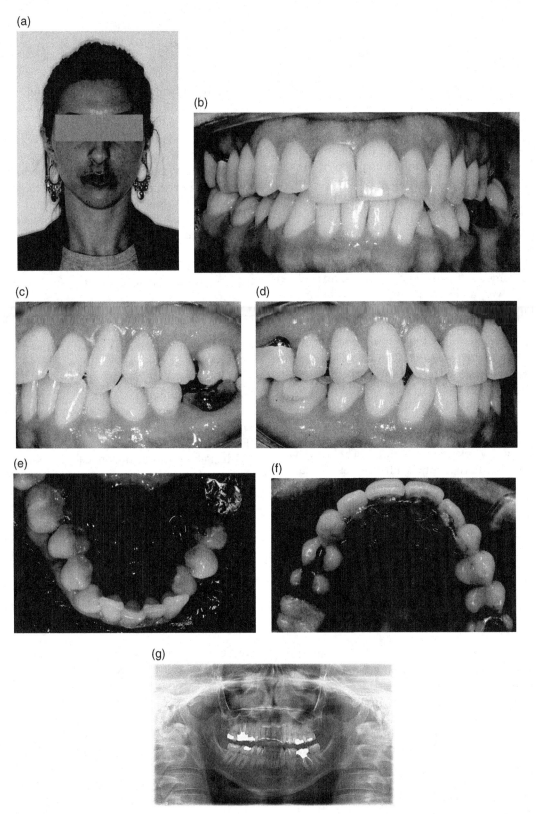

Figure 6.24 Case 1: A 31-year-old female class I malocclusion with inferior bilateral scissor bite treated previously in another office with conventional ortho only: (a) frontal facial view; (b) intraoral frontal view; (c) intraoral left view; (d) intraoral right view; (e) inferior occlusal view; (f) superior occlusal view; (g) initial OPT.

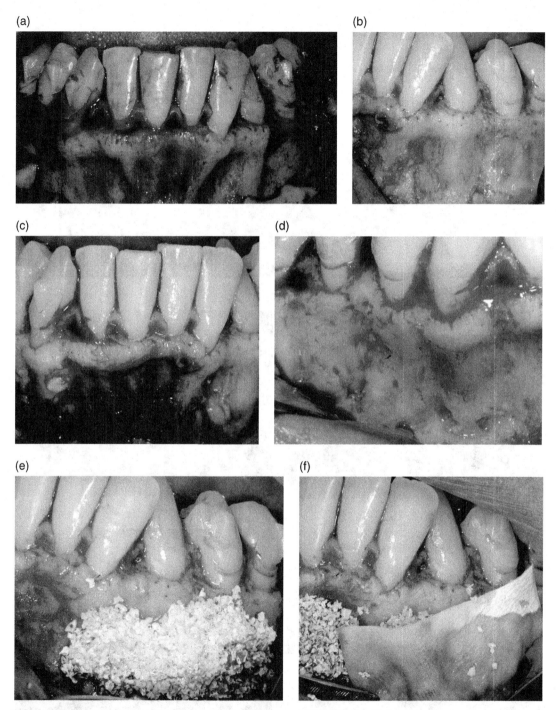

Figure 6.25 Surgical procedure performed in a segmental SFC fashion: (a) flap opening and bone exposure; (b) left side close-up – notice the fenestrations at the canine and the lateral incisor; (c) corticotomy at the lower incisors; (d) corticotomy at the right side; (e) positioning of the xenograft (left side); (f) positioning of a collagen membrane above the graft.

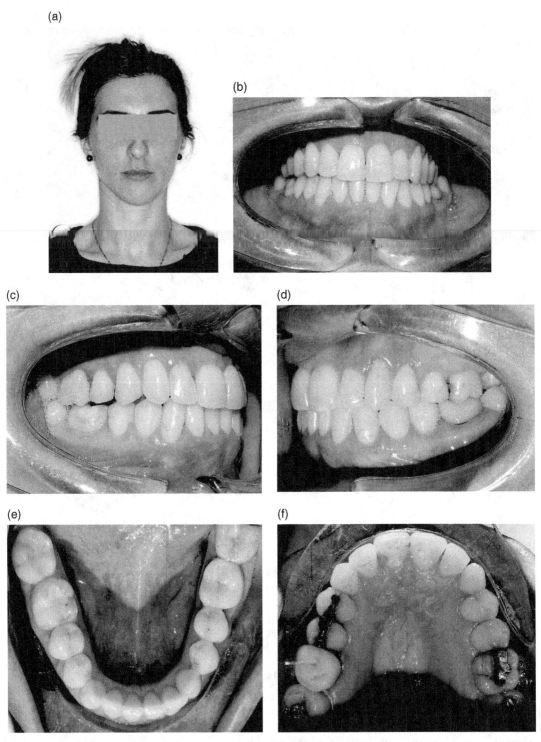

Figure 6.26 Case completed after 6 months of treatment: (a) facial view final frontal; (b) frontal intraoral view final; (c) intraoral view right side final; (d) intraoral view left side final; (e) inferior occlusal view final; (f) superior occlusal view final.

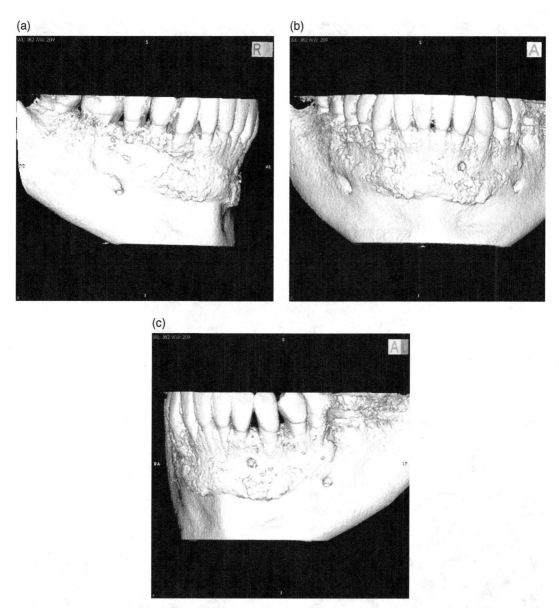

Figure 6.27 A 3D reconstruction 6 months after surgery. Presence of grafting material, suggesting a bone regeneration, can be appreciated. (a) Frontal 3D reconstruction of a CBCT at 6 months. (b) Lateral left 3D reconstruction of a CBCT at 6 months. (c) Lateral right 3D reconstruction of a CBCT at 6 months.

She refused orthognathic surgery and accepted an alternative treatment plan that included corticotomy-aided orthodontic treatment, placement of two osteo-integrated implants replacing the missing incisors. She declined the placement of four other implants replacing her missing molars, owing to financial reasons, and opted to have the lower second molars mesialized, replacing the first molars. This is very representative case of application of "ODC" explained in Table 6.1.

(a)

(b)

(c)

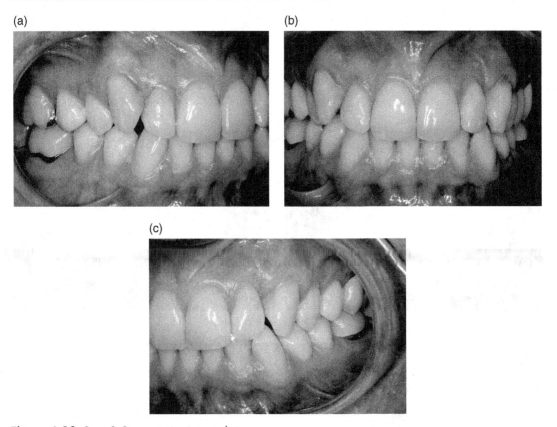

Figure 6.28 Case 2: Pre-operative intraoral view.

(a)

(b)

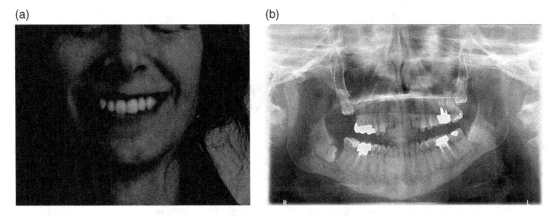

Figure 6.29 (a) Extraoral view of smile (b) pre-operative OPT.

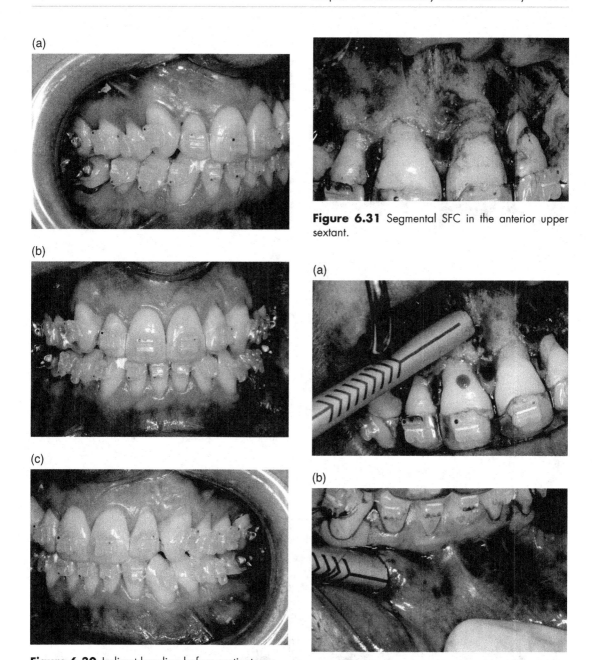

(a)

(b)

(c)

Figure 6.30 Indirect bonding before corticotomy.

Figure 6.31 Segmental SFC in the anterior upper sextant.

(a)

(b)

Figure 6.32 (a) Scraping instrument used for thinning alveolar bone in the anticipated direction of movements, over the roots and collecting bone at the same time. (b) Scraping instrument may be used in tunnel approach.

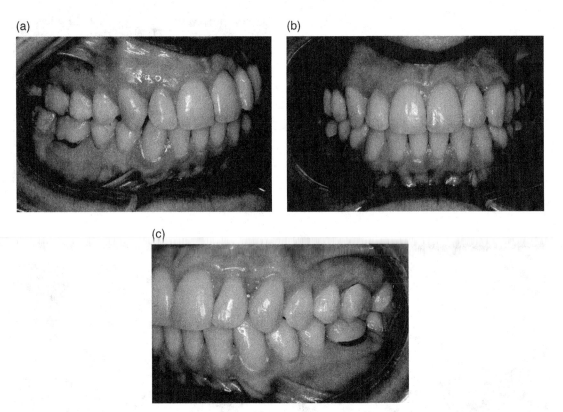

Figure 6.33 Final intraoral view at end of treatment. Treatment was completed in 22 weeks and nine appointments, including the surgical session.

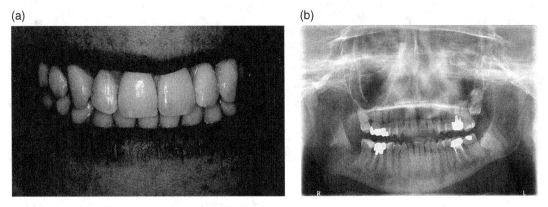

Figure 6.34 (a) Final extraoral smile detail. (b) Post-operative OPT.

(a)

(b)

(c)

(d)

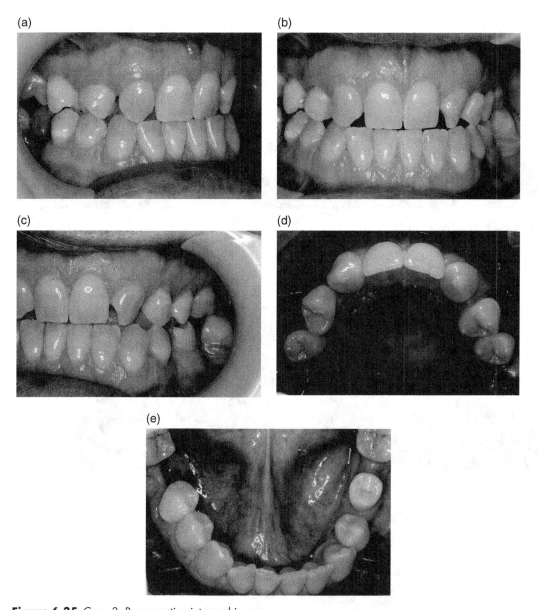

(e)

Figure 6.35 Case 3: Pre-operative intraoral images.

We had the following options: (a) perform the surgery in both full arches at day 1 and have the orthodontist trying to combine different mechanics attempting to take advantage of the window of opportunity; (b) plan several small surgeries in segmental and/or sequential fashion to trigger the RAP when it was most needed, according to the orthodontist's need, and amplify the window of opportunity.

(a)

(b)

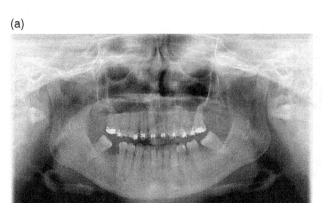
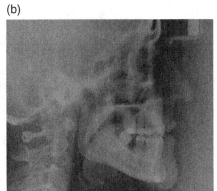

Figure 6.36 Initial radiograph.

(a)

(b)

(c)

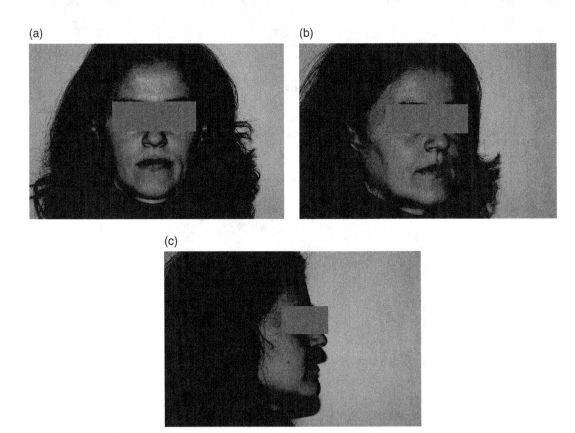

Figure 6.37 Extraoral pictures, showing a flat/concave profile.

(a)

(b)

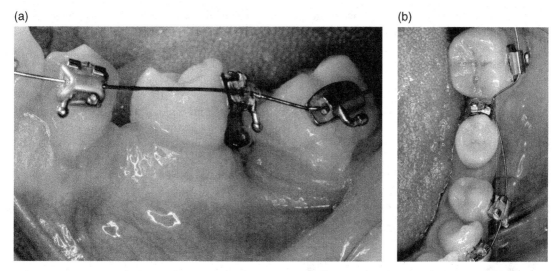

Figure 6.38 Details of the rotation of lower left second premolar.

(a)

(b)

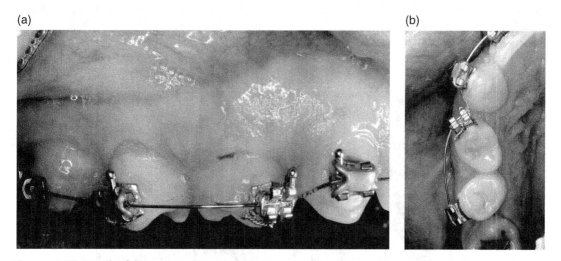

Figure 6.39 Details of the upper right premolar's rotations.

We opted for plan b, and planned to perform the surgeries following the orthodontic archwire sequence and treatment:

1. Flapless segmental corticotomy in the area of rotated teeth at leveling and aligning with nickel-titanium archwires (Figures 6.38–6.41).

2. SFC with bone graft to achieve transverse and sagittal maxillary expansion as soon as leveling was completed and the orthodontist was passing at a stainless steel archwire. Skeletal anchorage with bone plates in the zygomatic process was also planned in the same surgery.

The rationale for a skeletal anchorage in the zygomatic process was (a) to obtain indirect anchorage of the upper molars an avoid distal drifting, (b) to improve expansion of the arch and control opening of lateral incisor space for implant placement, and (c) place the skeletal anchorage far from the anticipated area of RAP (Figures 6.42–6.46; see website for Video 6.3).

3. Corticotomy with the Wilckos' approach (buccal and lingual flaps) in the posterior area of the mandible to mesialize the second molars and close the space when the sequence arrived at a rectangular stainless steel archwire (Figure 6.47).

She completed the treatment in 13 months, including final prosthetic restoration on implants (Figures 6.48–6.55).

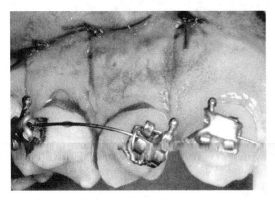

Figure 6.40 Minimally invasive flapless corticotomy in the area of the upper premolars. Both upper and lower procedures were done in a total time of approximately 10 min.

Case 4

The patient, a 15-year-old female, presented to her orthodontist with class II malocclusion and an impacted upper right canine

(a)   (b)

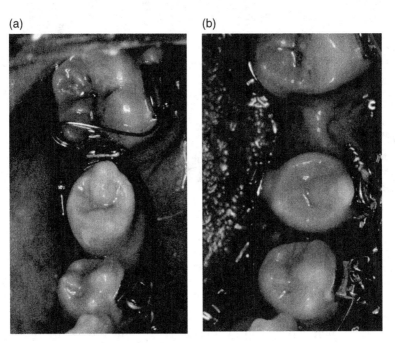

Figure 6.41 De-rotation: (a) pre-operation; (b) after 3 months.

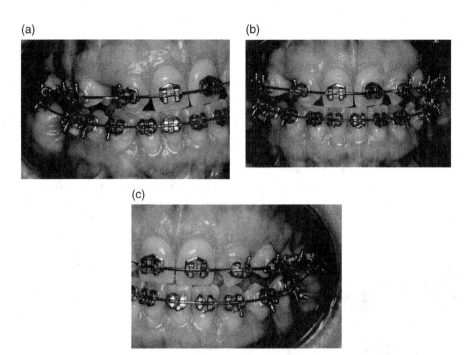

Figure 6.42 After leveling and aligning was completed, the patient was ready for upper expansion with SFC in the entire upper arch.

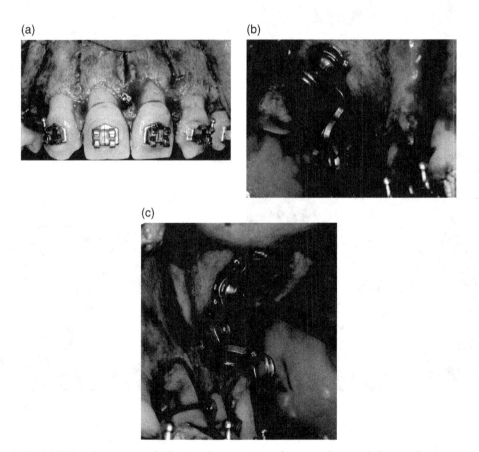

Figure 6.43 (a) SFC in the upper arch; (b, c) with positioning of two stainless steel plates in the zygomatic area for bone anchorage.

(Figure 6.54a–d). The decision was made to treat her malocclusion with conventional orthodontics to correct the malocclusion and to create an adequate space into the arch for the canine to be in occlusion. The canine was exposed 4 months after the beginning of treatment; 5 months later the orthodontist noticed no advancement of the exposed canine and an open bite on the right side (Figure 6.54e). At this point the canine was left out of the wire and an attempt was made to close the open bite. The bite was closed 4 months later (Figure 6.54f).

A surgical consultation was required to rule out ankylosis of the canine; a CBCT was taken to evaluate the position of the tooth (Figure 6.54g), which revealed a close proximity between the root of the canine and the root of the first premolar. When the bite was completely closed the patient underwent selective corticotomy around the "blocked-out" canine. At the time of surgery upon alveolar decortication (Figure 6.54h and i) the proximity of the roots as seen on the 3D X-ray was confirmed. The selective corticotomy was performed in an SFC manner, by creating a dome-shaped design around the root of the canine and a generous decortication above it; no grafting material was used. Since one of the reasons for the canine to suddenly stop could be the mechanical impeachment of the root of the premolar, the orthodontist was asked to

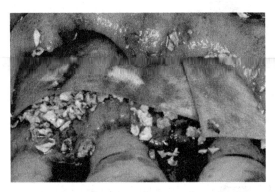

Figure 6.44 Xenogeneic bone graft and collagen membrane for GBR to enhance arch expansion in the area of corticotomy.

(a)

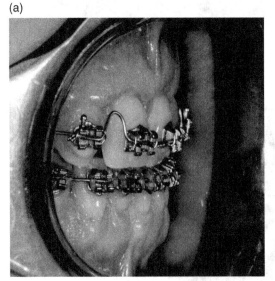

(b)

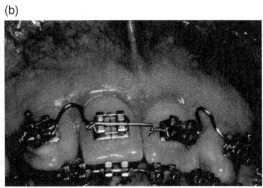

Figure 6.45 Expansion arch 0.016″ stainless steel is place at the end of surgery. The bone plates serve as indirect anchorage for the upper first molars, to avoid distal drifting and maximize sagittal expansion toward the anterior; 16 days later a positive overjet is achieved.

(a)

(b)

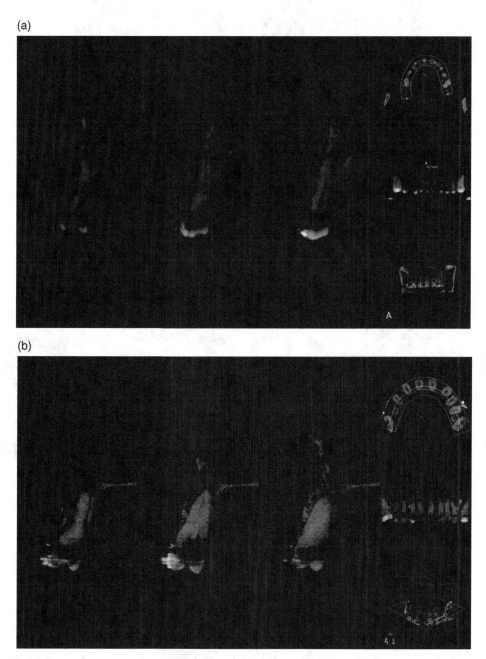

Figure 6.46 Pre- and post-operative CBCT showing buccal plate regeneration and increase in thickness.

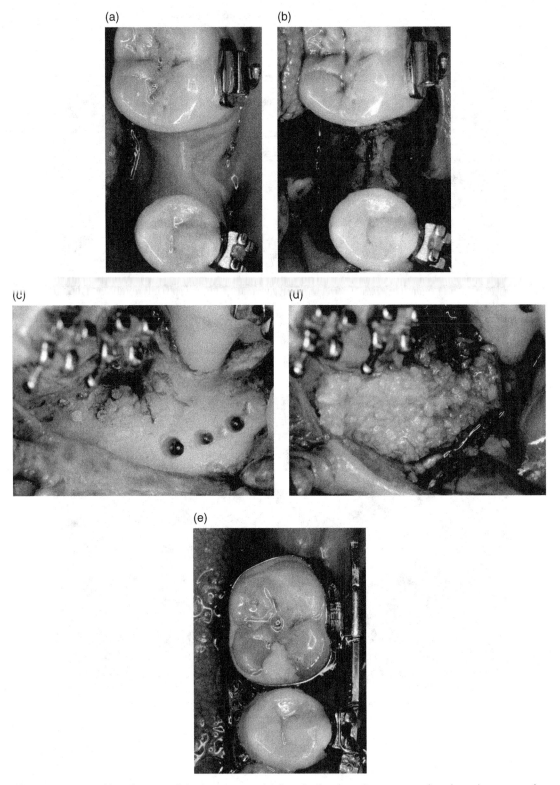

Figure 6.47 (a) Mesialization of the lower second left molar to close the space and replace the missing first molar. (b) Segmental corticotomy in the lower left molar area; buccal and lingual flaps are elevated. Note buccal lingual resorption of edentolous area. (c) Initial outlining of corticotomy with round burs on the buccal side. (d) Bone grafting. (e) Space closure.

(a)   (b)

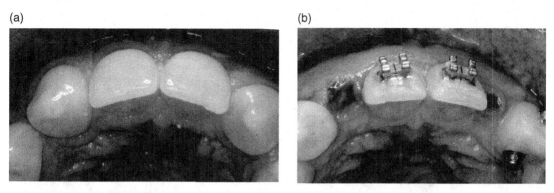

Figure 6.48 Opening of space at incisor level to allow implant placement: (a) pre-operatively; (b) after arch expansion.

(a)

(b)

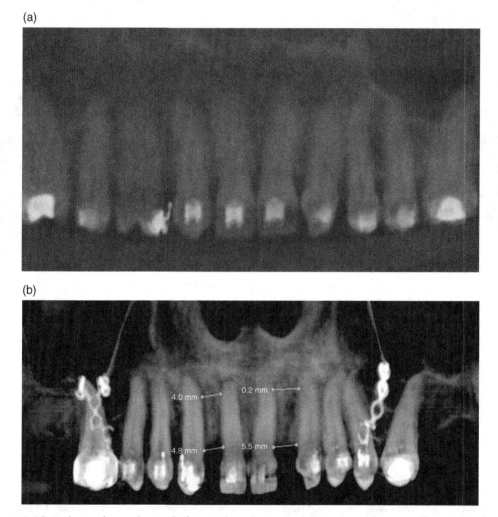

Figure 6.49 Radiographic evaluation before implant placement: (a) preoperative panorex from CBCT; (b) post-operative panorex from CBCT – note optimal 3D control of roots positioning and adequate space for proper implants placement.

(a)   (b)

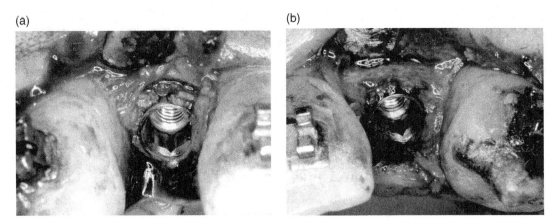

Figure 6.50 Implants positioning

(a)   (b)

(c)

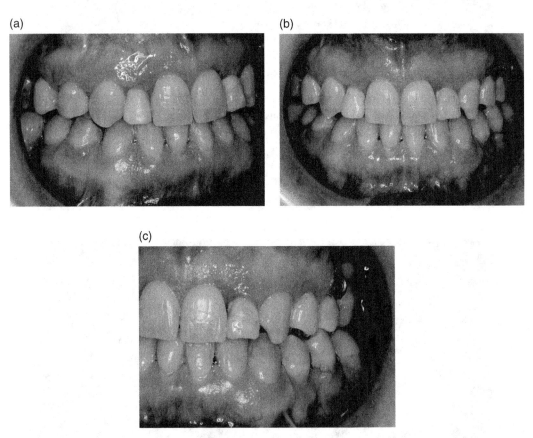

Figure 6.51 Final orthodontic treatment. Implant restorations on the lateral incisors are still on the provisional phase. This phase is important to achieve proper soft tissue contour around the implants (soft tissue sculpting).

(d)

(e)

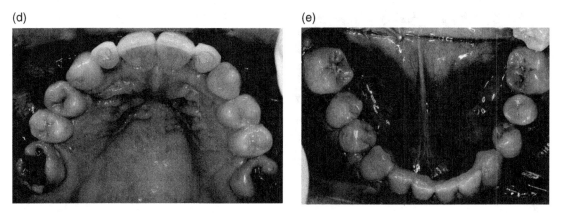

Figure 6.51 (*Continued*)

(a)

(b)

(c)

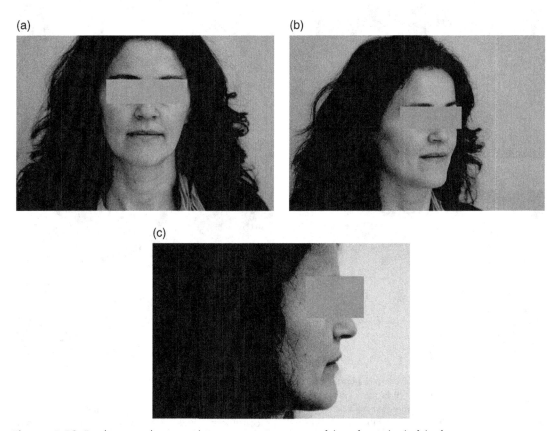

Figure 6.52 Final extraoral images showing an improvement of the inferior third of the face.

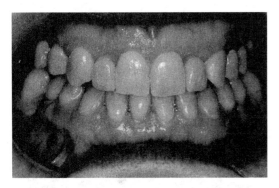

Figure 6.53 Definitive restoration of implants.

move the tip of the root of the premolar distally to the canine. Three months after surgery the canine was in occlusion and no further treatment was necessary (Figure 6.54j–m here). The fast movement confirmed that the canine was not ankylotic and a periodontal ligament was present, since this entity is necessary to have a faster movement with selective alveolar decortication (Sebaoun *et al.*, 2008).

Orthodontics: Dr Giulia Vitale, private practice, Salerno, Italy.

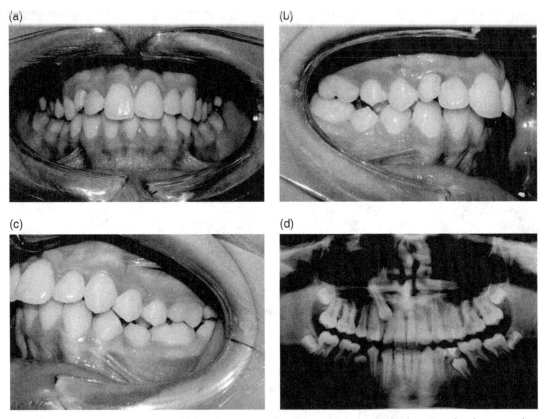

Figure 6.54 Case 4: A 15-year-old female presented to her orthodontist with class II malocclusion and an impacted upper right canine. (a) Frontal intraoral view. (b) Right intraoral view. (c) Left intraoral view. (d) Initial OPT. (e) In this picture an opening of the bite at the right side can be noticed. (f) The orthodontist left the canine out of the wire to obtain a closure of the bite. (g) 3D CBCT reconstruction showing the close proximity of the roots of the canine and the premolar. (h) Flap elevation and bone exposure. (i) Corticotomy design and alveolar decortication. (j) One month after surgery. (k) Follow-up 2 months after surgery. (l) Case completed 3 months after surgery. (m) Final intraoral X-ray.

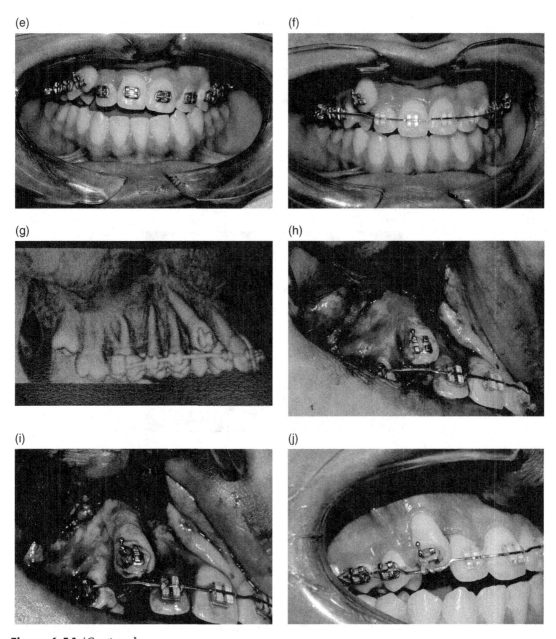

Figure 6.54 (*Continued*)

(k)

(l)

(m)

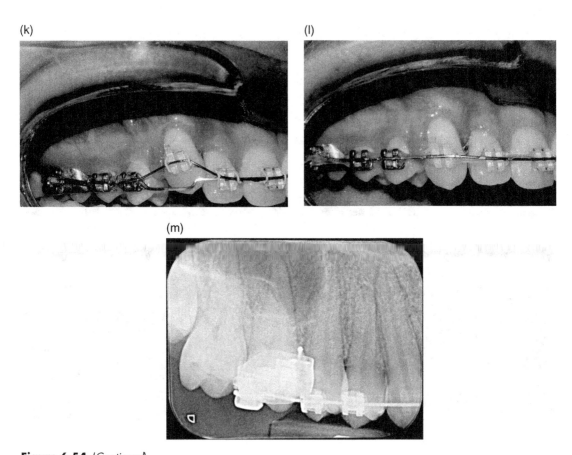

Figure 6.54 (*Continued*)

CONCLUSIONS

Considering corticotomy as just a method to accelerate orthodontic movement would be limitative. The most interesting effect is that this technique may help expand the basal bone, as confirmed by the clinical and histological findings. This will clinically translate into at least two main positive effects: (1) more space to accommodate crowded teeth and then less extraction of healthy premolars in growing patients; (2) a thicker, more robust periodontium, which may help to prevent recessions during or after orthodontic movement (Wilcko *et al.*, 2003). The concept can be stretched to the point that, according to Williams and Murphy (2008), " the alveolar 'envelope' or limits of alveolar housing may be more malleable than previously believed and can be virtually defined by the position of the roots." As we stated before, this is the beginning of bone engineering in orthodontics.

In a recent point–counterpoint article, Mathews and Kokich (2013) questioned the efficiency of PAOO®. They presented a concept of efficiency based on the acceleration and argued that, although the acceleration of tooth movement has been proven, shortening of orthodontic treatment has not been done yet. The ability of the orthodontist encompasses the use of the techniques they use. The use of corticotomy does not automatically make any orthodontist a good orthodontist, and a wrong use of the technique does not automatically make it a "bad technique." They also questioned the use of PAOO® from the cost–benefit point of view, concluding that this procedure in terms of efficiency does not seem to justify a surgical exposure to the patient.

It would be interesting to re-evaluate their concept of cost–benefit considering the application of PAOO® (which is a surgically reversible procedure), which may avoid another surgical (completely irreversible) procedure, such as extractions to solve crowding, or damage to the periodontal tissue.

In our clinical and research experience, which will be presented in Chapters 7 and 8, there are strong indications besides acceleration of treatment that make this technique an excellent tool in the hands of the orthodontist and an optimal option for the informed patient. Corticotomy has the potential to provide a solid platform for improvement in the efficiency and effectiveness of current-day orthodontic therapy and may offer the following advantages:

- Expands scope of orthodontics:
    - reduces orthodontic treatment time
    - improves range of movements
    - modifies differential anchorage between groups of teeth
    - diminishes risks of relapse.
- Eliminates the need for dental extractions in many patients.
- Reduces risks of periodontal side effects of orthodontics treatment:
    - less incidence of marginal bone resorption
    - expansion of alveolar basis and more bone support
    - shorter treatment time, and therefore less plaque accumulation on orthodontic armamentarium.
- Improved post-surgical outcomes:
    - less root resorption during active ortho-

dontic movement due to decreased resistance of cortical bone
    - change of periodontal biotype due to the addition of bone graft.
- Modifies lower third of face.
- Minimally invasive surgery (compared with orthognathic or osteo-distraction):
    - decreased postoperative discomfort
    - minimal complications
    - ability to perform surgery in an office setting
    - improved efficiency
    - decreased costs
    - no requirement for hospitalization.

References

Brugnami F, Caiazzo A, Ferro R et al. (2010) Il movimento Ortodontico Accelerato. *Ortodonzia Clinica*, **3**, 23–28.

Cassetta M, Di Carlo S, Giansanti M et al. (2012) The impact of osteotomy technique for corticotomy-assisted orthodontic treatment (CAOT) on oral health-related quality of life. *European Review for Medical and Pharmacoogical Sciences*, **16**, 1735–1740.

Dibart S, Sebaoun JD, Surmenian J (2009) Piezocision: a minimally invasive, periodontally accelerated orthodontic tooth movement procedure. *Compendium of Continuing Education in Dentistry*, **30** (6), 342–344, 346, 348–350.

Köle H (1959) Surgical operations on the alveolar ridge to correct occlusal abnormalities. *Oral Surgery Oral Medicine Oral Pathology*, **12**, 515–529.

Mathews DP, Kokich VG (2013) Accelerating tooth movement: the case against corticotomy-induced orthodontics. *American Journal of Orthodontics and Dentofacial Orthopedics*, **144**, 4–13.

Maurer P, Kriwalsky MS, Veras RB et al. (2008) Micromorphometrical analysis of conventional osteotomy techniques and ultrasonic osteotomy in the rabbit skull. *Clinical Oral Implant Research*, **19**, 570–575.

Mostafa YA, Tawfik KM, El-Mangoury NH (1985) Surgical–orthodontics treatment for overerupted maxillary molars. *Journal of Clinical Orthodontics*, **19**, 350–351.

Schaller BJ, Gruber R, Merten HA *et al.* (2005) Piezoeletric bone surgery: a revolutionary technique for minimal invasive surgery in cranial base and spinal surgery. Technical note. *Neurosurgery*, **57** (Suppl 3), E410–E411.

Sebaoun JD, Kantarci A, Turner JW *et al.* (2008) Modeling of trabecular bone and lamina dura following selective alveolar decortication in rats. *Journal of Periodontology*, **79**, 1679–1688.

Sivolella S, Berengo L, Bressan E (2011) Osteotomy for lower third molar germectomy: randomized prospective crossover clinical study comparing piezosurgery and conventional rotatory osteotomy. *Journal of Oral Maxillofacial Surgery*, **69**, e15–e23.

Spena R, Caiazzo A, Gracco A *et al.* (2007) The use of segmental corticotomy to enhance molar distalization. *Journal of Clinical Orthodontics*, **41**, 693–699.

Suya H (1991) Corticotomy in orthodontics, in *Mechanical and Biological Basics in Orthodontic Therapy* (eds E Hösl, A Baldauf), Hütlig Buch, Heidelberg, pp. 207–226.

Wilcko MW, Wilcko MT, Bouquot JE *et al.* (2001) Rapid orthodontics with alveolar reshaping: two case reports of decrowding. *International Journal of Periodontics and Restorative Dentistry*, **21**, 9–19.

Wilcko WM, Ferguson DJ, Bouquot JE *et al.* (2003) Rapid orthodontic decrowding with alveolar augmentation: case report. *World Journal of Orthodontics*, **4**, 197–205.

Williams MO, Murphy NC (2008) Beyond the ligament: a whole-bone periodontal view of dentofacial orthopedics and falsification of universal alveolar immutability. *Seminars in Orthodontics*, **14**, 246–259.

Orthodontically driven corticotomy: Tissue engineering to expand the basal bone, modify the periodontal biotype and lowering the risks of orthodontic damage to the periodontium

Federico Brugnami[1] and Alfonso Caiazzo[2,3]

[1]*Private Practice Limited to Periodontics, Oral Implants and Adult Orthodontics, Piazza dei Prati degli Strozzi 21, Rome, Italy*
[2]*Department of Oral and Maxillofacial Surgery, Boston University Henry M. Goldman School of Dental Medicine, Boston, MA, USA*
[3]*Centro Odontoiatrico Salernitano, Via Bottiglieri 13, Salerno, Italy*

INTRODUCTION

Orthodontic movements and gingival recession have always been a clinical concern. Wennstrom *et al.* (1996), in talking about tooth movement within the arch, stated that "a more lingual positioning of the tooth results in an increase of the gingival height on the facial aspect with a coronal migration of the soft tissue margin. The opposite will occur when changing to a more facial position in the alveolar process." When the tissue is apical to the cemento-enamel junction (CEJ) it is called gingival recession. Some unpublished data suggests that there is a higher incidence of gingival recession in patients orthodontically treated for transverse discrepancy (Graber *et al.*, 2005). On the other hand, other studies failed to correlate expanding movement and vestibular recessions. Bassarelli *et al.* (2005) studied stone models before and after treatment and found no higher incidence of increased length of clinical crown. One other study from the same group concluded that even in case of proclination of mandibular incisors there was no correlation between orthodontic treatment and development of vestibular recession. Anyway, they included a thin biotype as a predictor of gingival recession in proclination of mandibular incisors (Melsen and Allais, 2005). In both studies the analysis was performed right at the end of orthodontic treatment, thus limiting the possibility to intercept a late manifestation of apical migration of the gingival margin. One possible theory is that orthodontics per se is not creating a recession but it may create a marginal bone resorption if the tooth is moved outside the bony envelope of the alveolar process (Wennstrom, 1996). This may be observed, for example, in untreated patients with crowding. In these cases the discrepancy between the mesio-distal teeth's size and the space available may force some of the teeth outside the bony alveolar housing. Staufer and Landmeser (2004) showed that, in cases of more than 5 mm of crowding, gingival recession of more than 3.5 mm was 12 times more likely to occur. This may not be irreversible as previously thought. In a recent case report, a non-surgical correction of multiple recession "was accomplished by orthodontically moving teeth more into alveolar bone and by taking more careful oral hygiene measures" (Northway, 2013) (Figures 7.1–7.5).

This confirms the importance of achieving proper tridimensional positioning of the roots inside the bony alveolar housing after orthodontic treatment. Gingival recession may eventually become evident only if an inflammatory process (traumatic and/or infective) starts the disruption of the gingival attachment. Therefore, we may expect to visualize the incidence of

recessions only some time after treatment (Figure 7.6).

A more recent study by Renkema et al. (2013) evaluated the long-term development of labial gingival recession during orthodontic treatment and retention phase. In this retrospective case–control study on stone models the percentage of subjects with recession was consistently higher in cases than in controls. The presence of gingival recession was scored (Yes or No) on plaster models of 100 orthodontic patients (cases) and 120 controls at the age of 12 (T12), 15 (T15), 18 (T18), and 21 (T21) years. In the treated group, T12 reflected the start of orthodontic treatment and T15 the end of active treatment

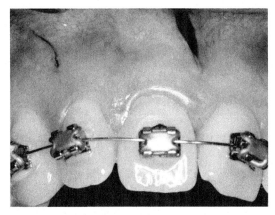

Figure 7.2 The patient was treated with the principle of Piezocision® (Chapter 5), with no bone graft.

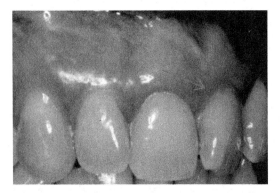

Figure 7.1 Upper left central incisor showing gingival recession. Although the recession may look small, its surgical treatment may give unpredictable results. Owing to the lack of inter-proximal mesial bone support caused by the rotation of the tooth, this defect falls in class III according to the Miller classification.

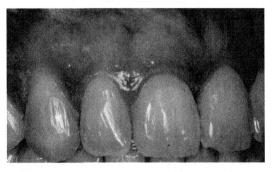

Figure 7.3 De-rotation of the tooth and spontaneous resolution of the muco-gingival defect, at the end of treatment.

(a)   (b)

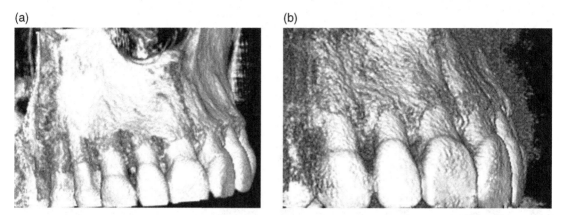

Figure 7.4 (a) 3D reconstruction area:The pre-treatment cone-beam computed tomography (CBCT) confirms the lack of bone support at the mesial line angle of the upper left central incisor. It also shows a very thin buccal plate in all the pre-maxilla, and some dehiscences. (b) The post-treatment CBCT shows the presence of bone support at the mesial line angle of the incisor, after his de-rotation and more proper 3D positioning of the root in the alveolar bony housing.

(a)   (b)

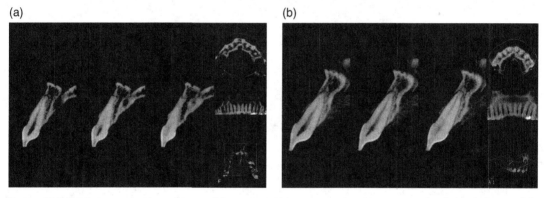

Figure 7.5 (a) Bidimensional axial view of the incisor. The pre-treatment shows a very thin buccal plate and the presence of a dehiscence. (b) The post-treatment showed a resolution of the dehiscence, due to a more centered 3D position of the root in the alveolar bony housing.

and the start of retention phase with bonded retainers. Overall, the odds ratio to have recessions for orthodontic patients compared with controls is 4.48 ($p < 0.001$; 95% confidence interval: 2.61–7.70). In particular, the lower incisors seem to be more at risk:

"Our results suggest that lower incisors are particularly vulnerable to the development of recessions in orthodontic patients. For example, 31% of the cases and 16.7% of the controls demonstrated at least 1

recession site at T21 (in all the teeth except lower incisors, ratio – 2:1), whereas 13% cases and 1.7% controls had at least 1 lower incisor with a recession at T21 (ratio – 8:1)".

They concluded that "orthodontic treatment and/or the retention phase may be risk factors for the development of labial gingival recessions," while "mandibular incisors seem to be the most vulnerable to the development of gingival recessions."

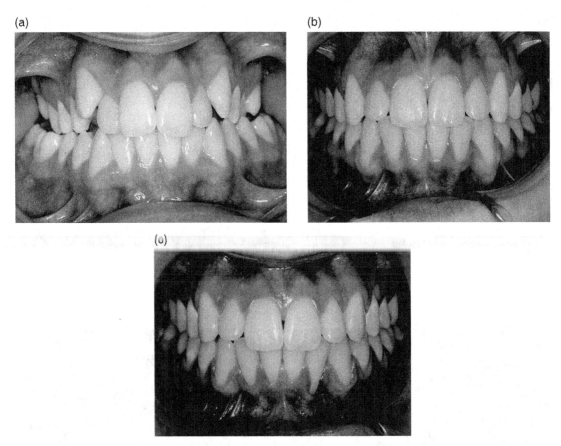

Figure 7.6 (a) A 14-year-old female presented with a sleletal class I, dental class II, with increased overjet, crowding and a transverse deficiency as seen in the frontal initial photograph. She was treated with rapid palatal expansion follow by low-friction attachment to expand the upper maxilla and solve the crowding. Owing to her flat profile and thin upper lip, it was decided to avoid extractions and over-proincline the incisors to solve the overjet. (b) At the end of treatment (26 months) a proper occlusion was achieved. The overjet went from −5 mm to −2 mm. Although the inclination of the lower incisors passed from a 1 inf – GoGn value of 90° to 102°, the periodontal tissue looked very thin, but no signs of gingival recession were yet visible. The periodontal situation remained stable at the 1 year follow-up. (c) At the 2 year follow-up, although the overjet rebounded to −2.5 mm and 1 inf – GoGn to 92°, gingival recession started to become evident. (Courtesy of Dr Roberto Ferro, Clinical Director "Unità Operativa Autonoma di Odontoiatria AULSS n 15 Regione Veneto" – Cittadella (Pd), Italy.)

RADIOGRAPHIC EVALUATION OF ORTHODONTIC SIDE EFFECTS

Most studies on alveolar bone changes in patients who have undergone orthodontic treatment have used bitewing and/or periapical radiography, thus restricting the assessments to proximal bone surfaces (Hollender *et al.*, 1980; Bondemark,1998; Janson *et al.*, 2003). Low-dose, high-quality CBCT is now becoming readily available, offering the possibility of evaluating bone changes in every dimension (Fuhrmann, 1996). During orthodontic tooth movement, teeth may be repositioned beyond the bony alveolar housing with resultant dehiscence and fenestration formation (Sarikaya *et al.*, 2002).

Baseline

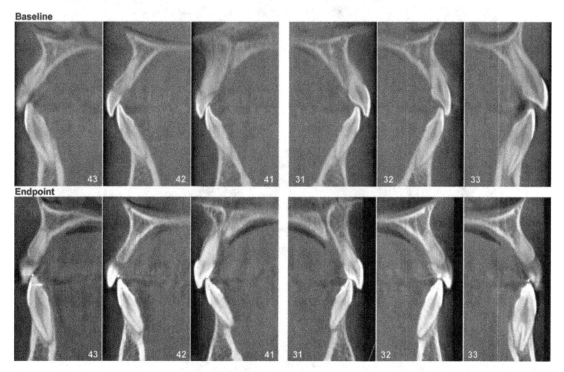

Endpoint

Figure 7.7 Sagittal images of mandibular frontal teeth (43–33) from a patient showing a large increase in the distance from the CEJ to the MBC between baseline and the study end point. Teeth numbered according to Federation Dentaire Internationale (FDI). (Reprinted from Lund *et al.* (2012), with permission from Wiley.)

Lund *et al.* (2012), using CBCT, investigated in 152 patients the distance between the CEJ and the marginal bone crest (MBC) at buccal, lingual, mesial, and distal surfaces from central incisors to first molars in adolescents before (baseline) and after extractive orthodontic treatment (study end point). Patients with class I malocclusion, crowding, and an overjet of 5 mm were examined with a CBCT unit using a 60 mm × 60 mm field of view and a 0.125 mm voxel size. Lingual surfaces, followed by buccal surfaces, showed the largest changes. Eighty-four percent of lingual surfaces of mandibular central incisors exhibited a bone-height decrease of >2 mm (Figure 7.7).

They concluded that "while some differences may be explained by reasons other than the orthodontic treatment per se, it seems likely that loss of marginal bone height, at least in the short-term, can be a side effect of extractive orthodontic treatment for a specific type of malocclusion, where retraction of teeth in anterior jaw regions causes remodeling of the alveolar bone." Garib *et al.* (2006) also showed a correlation between rapid palatal expansion and thinning of the vestibular plate up to almost 1 mm. This confirmed what was already stated before the advent of Periodontally Accelerated Osteogenic Orthodontics® (PAOO®): the buccal plate of the alveolus may be considered inviolable and any movement beyond that line might cause bony dehiscence and eventually a gingival recession (Engelking and Zachrisson, 1982). The revolutionary PAOO modifies this vision and the concept can be stretched to the point that, according to Williams and Murphy (2008), "the alveolar 'envelope' or limits of alveolar housing may be more malleable than previously believed and can be virtually defined by the position of the roots," as will be outlined by the following case (Figure 7.8).

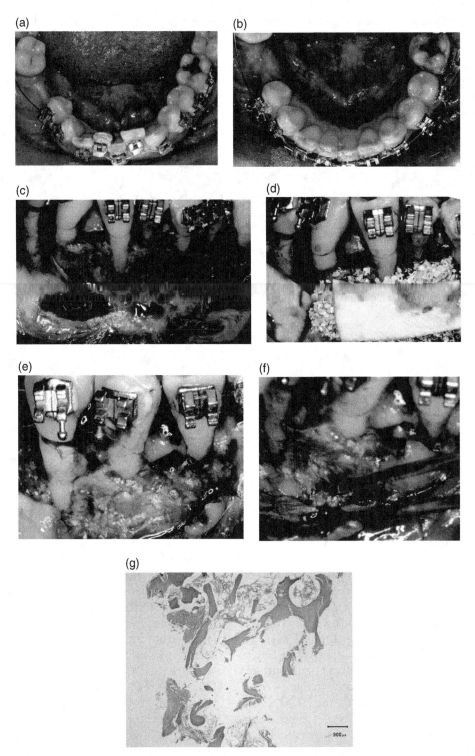

Figure 7.8 (a) Occlusal view at the beginning of treatment. (b) Decrowding 28 days after surgery. (c) Flap elevation and bone exposure recessions on several teeth should be noted. (d) Grafting material and membrane insertion. (e) At 6 months re-entry a coverage of the dehiscence treated with graft and membrane can be noted. (f) Biopsy of the site. (g) Histology showing a prominent bone marrow portion with some fibrous connective tissue and mature bone for 35% of the core area.

A 42-year-old white female presented with a class II division I malocclusion, deep bite, and severe crowding in the lower jaw. Clinical examination revealed an edentulous and severely atrophic mandibular alveolar ridge and missing teeth nos. 24 and 25.

As the patient desired rehabilitation of the edentulous areas with implant-supported restorations, she was informed that bucco-lingual ridge augmentation would be required. It was possible to perform the ridge augmentation, including the harvesting of autologous bone, and the corticotomy in one combined surgical procedure. The exposure of the alveolar bone level showed an unexpected, although not unusual, situation: large fenestrations (hidden recession) on teeth nos. 26 (lower right lateral) and 28 (first lower right premolar). A very thin buccal plate on the lower right canine (no. 27) and a smaller fenestration of the lower central left incisor (no. 24) were also noted. In the anticipated resolution of the crowding, teeth nos. 26 and 24 were expected to remain in the same position or slightly move buccally, tooth 27 to move buccally and tooth 28 to move mainly distally and slightly buccally.

Corticotomy was performed with a surgical round bur under copious irrigation, with a scalloped design around the roots of the teeth, until bleeding from the marrow was noticed. Bone thinning was refined with a manual bone-scraping instrument that also acted as collector of autologous bone graft needed to be placed over the deficient contiguous ridge. The autologous graft in the edentulous area was covered with a layer of xenogeneic bone (Endobone, Biomet Palm Beach Gardens, FL, USA) and with a resorbable membrane (Osseoguard, Biomet Palm Beach Gardens, FL, USA). The xenogeneic bone was also placed over the buccal plate in the anterior sextant where corticotomy was performed, with particular care to ensure coverage of the areas with dehiscence of the roots. In the region of tooth no. 26, a resorbable membrane was used to cover the osseous defect following the principles of conventional guided tissue regeneration (GTR) technique,

while the recession over no. 28 was left uncovered by both graft and membrane to act as a control.

Six months after surgery, an endosseous implant was placed into the augmented edentulous area. The design of the flap was extended mesially, offering a chance to visually control the right quadrant where corticotomy was performed: regeneration of the bony dehiscence overlying tooth no. 26 (lower right lateral) was evident, while the control (tooth no. 28, first lower right premolar) remained unchanged, confirming the importance of combination of the corticotomy with a regenerative procedure (guided bone regeneration (GBR) and/or GTR). The buccal plate on tooth no. 27 also appeared augmented in thickness despite a movement outside the original bony envelope.

In the area of tooth no. 27 a fragment of tissue was harvested with a blade. The result showed a prominent bone marrow portion with some fibrous connective tissue and mature bone for 35% of the core area.

RESEARCH EXPERIENCE

Aim of the study

Bone resorption occurs in the direction of tooth movement. The reduced volume of the alveolar bone, sometimes with minimal thickness and sometimes non-existent, is a complicating factor for orthodontic treatment. Previous 3D CBCT studies have shown a great incidence of bone marginal resorption in those areas where the movement was carried out toward the cortical plate (Lund *et al.*, 2010). Corticotomy has shown the ability to expand the alveolar basis (Wilcko *et al.*, 2008), potentially minimizing the risk of bone dehiscence and fenestrations as side effects of orthodontic movement outside the original bony envelope.

Material and methods

This retrospective evaluation included 20 adult patients (age 13–58 years, mean 45 years) treated in two private offices, with a combination of

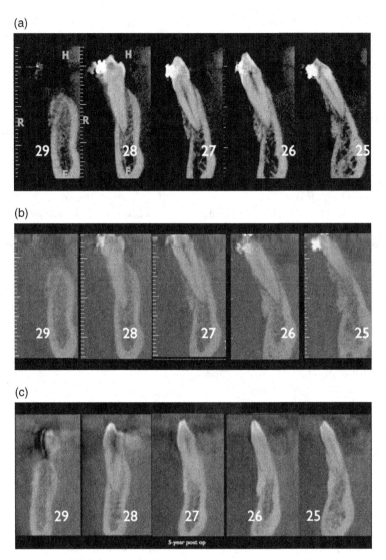

Figure 7.9 Axial views of a 5-year follow-up CBCT. (a) Inferior anterior group. Note the presence of the grafting material. (b) Grafting still covering most of the buccal cortex. Teeth numbered according to the American Dental Association (ADA). (c) Without the grafting material a fenestration would be present, highly increasing the risk of recession.

orthodontics and corticotomy, with or without bone graft. For the nature of their malocclusion, the treatment plan included a movement of one or more teeth, toward the cortical plate on the buccal (i.e., expansion of upper arch or proclination of the lower inferior) or lingual (i.e., extraction cases with anterior retraction) surfaces for a total of 142 teeth. In one case a 6-month re-entry was possible, allowing a visual comparison of treated and untreated areas, regeneration of previously missing buccal plate (dehiscence), and harvesting of a bone biopsy for histologic analysis (Figure 7.8f and g). In two cases a 5-year CBCT follow-up was available (Figure 7.9).

Radiographic examination

The CBCT examinations were performed not later than starting the active treatment and at the end of treatment. All examinations were made using a 9000 3D CBCT (Carestream Health, Inc., USA) unit equipped with a flat-panel detector. The exposed volume was 50 mm by 30 mm (voxel size 0.679 µm to 0.2 mm, depending on whether a "stitching" of three consecutive volumes were performed to represent the entire jaw), encompassing the teeth in the jaw where corticotomy had to be performed. Exposure parameters were: 70 kV, 8–10 mA (based on subject size), and a single 360° 24 to 72 s exposure time comprising a range of 235 to 468 projections. CBCT was performed to evaluate the thickness of bone and the 3D positioning of the roots in the alveolar ridge before treatment. Primary data reconstructions were made using the acquisition software (CS3D Imaging, Carestream Health, Inc., USA), resulting in perpendicular slices in axial, coronal, and sagittal planes of the image volume. Subsequently, a second reconstruction was made to obtain contiguous 0.5 mm thickness slices. The workstation consisted of an ASUS Computer, Intel® i5 CPU, with a graphics card (NVIDIA GeForce 9500 GT Series GPU 32-bit – NVIDIA Corporation, Santa Clara, CA, USA). Reformatting and measurements were made on 19-inch flat-panel monitor (resolution 1600 pixels × 1200 pixels).

Assessment of marginal bone level and buccal/lingual plate thickness

Reconstructions were made so that, for each individual tooth/root, that was inclined lingually or labially the axial slices became perpendicular to its long axis. This can be done irrespective of the angulation of the tooth relative to the alveolar process or the presence of crowding. Image slices, perpendicular to the axial slices, are automatically reconstructed. This results in optimal visualization of the MBC in relation to the CEJ in axial, coronal, and sagittal views, as described by Lund *et al.* (2010).

Using the axial view, one reference line was placed between the CEJs at the buccal and palatal/lingual surfaces. Parallel to that, three lines were placed at 4, 7, and 9 mm distance; one of the authors (FB) measured the thickness of the plate (to the nearest 0.1 mm). Only the teeth where the movement was carried out outside the original bony envelope were considered (Figure 7.10).

Post-treatment measurements were made without access to previous radiographs or protocols. The difference between post- and pre-treatment represented the change in alveolar thickness.

Results

The preliminary data of this ongoing project show, on average, a preservation of the height of the marginal crest in both groups. The thickness of bone plate toward which the movement was done was maintained or augmented only where bone graft was used (Figures 7.11 and 7.12).

Augmentation at the 4, 7, and 9 mm heights was observed in the grafted teeth. Average increase in thickness was 0.2 mm at the 4 mm height, 0.5 mm at the 7 mm height, and 0.6 mm at the 9 mm height. This is consistent with the tendency of the bone graft to be displaced apically on closure of the flap, especially on the marginal level (Figures 7.13–7.19).

In particular, several areas where bone was absent at pre-treatment (dehiscences and/or fenestrations) show a radiographic change suggesting a regeneration, despite the fact that the root was not repositioned in the center of the alveolus or the tooth movement was

(a)

(b)

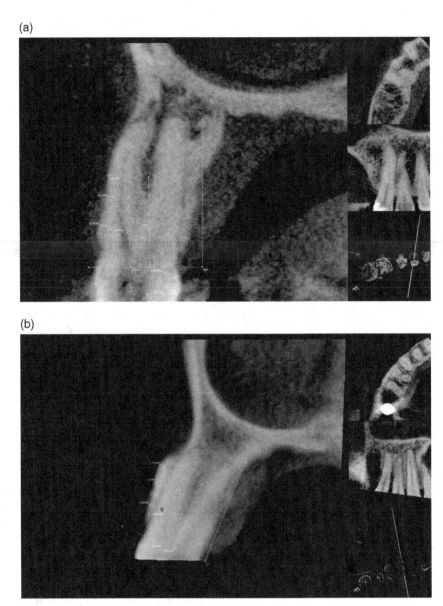

Figure 7.10 (a) Using the axial view, one reference line was placed between the CEJs at the buccal and palatal/lingual surfaces. Parallel to that, 3 lines were placed at the 4, 7 and 9 mm distance measuring the thickness to the nearest 0.1 mm by one of the authors (F.B.), of the plate were the movement was carried out. (b) Post-treatment measurements were made without access to previous radiographs or protocols. The difference between post and pre-treatment represented the change in alveolar thickness.

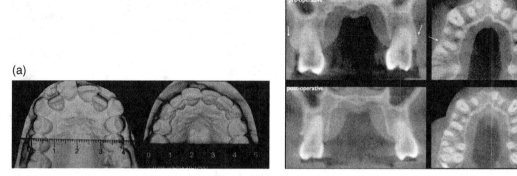

Figure 7.11 Pre- and post-operative CBCT without bone graft. (a) Pre- and post-operative models showing increased distance cusp-to-cusp distance at the second upper premolar level. (b) Pre- and post-operative CBCT of same case showing decrease of buccal thickness both in the axial and tranverse sections (white arrows pretreatment bone thickness; red arrows posttreatment bone thickness), at the second upper premolar level.

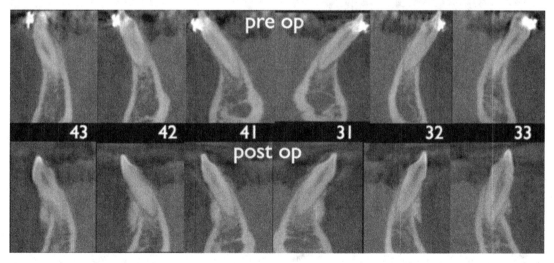

Figure 7.12 Pre- and post-operative CBCT with bone graft in the anterior lower sextant treated for decrowding. Note the increase in thickness. Teeth numbered according to the FDI.

directed outside the alveolar boundaries (Figure 7.20).

Bone graft seems stable, and the 5-year follow-up showed volume maintenance and radiographic changes in radio-opacity suggesting a maturation of the originally grafted particles into a more organized bone.

Preliminary conclusions

Corticotomy with bone graft seems to be an effective method to minimize the risk of marginal bone resorption and fenestration when a tooth is inclined or moved toward the cortical plane. When bone graft is used, an

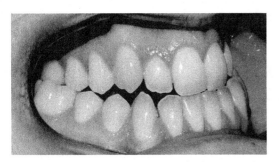

Figure 7.13 A 21-year-old female presented with skeletal and dental class III. A transverse and sagittal discrepancy was evident at both radiographic and clinical levels. She refused orthognathic surgery, but accepted an in-office less-invasive procedure, such as corticotomy and bone graft.

(a)

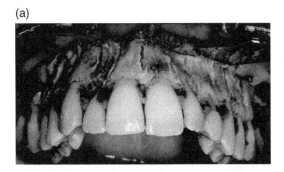

(b)

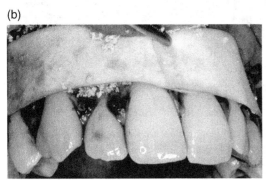

Figure 7.14 (a) Corticotomy and bone graft was performed in the upper jaw, with a single flap approach, anticipating an expansive centrifugal dental movement. (b) Application of a collagen membrane above the bone graft.

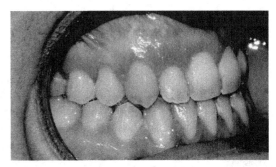

Figure 7.15 At the end of treatment, in the 11th month, sagittal and transverse discrepancy was corrected at dental level.

(a)

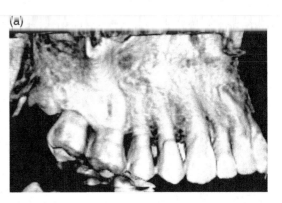

(b)

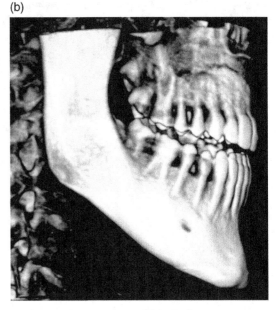

Figure 7.16 Radiographic 3D evaluation of pre-operative and post-operative CBCT showed a robust expansion of the alveolar basis: (a) pre-operative 3D evaluation (b) post-operative 3D evaluation.

(a)   (b)

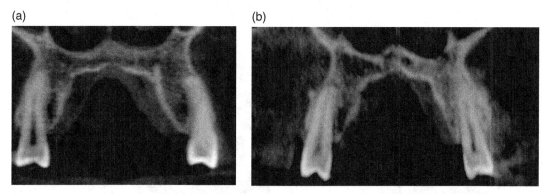

Figure 7.17 The 2D sagittal pre-operative and post-operative reconstruction showing an increase in thickness of 1–2 mm of the buccal plate, despite the movements outside the original alveolar boundaries. (a) Preoperative 2D sagittal reconstruction of the upper arch. (b) Post-operative sagittal reconstruction at the same level at the end of treatment; note the increase of 1–2 mm of the buccal plate.

(a)   (b)

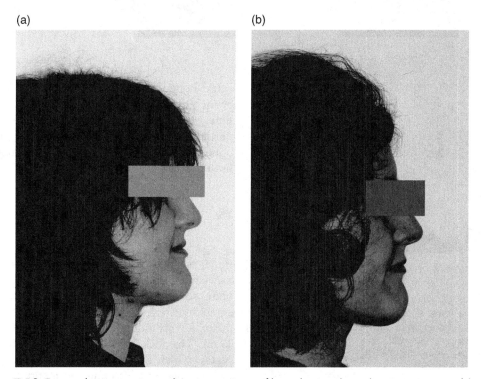

Figure 7.18 Extraoral pre-operative and post-operative profile evaluation showed an improvement of the lower third of the face, with a profile that was markedly concave to a convex one (orthodontic treatment by Dr Maria Francesca Valentino, Private Practice, Milan and Bari, Italy). (a) Pre-op lateral facial view. (b) Post-op lateral facial view. (c) Pre-op lateral facial view with smile. (d) Post-op lateral facial view with smile.

(c)

(d)

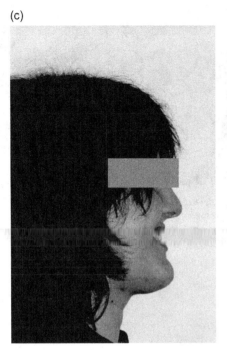
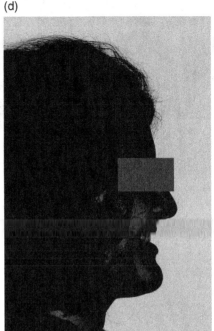

Figure 7.18 (*Continued*)

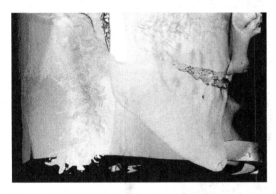

Figure 7.19 A 3D visualization of occlusion, bone, and soft tissues of the face; soft tissue transparency is set at 75%, allowing the 3D visualization of the skeleton of the lower third of the face. Note bone graft reconstructed premaxilla and the support to the upper lip and change in the profile seen in Figure 7.18c and d (reconstruction with OsiriX® v.3.3.1 32-bit).

increase in radiographic thickness of the external plate has also been noted, even when the movement is toward the cortical plate and outside the boundaries of the original alveolar ridge. Longer term follow-up showed stability of the grafted area, and the histologic evaluation showed presence of bone particles, partially surrounded by newly formed woven bone and partially encapsulated in connective tissue.

DEHISCENCES AND FENESTRATIONS

Bone resorption occurs in the direction of tooth movement, the reduced volume of the alveolar bone, sometimes with minimal thickness and sometimes non-existent, and is a complicating factor for orthodontic treatment (Handelman, 1996). The lack of facial or lingual cortical plates, which results in exposing the cervical root surface and affecting the marginal bone, represents an alveolar defect called dehiscence. When there is still some bone in the cervical region, the defect is termed fenestration (Lindhe *et al.*, 2003). Dehiscence and fenestration may be

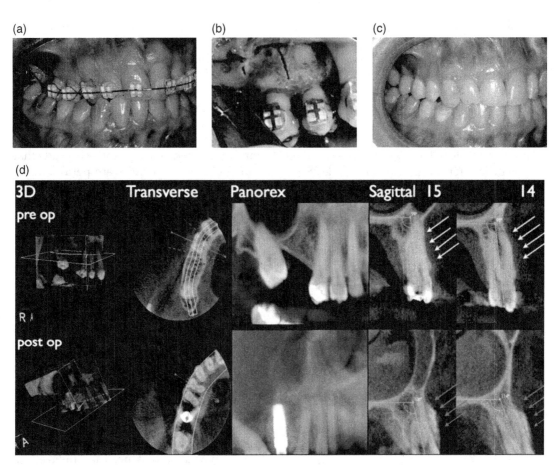

Figure 7.20 A 44-year-old woman presented with unilateral crossbite on the right side, where first and second molars were missing. The wisdom tooth was mesio-inclined, partially occupying the space that originally was of the second molar, and not in contact with the opposite dentition. She wanted to have her occlusion corrected and the first molar replaced by an osteo-integrated implant. A CBCT was performed to assess the bone volume available for implant placement. Upon review of the scan, it became evident that a fenestration was present at the level of first right premolar. A very thin buccal plate was also preset on the second right premolar. Both teeth were anticipated to move outside the bony envelope to correct the crossbite, potentially aggravating the already fragile bone architecture. It was considered a strong indication to perform corticotomy and bone graft to regenerate and protect the periodontium. The surgery was coordinated to perform both implant placement and corticotomy at the same time, diminishing the surgical exposure of the patient. The concept and the case will be explained in detail in Chapter 8 dedicated to "multidisciplinary treatment." (a) Crossbite at the right side at the beginning of treatment. (b) Close-up of the fenestration. (c) Resolution of the crossbite and definitive crown on the first upper molar. The third molar was also extruded, rotated, and uprighted to take the place of the second molar. Please note the good quality and the increased thickness of the periodontal tissues. (d) Composite picture of the preoperative and postoperative CBCT, showing the resolution of the fenestration and increased thickness of the buccal plate at both first and second premolars.

difficult to diagnose preoperatively without a 3D radiographic image. Recently, a study on modern American skulls showed that a dehiscence was present in 40.4% and fenestration in 61.6% of skulls examined (Rupprecht *et al.*, 2001). In a CBCT human study, "the most frequent dehiscence was seen in the mandibular anterior segment for all samples. The most frequent fenestration in the maxilla was seen at the first premolars for all groups (class I, 36.78%; class II, 24.75%; class III, 35.38%)" (Yagci *et al.*, 2012). The authors concluded: "For this reason, a CBCT investigation would be useful for assessment of premolar inclination to put the teeth in the center of the alveolus." If these data are translated to clinical applications, it may mean that a large number of patients undergoing orthopedic or orthodontic expansion mechanics or excessive proinclination may be at risk of developing gingival recession and periodontal damage, even with the most careful mechanics and controlled orthodontic movement.

INDICATIONS OF USE FOR CORTICOTOMY AND BONE GRAFT

Orthodontists routinely compare the length of the dental arch perimeter with the mesio-distal dimension of teeth. A measurement is taken relative to the occlusal surface of all teeth in the mesio-distal dimension, and a separate measurement is made relative to the ideal arch form. The difference between these two measurements enables the orthodontist to evaluate the amount of space available for alignment of teeth. If the space required is above a certain number, extractions may be indicated.

If it is below a certain number, inter-proximal reduction of tooth enamel (IRP or stripping) may be sufficient. From the periodontal perspective, however, space analysis does not evaluate the bucco-lingual (sagittal) dimension of the tooth nor the alveolar bone

perimeter compared with the roots dimension. Richman (2011) pointed out that conventional orthodontic space analysis does not evaluate the bucco-lingual dimension of the tooth associated with the alveolar bone present at that level. He examined 72 teeth from 25 consecutively treated patients with facial clinical gingival recession of more than 3 mm. He used CBCT and showed that although all of the teeth were periodontally healthy, they all had significantly prominent facial tooth contours and associated alveolar bone dehiscence. He also proposed a radiographic supporting bone index (RSBI), which is the sagittal difference between the alveolar bone width, measured 2–3 mm apical to the CEJ, and the width of the tooth measured at that level, as an aid to evaluate risk of periodontal damage after orthodontic treatment. Other authors proposed individual clinical reference points to establish the maximum possible arch expansion. Andrews, for example, uses the Wala ridge, which is defined as the band of keratinized soft tissue immediately above the mucogingival junction (Ball *et al.* 2010). According to L Andrews and his Six Elements Philosophy, there is an optimal distance from the teeth to the Wala ridge once the teeth are optimally inclined. Whenever the treatment required bodily movement of the teeth beyond the Wala ridge, the alveolar basis may need to be reshaped according to the principles of bone engineering described in this book. If the expansion is beyond a certain limit, maxillo-facial surgery may be required (see Chapter 3). The combination of corticotomy and bone graft to facilitate orthodontic movement and expand the alveolar basis, as seen previously in this chapter, may help to minimize or eliminate the risk of periodontal side effects during or after orthodontic treatment (Wilcko WM *et al.* 2001, 2003; Spena *et al.* 2007; Wilcko MT *et al.* 2008; Williams and Murphy 2008; Brugnami *et al.* 2010) (Figure 7.21; see website for Video 7.1).

(a)   (b)

(c)   (d)

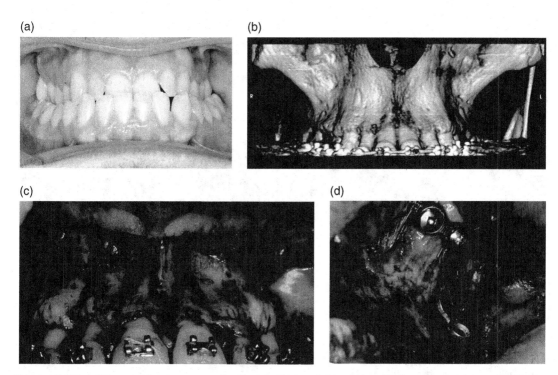

Figure 7.21 A 29-year-old man presented with a skeletal and dental class III. He refused orthognathic surgery and accepted an alternative solution based on a combination of orthodontic treatment with skeletal anchorage and corticotomy and bone graft. From the CBCT analysis of the upper jaw it was anticipated that a very thin buccal plate and a bone dehiscence on the upper right canine root was present. A full-flap muco-periosteal flap was elevated only in the buccal site, as described in Chapter 6. Care was taken to further elevate the flap in the molars area, in order to expose the zygomatic process of the maxilla to fixate the plate. Corticotomy was performed with high-speed surgical burs, under copious irrigation, and refined with the use of a piezoelectric scalpel to increase the inter-radicular depth of the cuts. Stainless steel bone plates were preferred over mini-implants in order to achieve a proper anchorage far from the area of RAP and the subsequent expected bone demineralization. Two plates were placed in the zygomatic process of the maxillary bone, above the roots of the upper right and left first molars, and two in the retromolar areas of the mandible. As already anticipated by CBCT analysis, an area of dehiscence over the root of the upper right canine was clinically evident. Bone thinning was accomplished with a scraping instrument. The bone scraping instrument acted also as an autologous bone graft collector. A first layer of autologous bone graft was place over the upper anterior sextant, with care on covering the dehiscence. A second layer of slow-resorbing xenograft material of bovine origin was placed over the autologous bone and a collagen membrane as a third layer. The rationale of this layer technique is to: (1) maximize the contact of autologous bone over the dehiscence and the outer layer of the buccal plate to optimize the chance of regeneration; (2) take advantage of slow properties of the xenogeneic bone and maintain the bulk of the graft; (3) apply the principle of GTR to enhance regeneration of bone and peridodontal tissues. (a) Intraoral pre-op view. (b) Pre-op 3D reconstruction. (c) Flap elevation and bone exposure. (d) Plate positioning. (e) Corticotomy design. (f) Harvesting of autogenous bone graft. (g) Bone graft harvested. (h) Positioning of the autogenous bone graft. (i) Collagen membrane in situ. (j) Note the xenogenic bone graft applied over the autogenous bone graft. (k) Patient at the time of plate removal, still in the finishing phase. Please note the correction of sagittal and transverse discrepancy and thickness of the periodontal tissues. (l) CBCT scan at the time of plate removal. Please note the resolution of the dehiscence and the increase of thickness of the buccal plate, suggesting periodontal regeneration. Frontal view. (m) 3D lateral view close-up compare to pre-operative CBCT scan (n). Orthodontics by Dr F. Pedetta, Pisa, Italy.

(e)

(f)

(g)

(h)

(i)

(j)

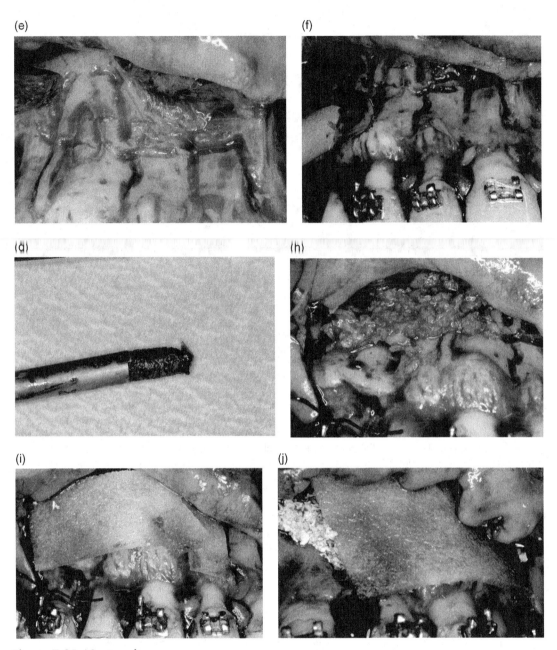

Figure 7.21 (*Continued*)

(k)

(l)

(m)

(n)

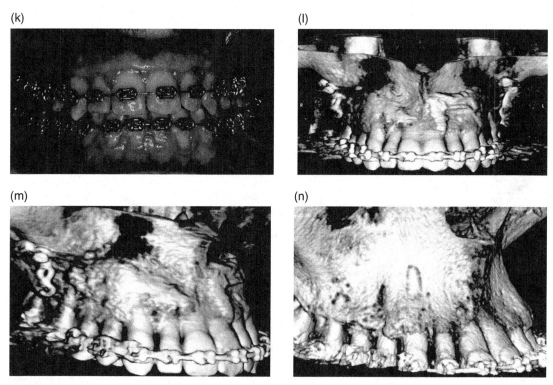

Figure 7.21 (*Continued*)

CASE PRESENTATION

Marco, a 13-year-old boy, presented for a second opinion after being diagnosed as an extraction case (Figures 7.22 and 7.23). He had dental crowding on the upper arch (−6 mm) and a buccally blocked out left canine (Figure 7.24). He and his father, a periodontist, were seeking an alternative, nonextractive therapy. Initial radiographs were showing a skeletal class I (A point–Nasion–B point angle: 4°), hyperdivergent skeletal pattern (Frankfort mandibular-plane angle (FMA): 33°), dental anterior open bite, lower incisors proclination (incisor mandibular plane angle: 94°), and a convex profile with a retruded maxilla (A to Na perpendicular, McNamara: −3 mm) (Figure 7.25). Evaluating the face in smiling profile is an integral part of a complete orthodontic diagnosis. Maxillary incisor labio-lingual inclination and anteroposterior (AP) position have a key effect on the

appearance of the smiling profile. To improve the prediction of the most proper position of the maxillary incisors, many cephalometric and profilometric measurements have been suggested. In order to evaluate the need for extractions, not only from the occlusal point of view, but from the facial esthetic as well, the Andrews and Andrews Six Elements of Oro-Facial Harmony have been used, for which the patient's forehead is used as a stable landmark to decide the maxillary incisor AP position in smiling profile (Andrews and Andrews, 2001). According to the authors, this philosophy of treatment would allow the clinician to take out the "art" from the decision process and to be as close as possible to "science." The first important part of this decision-making process is analyzing Element I, defined as "arch length and shape." According to Andrews, there are "clear and defendable guidelines for differentiating extraction from non-extraction arches." Marco's upper arch had

(a)   (b)   (c)

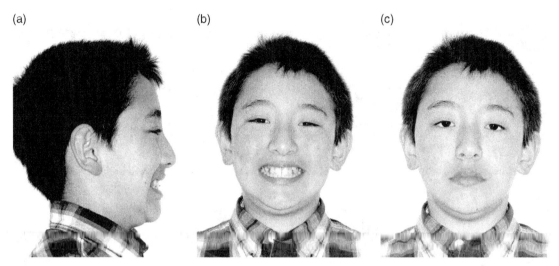

Figure 7.22 (a) Facial photograph pre-treatment lateral view. (b) Photograph with smile. (c) Facial photograph pre-treatment lateral view.

(a)   (b)

(c)

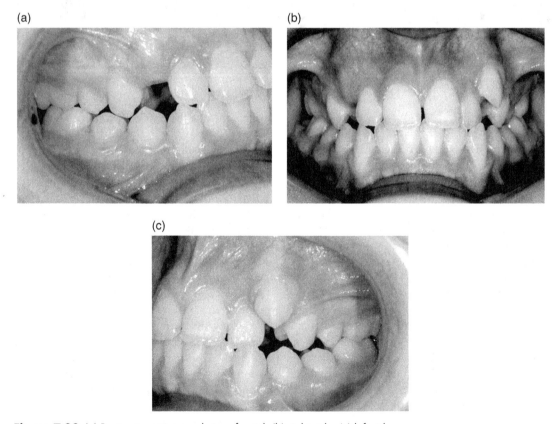

Figure 7.23 (a) Pre-treatment intraoral view, frontal; (b) right side; (c) left side.

(a)

(b)

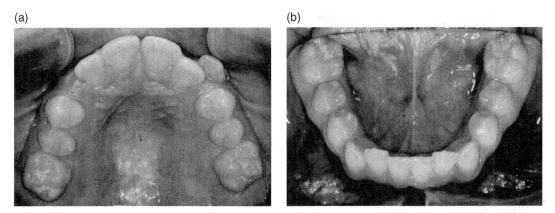

Figure 7.24 (a) Upper arch. (b) Lower arch.

(a)

(b)

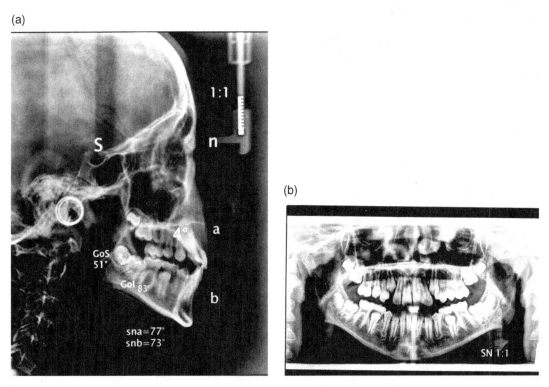

Figure 7.25 (a) Pre-op cephalometric radiograph. (b) Pre-op orthopantomography (OPT).

a crowding of 6 mm. Using the Andrews analysis (Figure 7.26), the central incisors should have had an optimal inclination of +7°. In this case, they should have been retracted by 2 mm.

This would have led to an additional 4 mm (2 mm × 2 = 4 mm) of crowding, making a virtual crowding of 10 mm (6 mm of actual crowding plus the additional 4 mm to allow for the proper

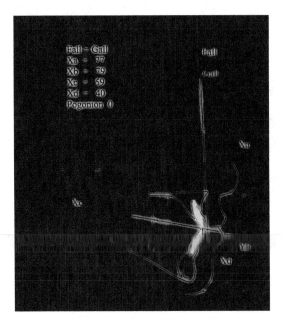

Figure 7.26 Andrews analysis. In green are the anticipated positions of the incisors; Fall represents the forehead anterior limited line, while the Gall represents the goal anterior limit line for the optimal position of upper incisors in patient profile. This line is individual and different for every patient, and in this patient they are almost coincident.

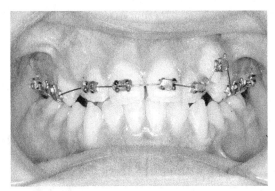

Figure 7.27 Patient on the day of surgery. Orthodontics by Dr F. Pedetta, Pisa, Italy.

inclination of the incisors). Defining the exact position of the incisors would allow us to know the optimal arch length for this particular patient. To complete the information that would enable us to determine the proper "arch shape," we then needed to define the width of the arch. To accomplish this goal, we had to measure the inclination of the buccal segments, keeping in mind that the optimal bucco-lingual inclination at the level of the molars should have been −9°. Knowing that every 5° = 1 mm of arch length, the inclination will determine an increase or decrease of the space available in the arch. In Marco's case, while the left segment had the correct position, the right buccal segment was palatally inclined. Ideally, it should have been inclined more buccally by 5°, leading to +1 mm of space gained. Once the optimal length and width of the upper arch were established, the virtual discrepancy between that mesio-distal diameter of Marco's

teeth and his ideal arch form accounted for 9 mm. This would normally be a candidate case for extractions, as correctly diagnosed by the first orthodontist. We had then to evaluate the needs for expansion (Element III, or optimal jaws width). Andrews says that once the virtual, ideal inclination of the upper molars is considered, we have to compare molar's cusp-to-cusp distance in the maxilla to the molar's fossa-to-fossa distance in the mandible. In Marco's case, we had to consider the 5° correction of the maxillary right molars. The inclination of the lower molars, by measuring the distance of their facial axis points to the Wala ridge, was considered correct. In this case we found a skeletal maxillary discrepancy of 3 mm (Element III). Assuming an ideal expansion of 3 mm, the virtual crowding would have fallen from 9 mm to 6 mm, still requiring extractions of premolars. In order to avoid extractions, one possibility would have been to retract the upper incisors only by 1 mm, instead of 2 mm. This would have diminished the discrepancy to 4 mm, making this a non-extractive case. Since the age of the patient and his skeletal maturation did not allow for maxillary expansion, one option was to overcome the skeletal transverse discrepancy according to the principles of bone engineering of this book, which was presented and accepted by the father of the patient. Corticotomy was performed 1 week after upper arch bracketing (Figure 7.27). Since at least 3 mm of bodily movement of the teeth toward the cortical plate

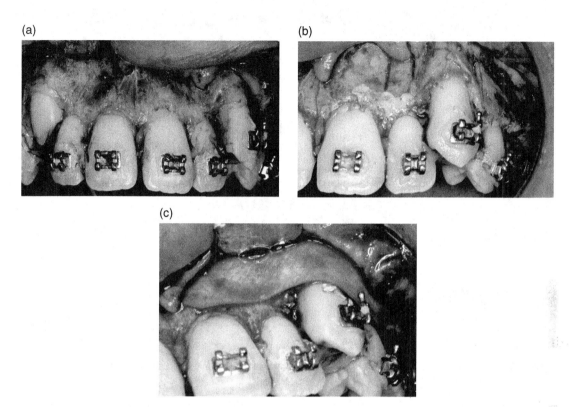

Figure 7.28 (a) Full-thickness mucoperiosteal single flap elevation. (b) Outline of interproximal corticotomy. (c) Regenerative procedure with xenogeneic bone graft and collagen membrane.

was required, and the vestibular plate was quite thin, as confirmed by the pre-operative CBCT, it was mandatory to consider a regenerative procedure associated with the corticotomy. Since the anticipated movement was the upper arch expansion, only the buccal flap was planned, according to the principle of single flap corticotomy (SFC) explained in Chapter 6 (see Table 6.1). Briefly, the design of the surgery was done in a segmental fashion, involving only the teeth that had to be moved the most. Therefore, the extent of the horizontal, intra-sulcular incision was from the mesial line angle of the first right molar to the mesial line angle of the first left molar, where two vertical incisions were also performed to obtain adequate surgical access. A full-thickness muco-periosteal flap was elevated, exposing the underling alveolar bone. Corticotomy was performed with surgical a piezoelectric scalpel. A xenogeneic bovine

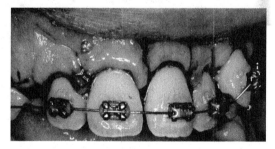

Figure 7.29 Nickel–titanium 0.014″ was reactivated at the end of surgery.

bone graft material was used to recontour the alveolar boundaries to the predetermined desired shape and width, and a collagen membrane was also utilized to optimize bone regeneration (Figure 7.28; and see website for Video 7.2), according to the principles of GBR. The orthodontic appliance was reactivated at the end of surgery (Figure 7.29), and stitches

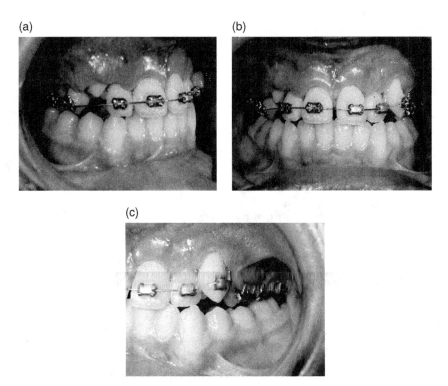

Figure 7.30 (a) Sutures removal at 1-week follow-up. (b) Note the extremely rapid extrusion of the left canine and (c) even of the unengaged right canine.

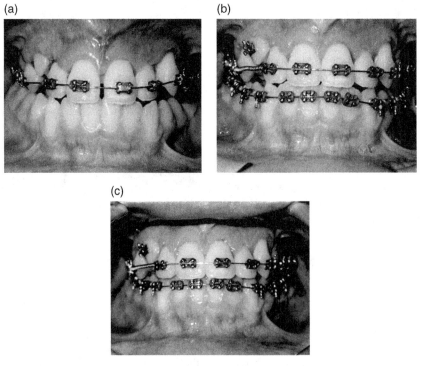

Figure 7.31 Periodontal follow-up at (a) 2 weeks, (b) 3 weeks, and (c) 5 weeks.

removed 1 week post-op (Figure 7.30). Figure 7.31 shows the periodontal follow-up at (a) 2 weeks, (b) 3 weeks, and (c) 5 weeks post-op. The inferior arch was bracketed at 3 weeks after corticotomy

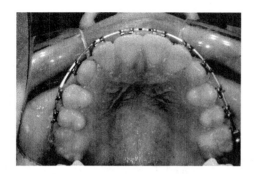

Figure 7.32 Progress 2 months into treatment: teeth have been aligned using the new Andrews2™ appliance and two sets of nickel–titanium wires, 0.014″ and 0.016″.

(4 weeks from beginning of treatment). The progress at 2 months is showing that the canine, which was buccally blocked out, was already aligned (Figure 7.32). At 4 months (Figure 7.33) crowding was completely solved and we were on the finishing phase, detailing the occlusion. Progress radiographs (Figure 7.34) show a good control on the upper central incisors, which has not been over-proinclined. The control on the vertical is also satisfactory, with FMA now being 30° (started at 33°). The final photographs show the case completed after 10 months of treatment (Figure 7.35). Optimal alignment of the teeth can be seen without elongation of the perimeter lines and a good overbite. Periodontal tissues look healthy, with good color and contour; the periodontal biotype, which appeared to be quite thin, appears to be thicker. Final radiographs show optimal root parallelism (Figure 7.36).

(a)   (b)

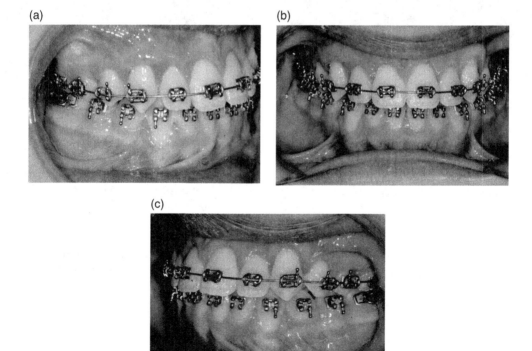

(c)

Figure 7.33 (a) Progress 4 months into treatment; correcting the upper left canine tip with 0.018″ nickel–titanium wire. Frontal view. (b) Left side. (c) Right side.

(a)

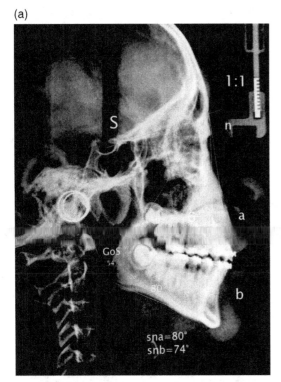

(b)

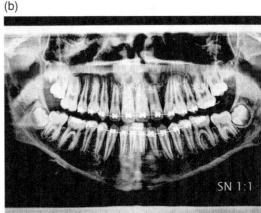

Figure 7.34 Progress radiographs; checking exact inclination of upper incisors: (a) cephalometric X-ray; (b) OPT.

The final extraoral photographs show good facial esthetic results (Figure 7.37) and CBCT follow-up showed a robust regeneration of the buccal plate in all the anterior sextant and coronal migration of the marginal bone level at the upper left canine (Figure 7.38; and see website for Video 7.3).

CONCLUSIONS AND RECOMMENDATIONS

The application of PAOO (corticotomy plus bone graft) may allow treatments that may be otherwise highly risky for the periodontium. There are strong indications besides acceleration of treatment that make this technique an excellent tool in the hands of the orthodontist and an optimal option for the informed patient. The orthodontist of the future will need to pay attention not only to the crown of the teeth, but also to the 3D positioning of the entire tooth, with a particular emphasis of position of the root in the center of the alveolar ridge.

In our opinion, all of the above considerations may be translated clinically in at least four practical applications to diminish or eliminate the risk or orthodontics side effects to the periodontium:

1. Cautions with bodily movement toward the cortical plate: if the movements bring the teeth beyond the Wala ridge or any other clinical landmark suggesting a root movement outside the alveolar process, corticotomy and bone graft may be required.

(a)

(b)

(c)

(d)

(e)

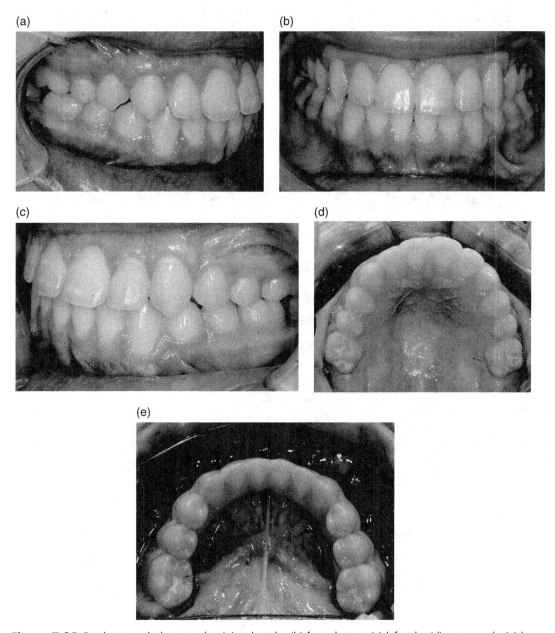

Figure 7.35 Final intraoral photographs: (a) right side; (b) frontal view; (c) left side, (d) upper arch; (e) lower arch. (Orthodontics by Dr F. Pedetta, Pisa, Italy.)

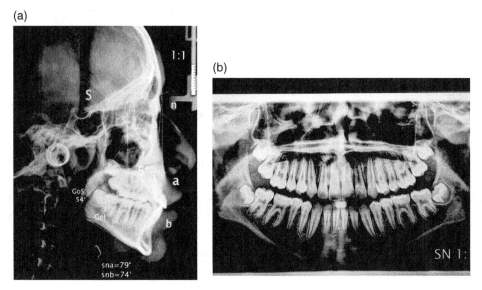

Figure 7.36 Post-treatment radiographs: (a) cephalometric X-ray; (b) OPT.

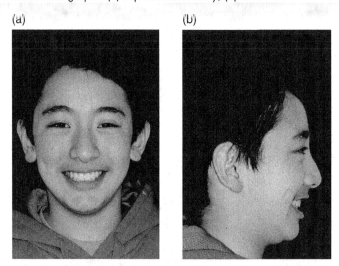

Figure 7.37 Final extraoral photographs: (a) frontal view; (b) lateral view.

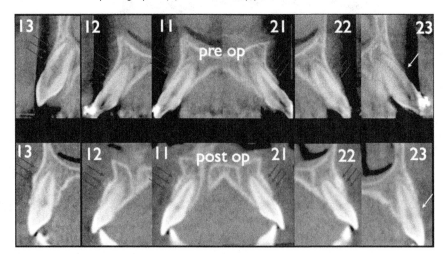

Figure 7.38 Composite picture of pre- and post-operative CBCT showing a robust increase in thickness of the buccal plate (red arrows) and regeneration of marginal bone at the upper left canine (white arrows) (orthodontic treatment by Dr Francesco Pedetta, Pisa, Italy).

2. A call for 3D pre-treatment radiographic evaluation in patients in which the treatment includes expansive movements. This is particularly relevant with a thin periodontium to evaluate the presence of fenestrations and/or dehiscences and to calculate the RSBI as proposed by Richman.
3. Use of corticotomy and bone graft regeneration when the bone is absent (dehiscence and fenestrations) or minimal (equal to or less than 1 mm).
4. Use of corticotomy and bone graft to correct transverse and sagittal discrepancy, keeping in mind that this procedure is not an alternative to orthognathic surgery: the maximum bone expansion is currently under scrutiny, but it should be considered not more that 2–3 mm, as outlined in Chapter 3.

ACKNOWLEDGMENTS

We would like to thank Dr Francesco Pedetta, Pisa, Italy, for the help in preparation of this chapter and Dr Francesca Angiero, Turin, Italy, for the histologic evaluation.

References

Andrews LF, Andrews WA (2001) *Syllabus of the Andrews Orthodontic Philosophy*, 9th edn. Lawrence F Andrews, San Diego, CA.

Ball RL, Miner RM, Will LA *et al.* (2010) Comparison of dental and apical base arch forms in class II division 1 and class I malocclusions. *American Journal of Orthodontics Dentofacial Orthopedics*, **138** (1), 41–50.

Bassarelli T, Dalstra M, Melsen B (2005) Changes in clinical crown height as a result of transverse expansion of the maxilla in adults. *European Journal of Orthodontics*, **27** (2), 121–128.

Bondemark L (1998) Interdental bone changes after orthodontic treatment: a 5-year longitudinal study. *American Journal of Orthodontics and Dentofacial Orthopedics*, **114**, 25–31.

Brugnami F, Caiazzo A, Ferro R *et al.* (2010) Il movimento ortodontico accelerato. *Ortodonzia Clinica*, **3**, 23–28.

Engelking G, Zachrisson BU (1982) Effects of incisor repositioning on monkey periodontium after expansion through the cortical plate. *American Journal of Orthopedics*, **82**, 23–32.

Fuhrmann R (1996) Three-dimensional interpretation of periodontal lesions and remodeling during orthodontic treatment. Part III. *Journal of Orofacial Orthopedics*, **57**, 224–237.

Garib DG, Henriques JF, Janson G *et al.* (2006) Periodontal effects of rapid maxillary expansion with tooth-tissue borne and tooth-borne expanders: a computed tomography evaluation. *American Journal of Orthodontics and Dentofacial Orthopedics*, **126**, 749–758.

Graber LW, Vanarsdall RL, Vig KWL (2005) *Orthodontics: Current Principles & Techniques*, 4th edition, Mosby, St Louis, MO.

Handelman CS (1996) The anterior alveolus: its importance in limiting orthodontic treatment and its influence on the occurrence of iatrogenic sequelae. *Angle Orthodontics*, **66**, 95–109.

Hollender L, Ronnerman A, Thilander B (1980) Root resorption, marginal bone support and clinical crown length in orthodontically treated patients. *European Journal of Orthodontics*, **2**, 197–205.

Janson G, Bombonatti R, Brandao AG *et al.* (2003) Comparative radiographic evaluation of the alveolar bone crest after orthodontic treatment. *American Journal of Orthodontics and Dentofacial Orthopedics*, **124**, 157–164.

Lindhe J, Karring T, Araujo M (2003) The anatomy of periodontal tissues, in *Clinical Periodontology and Implant Dentistry*, 4th edn (eds J Lindhe, T Karring, NP Lang), Blackwell Munksgaard, Copenhagen, pp. 3–48.

Lund H, Gröndahl K, Gröndahl HG (2010) Cone beam computed tomography for assessment of root length and marginal bone level during orthodontic treatment. *Angle Orthodontics*, **80**, 466–473.

Lund H, Gröndahl K, Gröndahl HG (2012) Cone beam computed tomography evaluations of marginal alveolar bone before and after orthodontic treatment combined with premolar extractions. *European Journal of Oral Science*, **120**, 201–211.

Melsen B, Allais D (2005) Factors of importance for the development of dehiscence during labial movement of mandibular incisors: a retrospective study of adult orthodontic patients. *American Journal of Orthodontics and Dentofacial Orthopedics*, **127** (5), 552–561.

Northway WM (2013) Gingival recession – can orthodontics be a cure? *Angle Orthodontist*, **83**, 1093–1101.

Renkema AM, Fudalej PS, Renkema AA *et al.* (2013) Gingival labial recessions in orthodontically treated and untreated individuals: a case–control study. *Journal of Clinical Periodontology*, **40** (6), 631–637.

Richman C (2011) Is gingival recession a consequence of an orthodontic tooth size and/or tooth position discrepancy? *Compendium*, **32** (1), 62–69.

Rupprecht RD, Horning GM, Nicoll BK *et al.* (2001) Prevalence of dehiscences and fenestrations in modern American skulls. *Journal of Periodontology*, **72** (6), 722–729.

Sarikaya S, Haydar B, Ciğer S *et al.* (2002) Changes in alveolar bone thickness due to retraction of anterior teeth. *American Journal of Orthodontics Dentofacial Orthopedics*, **122** (1), 15–26.

Spena R, Caiazzo A, Gracco A *et al.* (2007) The use of segmental corticotomy to enhance molar distalization. *Journal of Clinical Orthodontics*, **41**, 693–699.

Staufer K, Landmeser, H (2004) Effects of crowding in the lower anterior segment – a risk evaluation depending upon the degree of crowding. *Journal of Orofacial Orthopedics*, **65**, 13–25.

Wennstrom JL, Lindhe J, Sinclair F *et al.* (1996) Mucogingival therapy. *Annual Periodontoogy*, **1**, 671–701.

Wennstrom JL (1996) Mucogingival considerations in orthodontic treatment. *Seminars in Orthodontics*, **2**, 46–54.

Wilcko WM, Wilcko MT, Bouquot JE *et al.* (2001). Rapid orthodontics with alveolar reshaping: two case reports of decrowding. *International Journal of Periodontics and Restorative Dentistry*, **21**, 9–19.

Wilcko WM, Ferguson DJ, Bouquot JE *et al.* (2003) Rapid orthodontic decrowding with alveolar augmentation: case report. *World Journal of Orthodontics*, **4**, 197–205.

Wilcko MT, Wilcko WM, Bissada NF (2008) An evidence-based analysis of periodontally accelerated orthodontic and osteogenic techniques: a synthesis of scientific perspective. *Seminars in Orthodics*, **14**, 305–316.

Williams MO, Murphy NC (2008) Beyond the ligament: a whole-bone periodontal view of dentofacial orthopedics and falsification of universal alveolar immutability. *Seminars in Orthodontics*, **14**, 246–259.

Yagci A, Veli I, Uysal T *et al.* (2012) Dehiscence and fenestration in skeletal class I, II, and III malocclusions assessed with cone-beam computed tomography. *Angle Orthodontist*, **82**, 67–74.

Orthodontically driven corticotomy: Tissue engineering to enhance adult and multidisciplinary treatment

Federico Brugnami[1] and Alfonso Caiazzo[2,3]

[1]*Private Practice Limited to Periodontics, Oral Implants and Adult Orthodontics, Piazza dei Prati degli Strozzi 21, Rome, Italy*
[2]*Department of Oral and Maxillofacial Surgery, Boston University Henry M. Goldman School of Dental Medicine, Boston, MA, USA*
[3]*Centro Odontoiatrico Salernitano, Via Bottiglieri 13 Salerno, Italy*

INTRODUCTION

In Chapters 6 and 7 we described how the principles of tissue engineering applied to orthodontics may enhance treatment. In other words, it is the surgical insult that facilitates, improves, and hastens the tooth movement. In this chapter we would like to show how corticotomy-assisted orthodontics may enhance inter- or multidisciplinary treatment. Multidisciplinary treatment requires excellent communication and coordination between different specialists. Although this can be difficult to achieve at first, interdisciplinary collaboration may result in a very efficient execution that patients appreciate and benefit from. When appropriately coordinated, the goal of each different specialist is to facilitate the work of the other team members. For example, orthodontists can be of considerable assistance in periodontal and prosthetic treatment. Dental alignment of the arches can, in fact, facilitate the periodontist's and prosthodontist's objectives. This is done, for example, by aligning the natural dentition and making possible a path of insertion of a prosthesis, or establishing a physiologic alveolar crestal topography to facilitate periodontal surgery. Orthodontic tooth movement can then be a substantial benefit for the patient (Mihram and Murphy, 2008).

Many adults seeking routine restorative dentistry have, in fact, problems with tooth malposition that compromises either the final restorative outcome or the ability to clean the natural dentition. A particular emphasis on adult treatment will also be undertaken here not only because adult treatment is facing periodontal and/or restorative challenges that the youth treatment may not be facing, but also

Orthodontically Driven Corticotomy: Tissue Engineering to Enhance Orthodontic and Multidisciplinary Treatment,
First Edition. Edited by Federico Brugnami and Alfonso Caiazzo.
© 2015 John Wiley & Sons, Inc. Published 2015 by John Wiley & Sons, Inc.
Companion Website: www.wiley.com/go/Brugnami/Corticotomy

because adult orthodontics has recently become very popular, especially in the western part of the world. Many adults realize that correction of dental malocclusions in adulthood is certainly possible and has the benefit of preserving long-term dental and periodontal health besides causing significant esthetic enhancement. This rise in popularity has further been hastened by significant improvements in dental and surgical techniques and biotechnology. Orthodontic appliances have become smaller, less noticeable, and are easier to maintain during therapy. Invisible and/or lingual appliances are in high demand. In addition, dental implants have become a major part of the comprehensive treatment plans for adults with missing teeth.

The length of treatment still remains one of the major deterrents against universal acceptance of orthodontic treatment by the adult population. Corticotomy-assisted adjunctive orthodontics is the essence of multidisciplinary treatment: a periodontal procedure that enhances orthodontics in enhancing periodontal and prosthetic treatment.

CORTICOTOMY IN MULTIDISCIPLINARY TREATMENT

As previously seen, the concept of surgically accelerated orthodontics (SAO) can significantly reduce the total treatment time of orthodontic therapy, and when associated with bone graft, an expansion of the basal bone may be achieved. This may be translated clinically into less need for extractions, a better protection of periodontal health, and become a new powerful tool in adult complex cases needing an inter- or multidisciplinary approach. The major obstacle to a widespread application of corticotomy is the reluctance of the patients toward surgery. In most adult patients, which can be classified as mutilated dentition cases, many problems

may be associated with malocclusion, such as periodontal disease, missing dentition, resorbed edentoulous alveolar ridge, pathologic migration of the remaining teeth in the edentoulous space, complicating the path to an acceptable esthetical and functional rehabilitation of the mouth. Therefore, other oral surgical procedures, such as wisdom teeth extractions, bone augmentation, and/or implant placement may be already planned. Corticotomy may be combined and planned with these procedures in order to minimize the patient's surgical exposure. This approach may look somewhat cumbersome and time consuming at first, but has the potential to achieve optimal results that may be beneficial for many patients. It requires efficient communication between multiple clinicians who have expertise in varying fields. When appropriately coordinated and executed, the input of each specialist can help facilitate the work of other team members.

Orthodontics for prosthetics

Alignment of the alveolar arches by an orthodontist can, in certain select cases, be aimed to develop a path of insertion of a prosthesis or can be done to establish physiologic gingival margin topography to correct a gummy smile or asymmetry prior to esthetic prosthetic rehabilitation. Similarly, in patients where dental migration precludes prosthetic rehabilitation, orthodontic therapy has the potential to selectively move teeth into predesigned positions to allow for surgical implant placement and dental restoration. Many adult malocclusion cases are associated with tooth loss, bone resorption, and consequent need for implants and/or periodontal treatment and bone augmentation procedures. In such patients, reshaping and augmentation of bone by an endosseous implant placement by a surgical specialist can theoretically be used to obtain adequate anchorage and increase precision and predictability of tooth movement by the orthodontist.

Periodontics and orthodontics synergy: The two dental specialties that need a healthy periodontium

As already mentioned and demonstrated in different chapters, considering corticotomy just as a method to accelerate orthodontic movement would be limitative. One of the most interesting effects is that this technique may help (as confirmed here by the clinical and histologic findings) in expanding the basal bone. This will clinically translate into at least two main positive effects: (1) more space to accommodate crowded teeth and then less extraction of healthy premolars in growing patients; (2) a thicker, more robust periodontium, which may help minimize the risk of gingival recession during or after orthodontic movement. The concept can be stretched to the point that, according to Williams and Murphy (2008), "the alveolar 'envelope' or limits of alveolar housing may be more malleable than previously believed and can be virtually defined by the position of the roots." Please refer to Chapter 6 for a more detailed discussion on periodontal considerations during or after orthodontic treatment.

Adult orthodontics

Adult orthodontics is only expected to increase in prevalence. It is not uncommon for many adults to have a periodontium without optimal bone width and volume. The risk of creating root dehiscence in patients with such a thin periodontium is very high, even with slow, traditional orthodontic movement and light forces. Root fenestrations or dehiscences can be present even without the clinical manifestation of gingival recession. In these cases, a careful treatment planning using a multidisciplinary approach is critical for a successful recipe. Accelerated orthodontic movement techniques

can be successfully used to hasten dental movement, treat and prevent periodontal problems, and to regenerate ridge defects, thereby allowing delayed implant placement. In this chapter we would like to present a variety of different combinations of corticotomy in adult patients to facilitate the multidisciplinary treatment.

CASE PRESENTATION

Case 1. Mutilated dentition 1: Orthodontics and prosthodontics connection, enhancing the periodontal outcome

A 42-year-old white female presented with a class II, division I malocclusion, deep bite, and severe crowding in the lower jaw (Figure 8.1). She additionally complained of her smile, crowding of lower teeth, and wanting replacement of her missing lower teeth (Figure 8.2). Clinical examination revealed an edentulous and severely atrophic mandibular alveolar ridge (Figure 8.3) and missing teeth nos. 24 and 25. The patient also had ceramic dental restorations on teeth nos. 5 and 6 and an implant-supported ceramic restoration on tooth no. 11. Radiographically, there were no signs of periodontal or periapical disease. Clinically, periodontal heath was good, with only mild buccal gingival recession on teeth nos. 21, 23, and 28 (class I Miller classification).

The objective of the orthodontic therapy was to resolve lower crowding, correct deep bite, and level gingival margin of the anterior upper sextant to facilitate prosthodontist's work in achieving an optimal esthetic. No attempt to correct the skeletal and dental class II was planned.

The comprehensive dental treatment plan included augmentation of edentulous ridge, fixed restoration on implant for missing

(a)

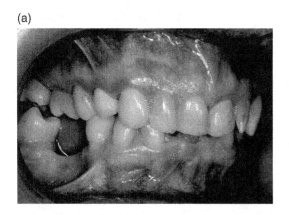

(b)

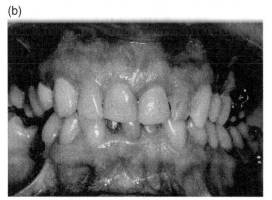

(c)

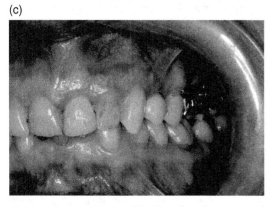

Figure 8.1 A 42-year-old white female presented with a class II, division I malocclusion, deep bite, severe crowding in the lower jaw, severely atrophic mandibular alveolar ridge and missing teeth nos. 24 and 25.

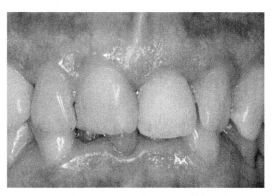

Figure 8.2 Case 1: Detail of the anterior sextant, showing mild crowding and gingival misalignment.

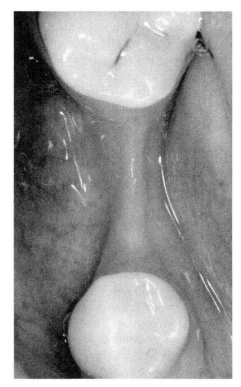

Figure 8.3 Occlusal view of edentulous ridge before augmentation.

lower right premolar, crowns on teeth nos. 6, 7, and 8 for esthetics.

She was given the two following options:

1. Conventional treatment, whereby the orthodontic treatment would be performed, followed by the augmentation procedure, and then the implant placement once the orthodontic movement had been completed later as a secondary procedure.
2. Corticotomy-Assisted Orthodontics.

The second treatment option was accepted, especially because it was possible to perform the ridge augmentation, including the harvesting of autologous bone, and the corticotomy in one combined surgical procedure.

Technical procedure

The patient was bracketed 2 weeks before surgery (Figure 7.8). She opted for ceramic brackets (Leone, Florence, Italy) in the upper arch and metal ones for the lower for esthetic reasons. Nickel–titanium 0.016″ wire was used in the upper arch and 0.012″ archwire was used in the lower arch. The periodontal procedure to accelerate the orthodontic movement was planned at the lower incisor level together with the ridge augmentation in the contiguous edentulous area and performed 2 weeks after bracketing. The symphysis area was also targeted as a source of autologous bone for the bone augmentation procedure. The patient was premedicated orally with 2 g of amoxicillin 1 h before surgery. A full-thickness muco-periosteal flap was elevated under local anesthesia using a sulcular incision extending from the distal line angle of the second lower right molar to the distal line angle of the first lower left premolar. Care was taken to preserve the papillae in the anterior area (lower incisors level). Autologous graft was then harvested from the same area using a manual bone-scraping instrument and placed over the deficient ridge. This area was then further augmented with xenogeneic bone (Endobone,

Biomet Palm Beach Gardens, FL, USA) and covered with a resorbable membrane (Osseoguard, Biomet Palm Beach Gardens, FL, USA). The xenogeneic bone was also placed over the buccal plate in the anterior sextant, with particular care to ensure coverage of the areas with dehiscence of the roots. In the region of tooth no. 26 a resorbable membrane was used to cover the osseous defect following the principles of conventional guided tissue regeneration (GTR) technique, while the recession at tooth no 28 no membrane or bone graft were used, the site was considered to be the control site (Figure 7.8c and d). The flap was then coronally repositioned and sutured in an interrupted fashion to obtain primary closure. The patient was placed on chlorhexidine 0.2% rinses twice a day, oral amoxicillin for 1 week, and nonsteroidal anti-inflammatory drugs (naproxen) for pain twice a day if needed. The orthodontic wires were replaced 1 week after surgery. The patient had no significant pain or discomfort during the first postoperative week. On postoperative day 7, a 0.014″ nickel–titanium archwire was placed. The patient was put on a soft diet for the following 10 days and was instructed to continue rinsing with the antimicrobial agent. On post-operative day 17 the archwire was changed to a 0.016″ and the patient advanced to a regular diet. The lower anterior dental alignment was almost completed 3 weeks post-operatively, and 6 weeks after surgery the anterior crowding was completely resolved (Figure 7.8). Soft tissue architecture and the periodontium continued to remain healthy, and the area of teeth nos. 29 and 30 retained the horizontal augmentation. Six months after surgery, an endosseous implant was placed into the augmented area. At the re-entry time, an adequately regenerated area was evident, with enough bony width and height to place an implant (Figure 8.4).

A bone core biopsy as a part of the implant placement as described by Brugnami *et al.* (1996) was performed (Figure 8.5). The specimen was fixed in formalin and decalcified in Mielodec Bio-Optica for 90 min. After being embedded in

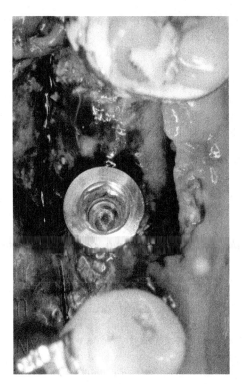

Figure 8.4 At the re-entry time, an adequately regenerated area was evident, with enough bony width and height to place an implant.

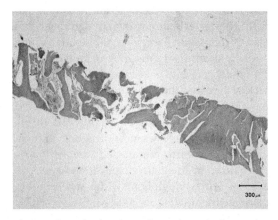

Figure 8.5 The histology showed residual particles of the graft that were completely surrounded by a newly regenerated mixture of woven and lamellar bone. Histomorphometry results indicated 62% of the area occupied by bone.

paraffin and cut to a 3 µm thickness, the sections were stained with hematoxylin and eosin, and then examined using light microscopy. The Image J software was used to calculate the percentage of mineralized tissue at a 4× magnification. The histology showed residual particles of the graft that were completely surrounded by a newly regenerated mixture of woven and lamellar bone. Histomorphometry results indicated that 62% of the area is occupied by bone. Despite the movement outside the original bony envelope that eventually takes place in the decrowding treatment because of the very nature of the straight-wire technique, a regeneration of the bony dehiscence overlying tooth no. 26 was evident in the anterior area while the control (tooth no. 28) remained unchanged (Figure 7.8e), confirming the importance of combination of the corticotomy with a regenerative procedure (bone graft alone or with guided bone regeneration (GBR)/GTR). The buccal plate on tooth no. 27 also appeared augmented in thickness. In the area of tooth no. 27, where the bone graft was not originally covered with the membrane, a fragment of tissue was harvested with a blade (Figure 7.8f) and processed as described previously. The result showed a prominent bone marrow portion with some rare fibrous connective tissue and mature bone for 35% of the core area (Figure 7.8g). Although we should refrain from making definitive conclusions based on analyzing one histologic sample, we can make some preliminary hypothesis:

1. Particulate graft alone may be enough to regenerate some bone (in the inner side, facing the tooth), while some of the original graft becomes encapsulated in fibrous connective tissue (in the outer side, facing the soft tissues).
2. Approximately two-thirds of the graft facing the tooth may turn into new bone.
3. Some of the the graft facing the flap may be encapsulated by fibrous connective tissue. This part will not contribute to the regeneration of periodontal attachments and may act as a (modified) connective tissue graft. In other words, it does not regenerate the periodontal

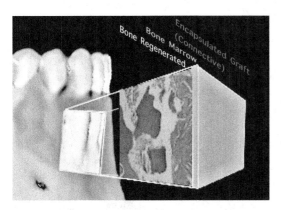

Figure 8.6 According to the histologic sample harvested in the area, the inner portion of the graft may turn into newly regenerated bone, with some portion of bone marrow, while the outer layer most likely becomes encapsulated by fibrous connective tissue. This is not necessarily a negative result, since it may be speculated that the slow resorption particles of the graft may act as a filler and contribute to a long-term stability of the soft tissues.

attachment, but may thicken the soft tissue, changing the periodontal biotype. It may be speculated that the slow resorption particles of the graft may act as a filler and contribute to a long-term stability of the soft tissues (Figure 8.6).

4. The difference in mature bone percentage between the implant area and the buccal plate of no. 27 (62% versus 35%) may be explained by the difference in harvesting (trephine for a depth to 6–7 mm versus blade for a superficial layer only), but also by the presence/absence of the membrane. This is an interesting topic that may require further investigation and clarification. The original PAOO technique, in fact, does not include the use of a membrane and the re-entry at 10 years shown by the Wilcko brothers definitely has proven their way of grafting to be very effective (Wilcko MW *et al.*, 2001; Wilcko MT *et al.*, 2008).

The main differences between the PAOO and our single-flap corticotomy (SFC) is the quantity of bone graft used: 0.5–1 cm^3 per tooth and 0.5 cm^3 for quadrant respectively. To overcome the difference in quantity, we suggest the use of a membrane.

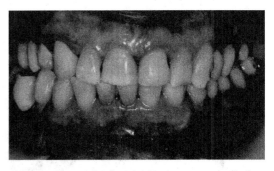

Figure 8.7 End of orthodontic treatment, before definitive prosthetic treatment; note the resolution of deep bite and crowding and alignment of cervical margins of upper anterior sextant.

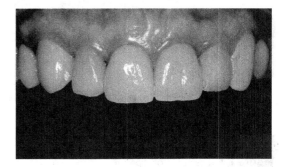

Figure 8.8 Delivery of final restorations. Note excellent final esthetic as a result of combination of optimal prosthetic work and gingival health and harmony (prosthetic work by Dr Graziano Brugnami, private practice, Rome, Italy; technical work by odt. Mauro Merletti, Rome, Italy).

5. In SFC the use of membrane may be required in cases where the surgery is attempting to solve skeletal transverse or sagittal discrepancy (i.e., palatal expansion and/or minor class II or class III). It may be less crucial in protecting the periodontium in decrowding cases.

Six months after implant placement a provisional crown was delivered. The case was de-bracketed when de-crowding, deep bite correction, and proper alignment of the cervical margin of the anterior sextant were achieved (Figures 8.7 and 8.9).

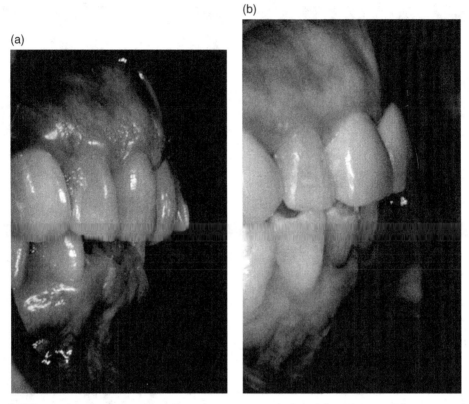

Figure 8.9 Pre- and post-operative detail of overbite correction, before definitive crown delivery on teeth nos. 7, 8, and 9; note the difference in thickness of the periodontal tissues of the lower anterior sextant.

Final functional and esthetic adjustments were accomplished with the delivery of the final prosthetic (Figure 8.8).

Case 2. The summer break case: An alternative to veneers to correct esthetics in the anterior area

The patient, a healthy 21-year-old woman who was dissatisfied with her smile, presented with a slight crowding of the anterior superior teeth and overlapping central incisors (Figure 8.10).

This college student on summer break wanted to resolve this rather mild esthetic problem before returning to college in the fall.

The medical/dental history and intraoral examination found no medical contraindication to treatment. The periodontium was healthy, with no recession or bone resorption, as confirmed by interproximal radiography.

Various treatment modalities were proposed to the patient, including porcelain veneers and conventional orthodontic movement. Also, in an effort to accelerate the treatment, a lingual approach was proposed, combined with the minimally invasive Piezocision™ technique, which, as described in Chapter 5, consists of small corticotomies done through vertical incisions of the soft tissues without the reflection of a flap. Considering the relatively short amount of time available, the patient opted for the latter solution.

Case management

The two-dimensional lingual brackets were applied from premolar to premolar via an indirect technique. A slight interproximal reduction of the upper front teeth was performed, and a lingual 0.014″ nickel–titanium arch was placed (Figure 8.11).

In the same session, the Piezocision technique as described by Dibart *et al.* (2009) was performed. After achieving anesthesia through local infiltration, vertical full-thickness incisions were made at mid-root level, interproximally between each tooth from the upper right first premolar to the upper left first premolar (Figure 8.12; and see website for Video 8.1).

The localized bone decortications were done through the vertical gingival opening with a piezoelectric knife to a depth of 3 mm (Figure 8.13).

Grafting of the area was not performed because a preoperative cone-beam computed tomography (CBCT) examination showed no presence of bony fenestrations, dehiscences, or thin buccal walls and because of the very limited

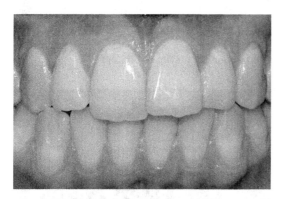

Figure 8.10 Case 2: Patient presented a very mild crowding and central incisors overlapping in the upper anterior sextant.

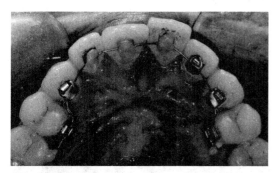

Figure 8.11 After a light interproximal reduction (IPR or stripping) a lingual 0.014″ nickel–titanium arch was applied.

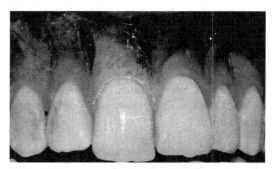

Figure 8.12 Using the Piezocision technique, vertical full-thickness incisions of the mucosa were performed in the interproximal area from canine to canine.

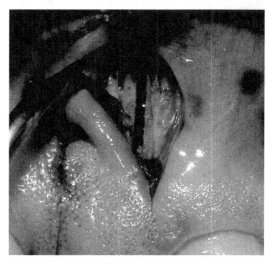

Figure 8.13 Corticotomies 2–3 mm deep were performed through the incisions of the mucosa.

amount of movement requested. Incisions were closed with single, interrupted resorbable sutures, and the patient was discharged. Patient instructions included a post-operative pain medication (naproxen sodium 550 mg twice a day) as needed and rinsing with chlorhexidine gluconate 0.2% from the day following the intervention for 1 week. Antibiotic coverage was not prescribed (Caiazzo *et al.*, 2011).

Clinical outcomes

At the 7-day follow-up visit, the patient reported a normal course, with no pain, discomfort, or swelling (Figure 8.14).

At the 18-day follow-up, the crowding was almost completely resolved (Figure 8.15).

The orthodontic appliance was maintained for stabilization. The patient left for a vacation and returned for the 30-day follow-up

(Figures 8.16 and 8.17). The crowding was completely resolved, the patient was de-bracketed, and a thermoformed contention was delivered.

When the patient was seen at 6 months post treatment, she was very satisfied with the esthetic result (Figure 8.18).

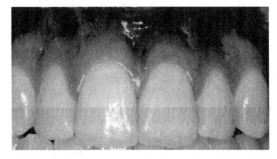

Figure 8.16 After 12 more days of stabilization, for a total of 30 days, the crowding was completely resolved and the patient de-bracketed.

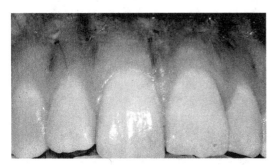

Figure 8.14 One week follow-up: the vertical cuts in the mucosa are completely healed.

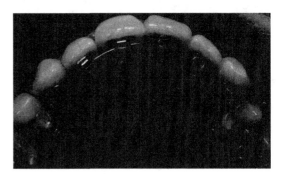

Figure 8.17 As Figure 8.16.

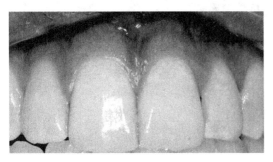

Figure 8.15 At the 18-day follow-up, the crowding was almost completely resolved.

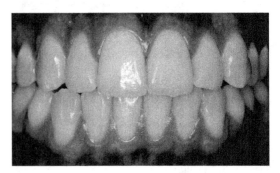

Figure 8.18 Six-month follow-up, showing stability of results and nice soft tissues healing.

Case 3. Mutilated dentition 2: Adjunctive corticotomy-enhanced segmental orthodontics to intrude overerupted molars and allow teeth replacement in the opposite arch

The following is a case in which different surgical procedures were used at once: corticotomy with anchorage plate positioning, wisdom tooth extraction, and periodontal surgery.

The patient was a 39-year-old female with missing lower right molars. She was referred by a general dentist because the upper right molars and the second premolar extruded, preventing a possible restoration on implants. At the oral and radiographic examination she also presented with 4–5 mm probing on the upper molars, and an impacted third molar. In the opposite arch enough bone volume was present to allow implants placement.

Two different comprehensive treatment options were proposed:

1. Crown lengthening, on teeth nos. 2, 3, and 4, with root canals and crowns to reduce the vertical height of the extruded teeth, and wisdom tooth extraction.
2. Orthodontic intrusion of the entire posterior right sextant with the aid of bone anchorage and corticotomy, combined with periodontal surgery and wisdom tooth extraction.

She opted for the second possibility.

Considering the mild periodontal pocketing, a scalloped crestal incision was preferred over the intrasulcular approach, to remove the inner secondary flap and facilitate pocket elimination. Vertical releasing incisions were place at the mesial line angle of the first premolar; a full muco-periosteal flap was elevated in both the palatal and the buccal sides. On the buccal side, the elevation was extended apically to expose the zygomatic buttress to allow the placement

of bone anchorage far from the anticipated area of corticotomy. After scaling and root planing, extraction of the wisdom tooth was carried out. One osteo-synthesis stainless steel plate was performed, bent, and screwed in place in the zygomatic process of the maxilla, above the apex of the first molar. Bone anchorage was placed only on the buccal side because the inclination of the molar was originally toward the palate, and subsequently a contra-inclination toward the buccal, while intruding the teeth, was desired. The corticotomy with burs and piezoelectric scalpel was then performed both on the buccal and palatal sides. Considering the movement inside the bony envelope, bone graft was not placed. Flaps were re-approximated and traction with closed 200 g nickel–titanium coils was started. Incisions were closed with single, interrupted resorbable sutures, and the patient was discharged.

Patient instructions included a postoperative pain medication (naproxen sodium 550 mg twice a day) as needed and rinsing with chlorhexidine gluconate 0.2% from the day following the intervention for 1 week. Antibiotic coverage was not prescribed.

Sutures were removed 2 weeks postsurgically and the patient was referred back to the dentist for placement of implants in the lower jaw. It is important to emphasize that the timing of the delivering the provisional fixed restoration on the opposite arch is crucial to avoid relapse, or force the patient to hold a contention for a long time. Since the anticipated intrusion time was just slightly longer than osteointegration, it was important to plan implants placement right after the intrusion was started, to ensure provisional delivery at the end of the orthodontic traction.

Intrusion was completed in 4 months. Before de-bracketing and removal of plate, the patient was referred back to the dentist for impressions and provisional restoration. Then the patient was de-bracketed and the plate removed (Figures 8.19–8.26).

(a)

(b)

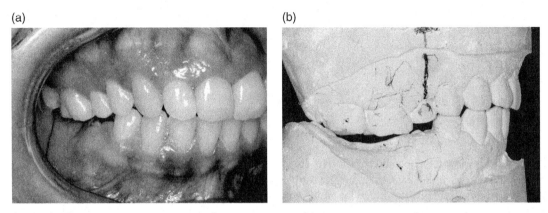

Figure 8.19 Case 3: Pre-operative view showing extrusion of the upper posterior right sextant that is preventing prosthetic rehabilitation of this case.

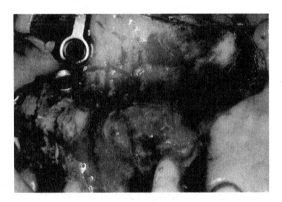

Figure 8.20 Corticotomy on the buccal side and positioning of a bone anchorage device in the zygomatic process of the maxillary bone, far on the area of corticotomy.

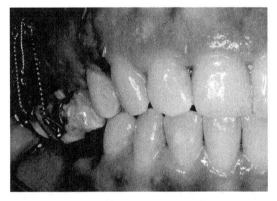

Figure 8.22 Orthodontic traction with 2 × 150 g nickel–titanium closed coils.

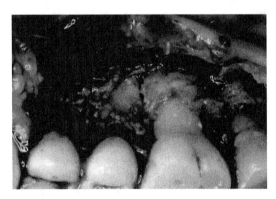

Figure 8.21 Corticotomy on the lingual side.

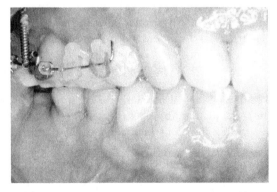

Figure 8.23 Once the intrusion was achieved, an active contention was maintained until delivery of provisional restoration in the opposite arch.

(a)

(b)

(c)

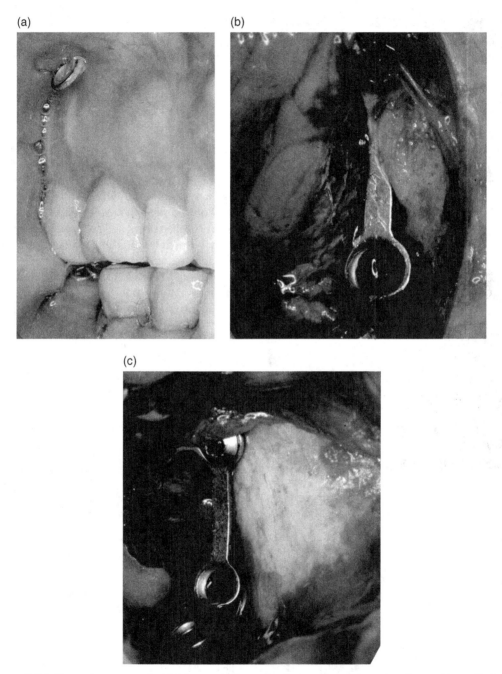

Figure 8.24 Bone plate removal. (a) Note overall good soft tissue reaction to the plate, with small plaque accumulation and no visible sign of inflammation. (b) Good reaction of tissue to the plate is confirmed by new bone apposition on the neck of the anchorage device compared with (c) time of placement.

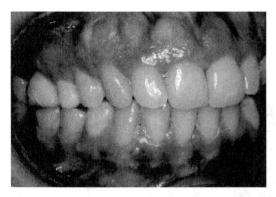

Figure 8.25 Case 4: End of treatment. Note cervical alignment of posterior right sextant and enough inter-arch space to allow proper prosthetic rehabilitation

(a)

(b)

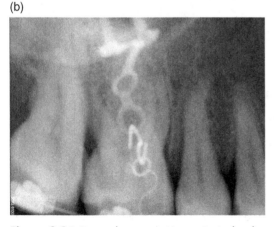

Figure 8.26 Pre- and post-operative periapical radiographs showing the amount of intrusion, with maintenance of interproximal bone level and no sign of roots resoprtion.

Case 4. Mutilated dentition 3: Adjunctive corticotomy-facilitated segmental orthodontics to enhance periodontics and prosthodontics

The patient, a 67-year-old woman, was seeking comprehensive dental treatment (Figure 8.27). She presented with a chronic generalized adult moderate periodontitis with localized advanced periodontitis on teeth nos. 3, 5, 9, 14, 31, and 32. Tooth no. 3 also presented an incongruous restoration, with violation of the biologic width and furcation anatomy and considered hopeless.

Teeth nos. 1, 2, 13, 15, 16, and 30 had been missing for long time. Long-term edentulous space contributed to migration of contiguous teeth. In particular, no. 31 was mesially inclined, aggravating the mesial infrabony defect and allowed extrusion of no. 3. The left upper central incisor pathologically migrated due to loss of periodontal support and trauma from occlusion. The upper right first premolar

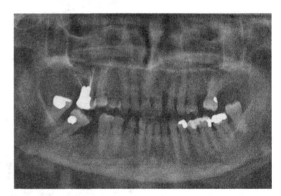

Figure 8.27 Case 5: Pre-operative panorex showing chronic generalized adult moderate periodontitis with localized advanced periodontitis on teeth nos. 3, 5, 9, 14, 31, and 32. Tooth no. 3 also presented an incongruous restoration, with violation of the biologic width and furcation anatomy and considered hopeless. Teeth nos. 1, 2, 13, 15, 16, and 30 had been missing for a long time. Long-term edentulous space contributed to migration of contiguous teeth.

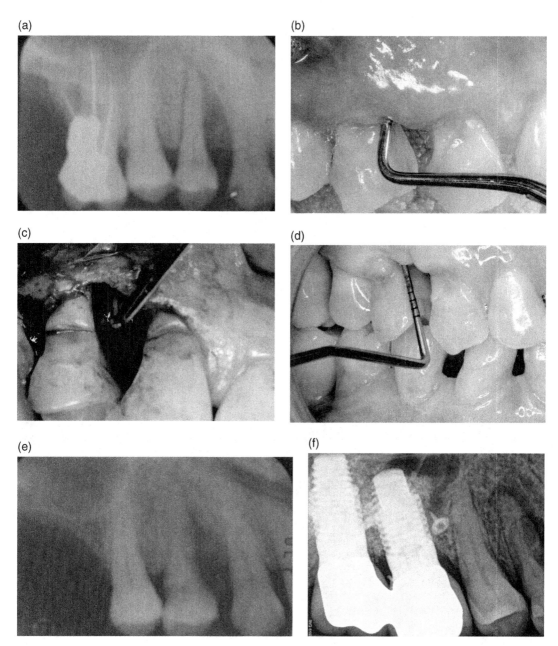

Figure 8.28 Case 6: Upper right quadrant. (a) Periapical radiograph showing: on tooth no. 3, distal bone resorption to the apex of the distal root, and an incongruous restoration invading the furcation; on tooth no. 5, a mesial infrabony defect up to the apex. (b) Periodontal condition of tooth no. 5, with probing depth at the mesial buccal line angle of more than 10 mm. (c) Intra-surgical view of the infrabony defect on tooth no. 5, with a vertical component of +10 mm. (d) Post-surgical clinical view of periodontal condition of no. 5 with reduction of probing to 6 mm, and clinical attachment level to 7 mm. (e) Post-surgical radiograph showing partial resolution of vertical infra bony defect mesial to no. 5 and healing of area of no. 3. Note sinus proximity that would prevent implant placement without sinus lift augmentation. (f) Final radiograph of restorations on osteointegrated implants.

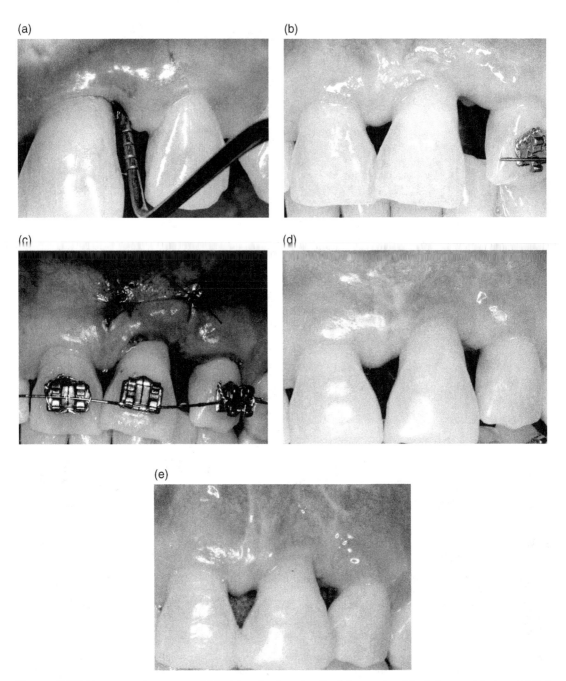

Figure 8.29 Upper anterior sextant. (a) Probing depth at the distal line angle of the left central incisor. (b) Soft tissue healing after regenerative procedure. Note soft tissue shrinkage and loss of interdental papillae between nos. 9 and 10. (c) Corticotomy-facilitated orthodontic intrusion. (d) Intrusion completed. Note papilla regeneration between nos. 9 and 10. (e) Composite splinting of tooth no. 9 with contiguous teeth.

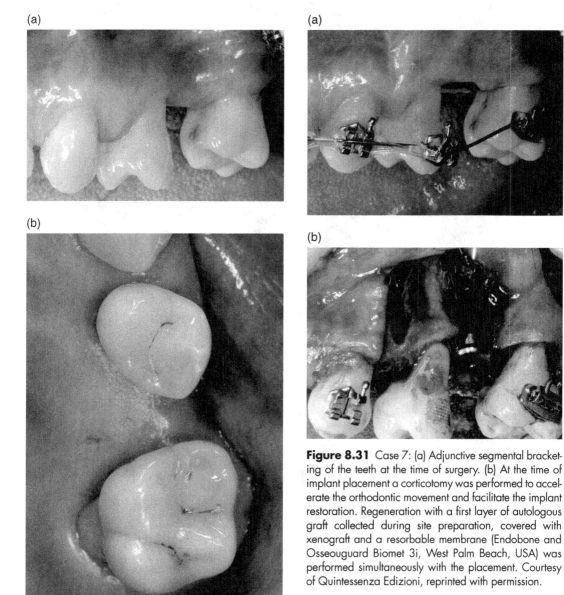

(a)

(b)

Figure 8.30 Upper left sextant. (a) Buccal view of the upper right first upper left first premolar and of the first molar. Both rotated and migrated in the edentulous space, preventing any possible replacement without repositioning in the original position. (b) Occlusal view. Courtesy of Quintessenza Edizioni, reprinted with permission.

(a)

(b)

Figure 8.31 Case 7: (a) Adjunctive segmental bracketing of the teeth at the time of surgery. (b) At the time of implant placement a corticotomy was performed to accelerate the orthodontic movement and facilitate the implant restoration. Regeneration with a first layer of autologous graft collected during site preparation, covered with xenograft and a resorbable membrane (Endobone and Osseouguard Biomet 3i, West Palm Beach, USA) was performed simultaneously with the placement. Courtesy of Quintessenza Edizioni, reprinted with permission.

and the first molar both rotated and migrated in the edentulous space, preventing any possible replacement without repositioning them in the original position. The lower right second molar inclination also was preventing proper implant placement and replacement of the missing first molar. Both lower wisdom teeth were extruded.

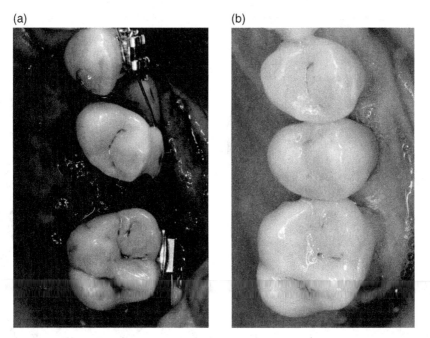

Figure 8.32 Occlusal view of movement: (a) at the end of surgery and (b) at the delivery of final prosthetic (restorative work by Dr Graziano Brugnami, Rome, Italy).

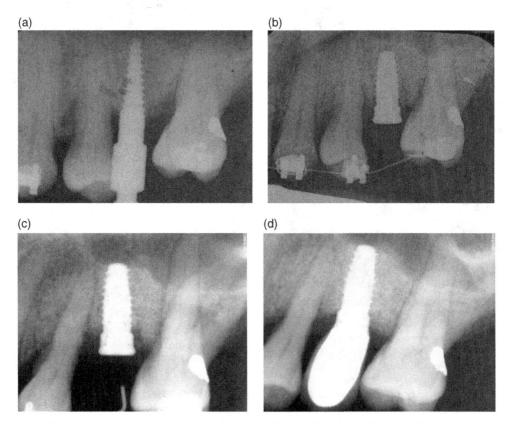

Figure 8.33 Radiographic series: (a) bone expansion at the tie of implant placement; (b) implant placement; (c) 6 months after placement; (d) final prosthetic on implant.

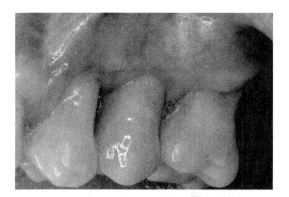

Figure 8.34 Buccal view of final result.

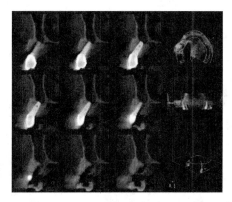

Figure 8.35 Post-operative CBCT showing the implant completely surrounded by bone.

(a)

(b)

(c)

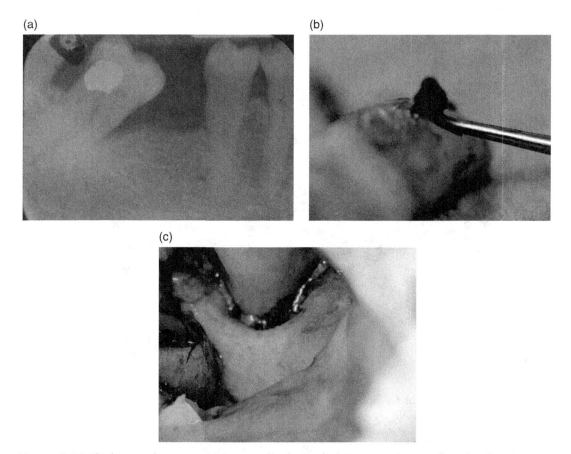

Figure 8.36 The lower right sextant. (a) Periapical radiograph showing no. 31 mesially inclined, aggravating the mesial infrabony defect. The lower right second molar inclination also was preventing proper implant placement and replacement of the missing first molar. (b) Extraction of no. 32 and periodontal regeneration on no. 31 were performed at the same time. Viable periodontal cells were harvested from extracted no. 32 and placed over the scaled root of no. 31 in an attempt to boost the periodontal regeneration. (c) View of semi-crater infrabony defect at the mesial line angle of no. 31.

(a) 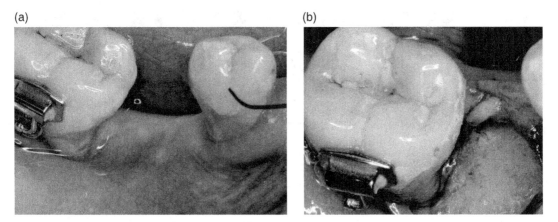 (b)

Figure 8.27 (a) Six months after periodontal regeneration, corticotomy to enhance molar uprighting was combined with implant placement. (b) Note periodontal regeneration at the mesial line angle.

(a) 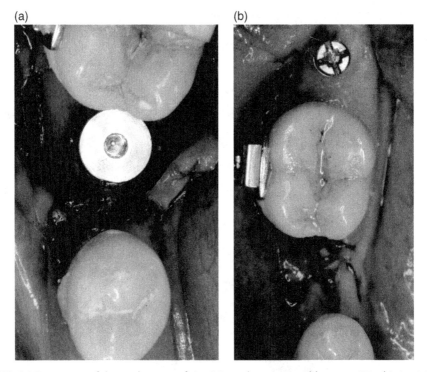 (b)

Figure 8.38 (a) Positioning of the implant are of no. 30 as close as possible to no. 31. (b) A mini-implant for temporary anchorage device (TAD) was placed distal to no. 31 to facilitate the uprighting.

The comprehensive treatment plan included: scaling and root planing, oral hygiene instructions and motivation for phase I therapy, extraction of hopeless tooth no. 3 and wisdom teeth nos. 17 and 32.

Re-evaluation for phase II periodontal surgical therapy included periodontal regeneration for teeth nos. 5, 9, 14, and 30.

Adjunctive orthodontic therapy to correct misalignment of teeth nos. 9, 12, 14, and 30 and

(a)   (b)

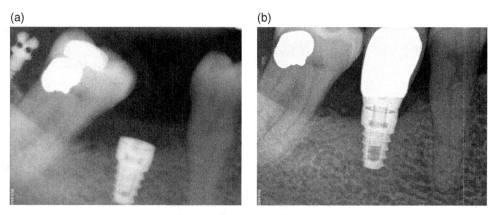

Figure 8.39 (a) Radiograph showing the most distal possible insertion path of the implant and the TAD in the retromolar area. (b) Final restoration of the implant. The distal uprighting of no. 31 allowed a good emergence profile of the restoration. Compare also periodontal regeneration with Figure 8.36a.

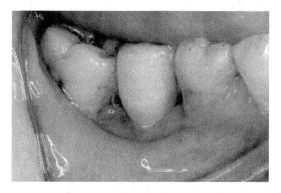

Figure 8.40 Clinical view of final restoration on no. 30 and good periodontal and peri-implant soft tissue conditions.

facilitate prosthetic rehabilitation, was used for sinus lift augmentation and placement of two integrated implants in the upper right quadrant, implant placement and concomitant ridge augmentation at tooth no. 13, and implant placement at area of tooth no. 30. Corticotomy was added to enhance adjunctive orthodontic therapy and planned at the same time of other contiguous surgical procedures.

Comprehensive periodontal–prosthetic–orthodontic treatment was completed in a year. The patient was then placed in maintenance and supportive periodontal therapy.

This case is illustrated in Figures 8.28–8.41.

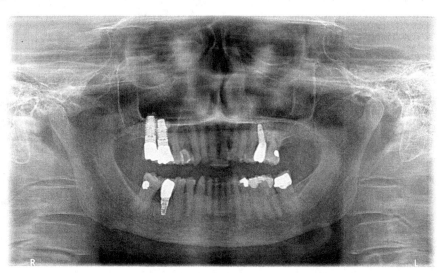

Figure 8.41 One year follow-up orthopantomography (OPT), showing the excellent full mouth rehabilitation.

Case 5. Mutilated dentition 4: Segmental corticotomy to treat unilateral crossbite with crowding, rotations, and missing dentition

A 44-year-old woman with missing dentition, crowding, and unilateral crossbite presented for functional and esthetic rehabilitation. She was periodontally healthy and had a thin periodontal biotype. Missing teeth nos. 2, 3, and 13 were extracted for caries several years before. Tooth no. 1 was out of the occlusion and rotated of 45°. Also, nos. 9 and 12 were rotated. See Figure 8.42.

The treatment plan included placement of an osteointegrated implant in the area of no. 3 and orthodontic treatment to solve crowding and unilateral crossbite, and extrusion of no. 1 to replace no. 2.

A pre-treatment CBCT scan revealed enough width and height to place a dental implant, but also a very thin buccal plate on the teeth that had to be moved outside the bony envelope to correct the crossbite. In particular, there was a dehiscence on tooth no. 5. In light of these findings, and considering the type of anticipated orthodontic movement, corticotomy and bone graft were considered to be necessary to prevent further damage to the periodontium (see Figures 6.37–6.41). The surgery was coordinated to perform both implant placement and corticotomy (see website for Video 8.2) at the same time, diminishing the number of surgical procedures. The orthodontic objective was right upper arch expansion to solve unilateral crossbite and resolution of misalignment (crowding and rotations). We therefore designed the surgery according to the principle of orthodontically driven corticotomy (ODC) explained in Chapter 7, and selected the following approaches (see also Table 6.1):

1. Segmental SFC with bone graft and GBR, in the right posterior upper sextant, to expand the alveolar basis, regenerating and strengthening the periodontium and also to modify

the differential anchorage between the right and left semi-arches. A true unilateral crossbite is, in fact, more problematic than bilateral crossbite, and requires unilateral expansion, which cannot be achieved using

(a)
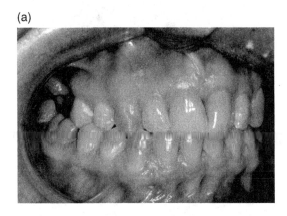

(b)
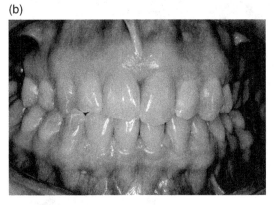

(c)
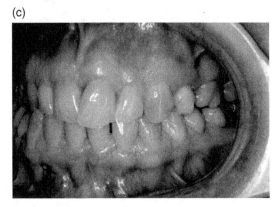

Figure 8.42 Case 5: Pre-operative photographs.

(d)

(e)

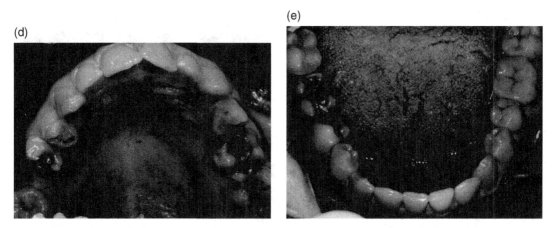

Figure 8.42 (*Continued*)

(a)

(b)

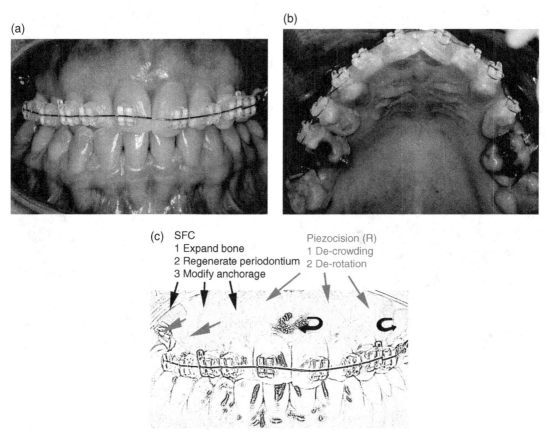

(c) SFC
1 Expand bone
2 Regenerate periodontium
3 Modify anchorage

Piezocision (R)
1 De-crowding
2 De-rotation

Figure 8.43 (a, b) Upper bracketing. (c) Schematic drawing representing rationale of different surgical approaches.

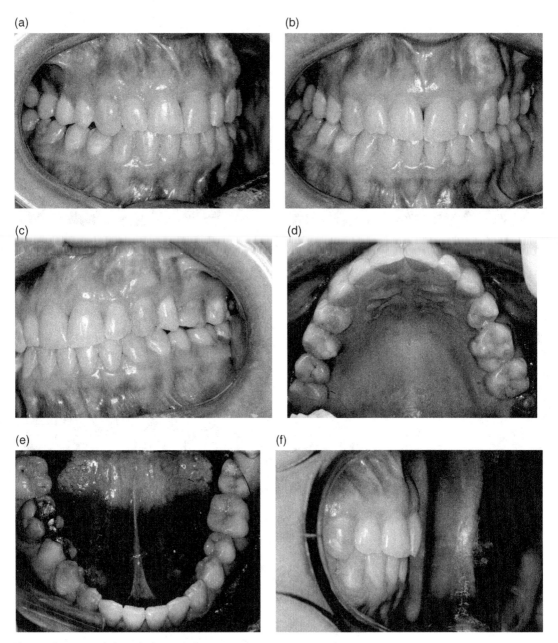

Figure 8.44 Final clinical photographs.

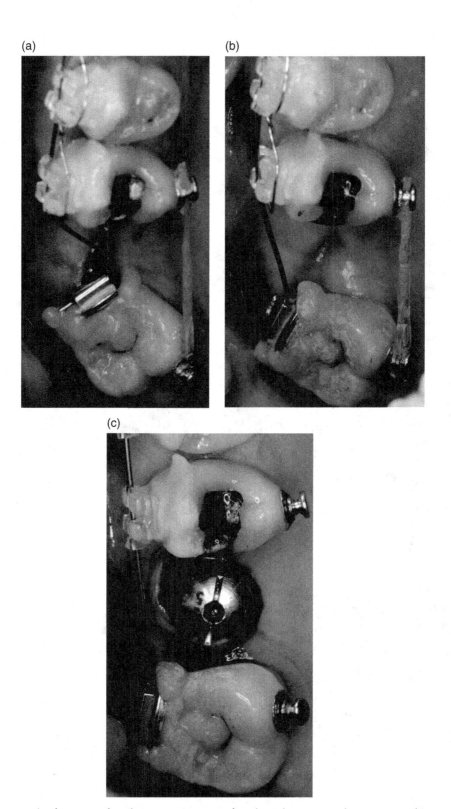

Figure 8.45 Details of rotation of tooth no. 1: (a) at time of implant placement and corticotomy; (b) 1 month follow-up; (c) 2 month follow-up at second stage surgery on implant; (d) provisional restoration – at this point the implant can be used as absolute anchorage; (e) definitive restoration (prosthetic work by Dr Riccardo Milo di Villagrazia, Rome, Italy).

(d)   (e)

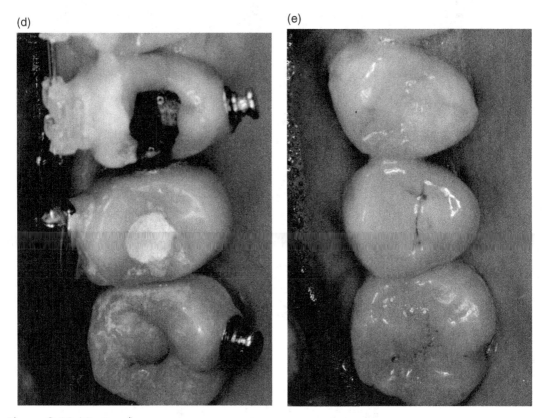

Figure 8.45 (*Continued*)

(a)   (b)

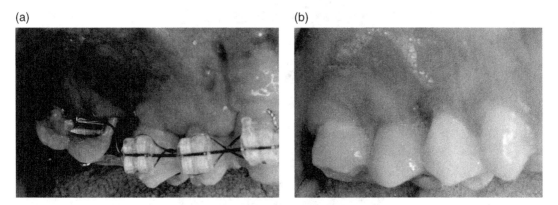

Figure 8.46 Buccal view of the same area as in Figure 8.45.

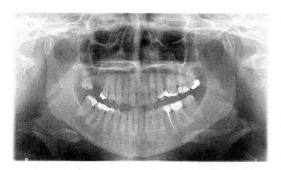

Figure 8.47 OPT at the beginning of treatment.

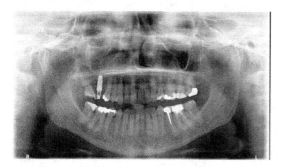

Figure 8.48 OPT at the end of treatment.

the conventional expansion appliances. Overcorrection on the unaffected side is a common consequence that may lengthen the overall treatment time and is difficult to correct (Brin *et al.*, 1996).

2. Segmental Piezocision in the anterior upper sextant, to facilitate de-crowding and de-rotation.

Both procedures were performed at the same time in combination with implant placement in the edentulous area of the right upper first molar (Figure 8.43; and see website for Video 8.2).

Arch sequence was as follows: 0.016″ and 0.018″ nickel–titanium, followed by 0.016″ and 0.020″ stainless steel, 0.019″ × 0.025″ nickel–titanium and 0.019″ × 0.025″ stainless steel.

The comprehensive dental rehabilitation, which included replacement of some old amalgam restorations, was complete in a year (Figures 8.44–8.48).

Case 6. Corticotomy in periodontal patients: Enhancing orthodontic treatment to facilitate periodontal maintenance

A 63-year-old periodontal patient, wanting to solve her upper and lower arch crowding and maintain her natural dentition, was seeking a second opinion and an alternative to proposed extractions and implants. She was diagnosed with a generalized moderate to severe chronic adult periodontitis with localized advanced periodontitis in the upper and lower anterior sextants (Figure 8.49).

In particular, the lower left lateral (no. 23) had a 10 mm probing depth at both lingual and buccal distal line angles, 85–95% bone loss, and mobility 2+. The upper central right incisor (no. 7) had a 4–5 mm probing depth, bone loss of approximately 80%, and mobility Miller class 2, and the right lower second molar (no. 31) had a probing depth of 8 mm distally with a furcation involvement of grade 2. The generalized prognosis with periodontal therapy was fair to good, and guarded for no. 31, guarded to poor for tooth no. 7, and poor to hopeless for no. 23.

From the orthodontic and occlusal point of view, she had severe upper and lower crowding, and posterior bilateral crossbite (Figure 8.50).

She accepted a treatment plan that included comprehensive periodontal treatment, corticotomy-assisted orthodontics to solve crowding and transverse discrepancy, and extraction of no. 23. After initial phase 1 periodontal therapy she showed excellent oral hygiene and compliance. She had a quadrant of periodontal surgery in the right lower quadrant to perform a rhizectomy of the distal root of the second molar. A second periodontal surgery in the anterior lower quadrant was scheduled in combination with SFC and extraction of lower left lateral incisor (no. 23) (Figure 8.51).

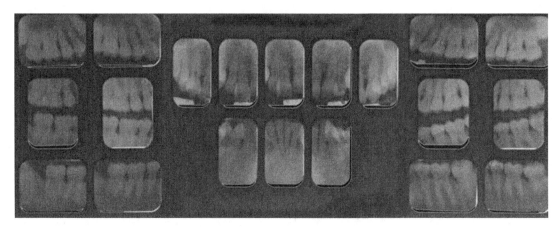

Figure 8.49 Case 6: Full mouth radiograph showing a generalized moderate to severe chronic adult periodontitis with localized advanced periodontitis in the upper and lower anterior sextants.

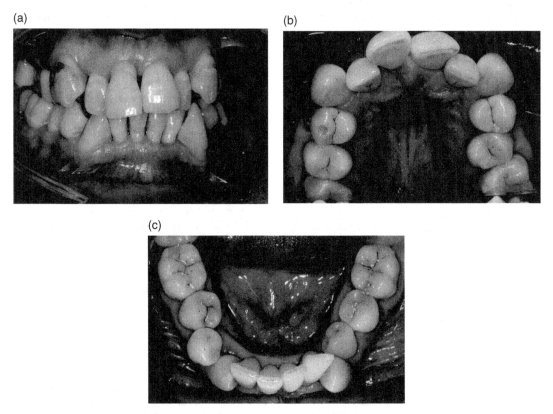

Figure 8.50 From the orthodontic and occlusal point of view the case presented a severe upper and lower crowding with posterior bilateral crossbite.

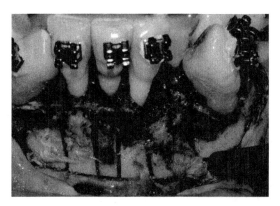

Figure 8.51 The periodontal surgery in the anterior lower quadrant was scheduled in combination with SFC and extraction of no. 23.

(a)

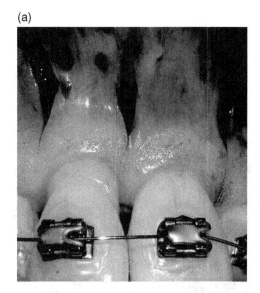

(b)

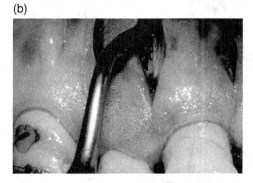

Figure 8.53 Flapless corticotomy in the upper anterior sextant.

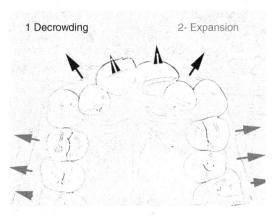

Figure 8.52 Schematic drawing of timing of corticotomy application, according to the ODC principles. (1) In black: Piezocision performed in the anterior upper sextant with elastic nickel–titanium archwires (0.012–0.016″). (2) In red: Piezocision in the posterior sextants, to facilitate correction of the posterior crossbites once alignment of the anterior was completed and was possible to pass at rectangular wires (0.019″ × 0.025″ nickel–titanium, followed by 0.019″ × 0.025″ stainless steel).

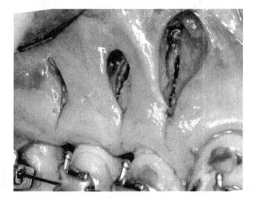

Figure 8.54 Flapless corticotomy in the upper posteriors sextants.

(a)

(b)

(c)

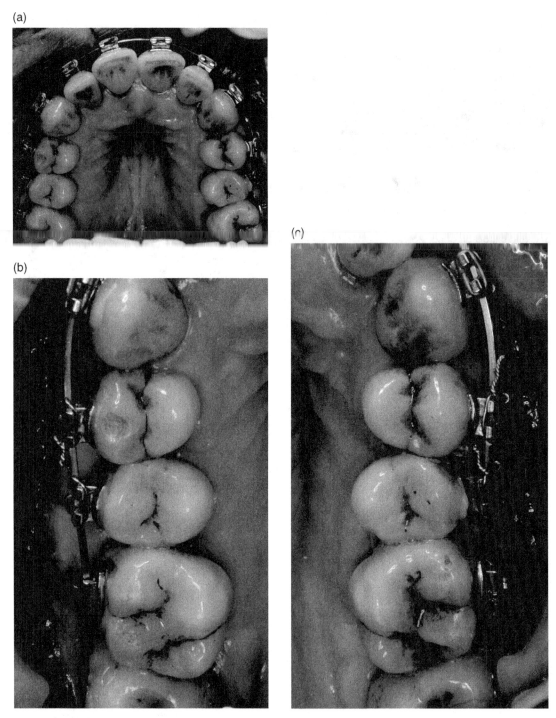

Figure 8.55 (a) Occlusal view at the resolution of anterior crowding. (b) Detail of upper right quadrant with insertion of rectangular wire. (c) Detail of the upper left quadrant.

(a)

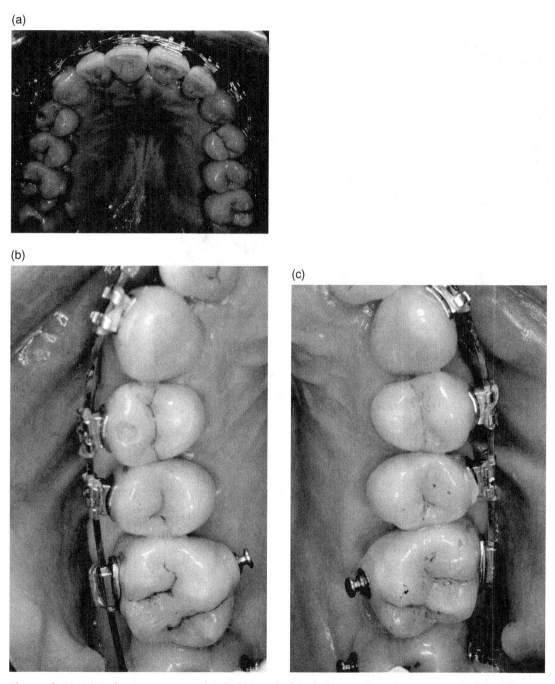

(b)

(c)

Figure 8.56 (a) Arch expansion completed. (b) Detail of the right upper quadrant. (c) Detail of the left upper quadrant.

(a)

(b)

(c)

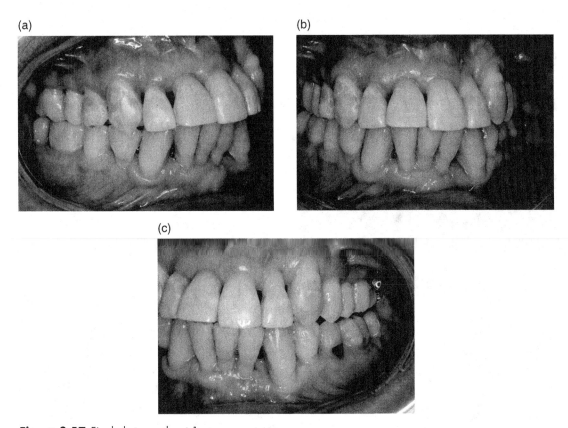

Figure 8.57 Final photographs at 1 year.

In the upper jaw the treatment objectives were: (1) resolution of the crowding and mis-alignment and (2) solve the transverse discrep-ancy (Figure 8.52).

The design of the surgeries, following the ODC principles, were planned accordingly:

1. Piezocision was performed in the anterior upper sextant at first, to facilitate the use of elastic archwires (0.012″ to 0.016″) in solv-ing the crowding (Figure 8.53).
2. Once alignment of the anterior teeth was completed and it was possible to pass to a rectangular wire (0.019″ × 0.025″ nickel–titanium, followed by 0.019″ × 0.025″

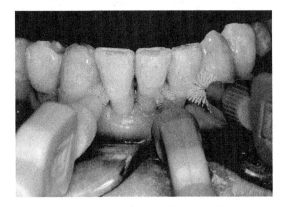

Figure 8.58 Improved possibility to perform proper oral hygiene.

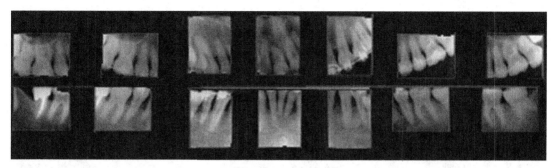

Figure 8.59 Full mouth final radiograph.

(a)   (b)

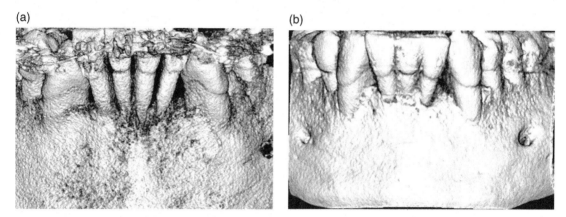

Figure 8.60 (a) Pre-operative lower jaw 3D reconstruction, showing a generalized advanced bone loss at the incisors. (b) Post-operative lower jaw 3D CBCT reconstruction, showing a generalized improvement of bone support at the incisors level.

(a)   (b)

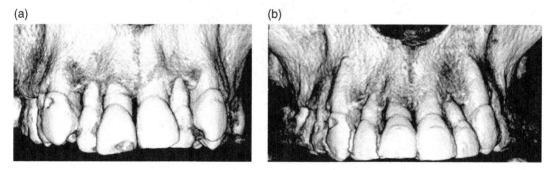

Figure 8.61 (a) Pre-operative maxilla 3D reconstruction, showing a generalized advanced bone loss at the incisors. (b) Post-operative maxillary 3D reconstruction, showing a generalized improvement of bone support at the incisors level.

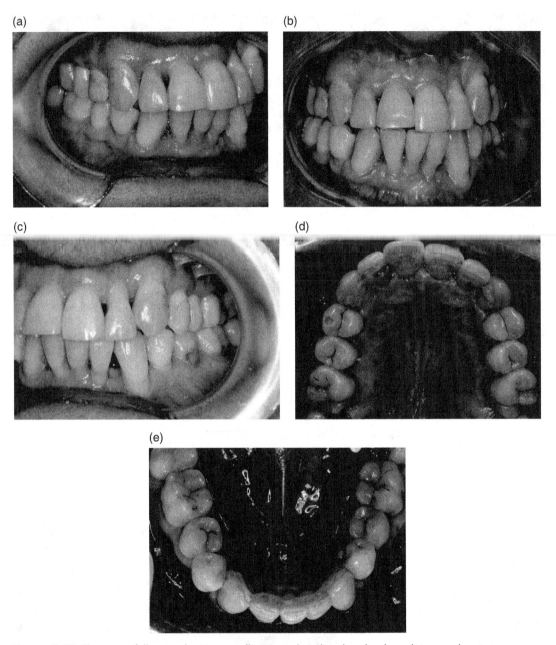

Figure 8.62 Three-year follow-up showing excellent periodontal and occlusal conditions and maintenance.

stainless steel), Piezocision was performed in the posterior sextants to facilitate correction of the posterior crossbites. A flap approach with bone graft may have been indicated in this case, since CBCT analysis showed a maintenance of attachment level, but a decrease in thickness of buccal plate, confirming the importance of combination of corticotomy and graft use in the expansion cases. A flap approach may allow a

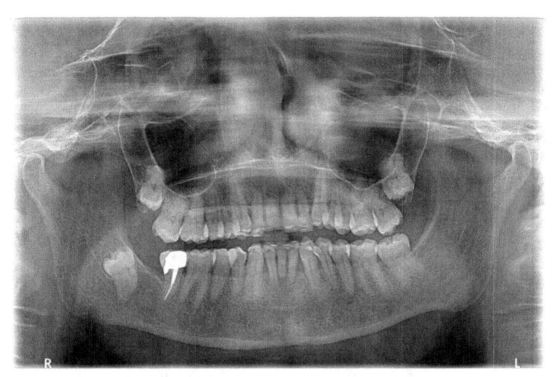

Figure 8.63 Three-year follow-up OPT.

more precise and controlled positioning at the graft, especially close to the cervical margin, as indicated in Chapter 6 (Figures 8.54–8.56). The case was completed in a year (Figure 8.57).

The patient was placed in supportive periodontal therapy with recall appointments every 2 months during orthodontic treatment and every 3 months at de-bracketing. Alignment and de-crowding facilitated proper oral hygiene by the patient (Figure 8.58).

Post-operative radiography showed a good maintenance of periodontal support (Figure 8.59), and pre- and post-operative CBCT scan comparisons showed a good maintenance of alveolar process (Figures 8.60 and 8.61).

Three-year follow-up showed an excellent periodontal maintenance, a small relapse at the level of no. 7, and closure of left posterior open bite (Figures 8.62 and 8.63).

Case 7. Managing partial edentulism in a growing patient: An alternative to life-long commitment to prosthetics

The patient is a 16-year-old female with missing first molars in four quadrants, extracted several years before because of decay (Figure 8.64). She was seeking dental treatment and restoration of her occlusion. In this case we had two different options to manage the edentulous spaces. The first option would be opening the spaces and replacing the missing teeth either with conventional fixed bridges or with osteintegrated implants. The second option was to close the spaces to bring the second molars to the site of the first molars and have the patient occluding only on natural teeth.

The first option, in the case of osteintegrated implants, would force the patient to wait

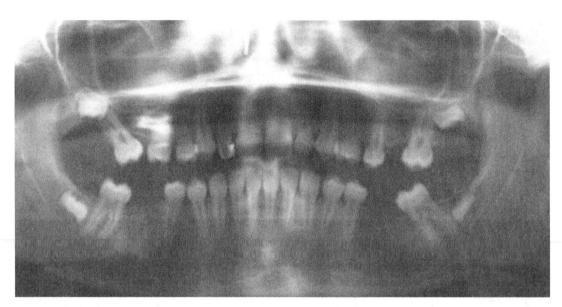

Figure 8.64 Case 7: Initial OPT.

(a)   (b)

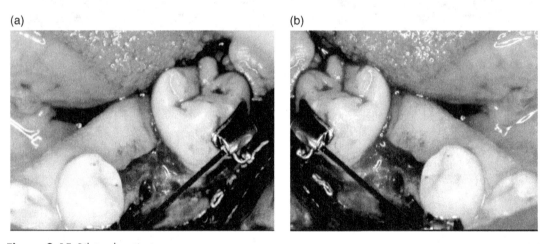

Figure 8.65 Bilateral corticotomy.

until completion of skeletal growth to completely restore her occlusion. With conventional
fixed bridges she would need continuous care
of the restorations, and in the long term this
solution would be less reliable.

Decision was made to close the spaces and
leave her occlusion only on natural teeth. To
obtain a correct bodily movement of the lower
second molars, bilateral segmental corticotomy
was proposed. In this case we would take
advantage of the faster movements obtained

with the surgical insult and of the differentiated
anchorage (Spena *et al.*, 2007).

The patient was bracketed and orthodontic
movements were started; once ready for surgery, a bilateral segmental corticotomy was
performed under local anesthesia at the first
and second molar sites. The surgical insult was
carried out in a dome-shaped design with
decortication of the area buccally and lingually.
On the lingual side, only parallel grooves were
performed in between the teeth (Figure 8.65).

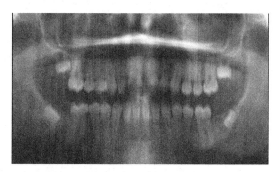

Figure 8.66 Final OPT showing closure of the first molar spaces in 6 months, with perfect roots alignments and no tipping of the crowns.

At 24 weeks after beginning of treatment, closure of the spaces was obtained with no tipping of the mesialized teeth (Figure 8.66).

CONCLUSIONS

Adult orthodontics is only expected to increase in prevalence. It is not uncommon for many adults to have a periodontium without optimal bone width and volume or missing teeth associated with malocclusion or misalignment that may prevent teeth replacement. An efficient multidisciplinary approach to a complex case may result not only in a faster treatment, but also in a better treatment. The periodontally accelerated orthodontic movement technique can be used to give a faster dental movement, to treat and prevent periodontal problems, and to regenerate ridge defects, allowing implant placement. If surgically assisted, corticotomy-facilitated orthodontic mechanics are to be considered in these cases, then careful treatment planning using a multidisciplinary approach is critical for a successful recipe. In these patients, accelerated orthodontic movement techniques can also be successfully combined with other surgical procedures used to hasten dental movement, to treat and prevent periodontal problems by facilitating orthodontic movement, and to allow and/or facilitate implant placement or conventional prostheses by facilitating orthodontic alignment and developing a correct path of insertion of the implants and prosthesis.

References

Brin I, Ben-Bassat Y, Blustein Y et al. (1996) Skeletal and functional effects of treatment for unilateral posterior crossbite. *American Journal of Orthodontics and Dentofacial Orthopedics*, **109**, 173–179.

Brugnami F, Then P, Moroi H et al. (1996) Histologic evaluation of human extraction sockets treated with demineralized freeze-dried bone allograft (DFDBA) and cell occlusive membrane. *Journal of Periodontology*, **67**, 821–825.

Caiazzo A, Casavecchia P, Barone A et al. (2011) A pilot study to determine the effectiveness of different amoxicillin regimens in implant surgery. *Journal of Oral Implantology*, **37** (6), 691–696.

Dibart S, Sebaoun JD, Surmenian J (2009) Piezocision: a minimally invasive, periodontally accelerated orthodontic tooth movement procedure. *Compendium of Continuing Education in Dentistry*, **30** (6), 342–344, 346, 348–350.

Mihram WL, Murphy NC (2008) The orthodontist's role in 21st century periodontic–prosthodontic therapy. *Seminars in Orthodontics*, **14**, 272–289.

Spena R, Caiazzo A, Gracco A et al. (2007) The use of segmental corticotomy to enhance molar distalization. *Journal of Clinical Orthodontics*, **41**, 693–699.

Wilcko MW, Wilcko MT, Bouquot JE et al. (2001) Rapid orthodontics with alveolar reshaping: two case reports of decrowding. *International Journal of Periodontics and Restorative Dentistry*, **21**, 9–19.

Wilcko MT, Wilcko MW, Bissada NF (2008) An evidence-based analysis of periodontally accelerated orthodontic and osteogenic techniques: a synthesis of scientific perspectives. *Seminars in Orthodontics*, **14**, 305–316.

Williams MO, Murphy NC (2008) Beyond the ligament: a whole-bone periodontal view of dentofacial orthopedics and falsification of universal alveolar immutability. *Seminars in Orthodontics*, **14**, 246–259.

Treatment efficiency with the use of skeletal anchorage and corticotomy

Birte Melsen[1] and Cesare Luzi[1,2,3]

[1]Department of Orthodontics, School of Dentistry, Aarhus University, Aarhus, Denmark
[2]University of Ferrara, Ferrara, Italy
[3]Private Practice Limited to Orthodontics, Rome, Italy

SKELETAL ANCHORAGE SYSTEMS

Skeletal anchorage was introduced into orthodontics when the limits of conventional orthodontic anchorage were encountered. These limits were evident when the number of teeth available was insufficient for the establishment of a reactive unit that could serve as anchorage, or when all teeth had to be displaced in the same direction and no equilibrium could be obtained. It is often when faced with a desperate situation that humans becomes inventive. The first study of the reaction to metal inserted into bone was done by Humphry (1878), who inserted metal ligatures in the mandibular ramus in order to study the modeling of the growing mandible. With the same purpose, metal indicators were used by Bjork and Skieller (1972) to differentiate between displacement and modeling of the individual bones of the craniofacial skeleton.

Already, Gainsforth and Higley (1945) had showed an interest in the tissue reaction to loading of metal inserted into bone. They applied forces to vitallium screws immediately after insertion into the mandible. The failure rate was 100%, and almost 25 years passed before Linkow (1970) suggested using metal blade implants for prosthodontics as anchorage. This approach did, however, have a limited indication and did not catch much attention. Sherman (1978) caught up on these results and recommended that a healing period would lead to higher stability. The interest in tissue reaction around loaded metal devices was most likely a spinoff from the development of dental implants (Albrektsson et al., 1986), and several researchers (Steinberg, 1978; Roberts et al., 1984) performed histological studies of the bone surrounding implants inserted in femora of rabbits.

The development of the dental implants had a direct impact on orthodontics, and the first application of intraoral extra-dental anchorage that allowed for an otherwise impossible treatment was done by Roberts *et al.* (1989), who, following loss of a first lower molar, inserted a small dental implant in the retromolar region and used it as anchorage for the mesial displacement of the second and third molars without adverse force systems to the anterior teeth that were in a desirable position (Roberts *et al.*, 1990). This application of skeletal anchorage was widening the spectrum of orthodontics as such a displacement could not be done with conventional appliances. During the same period, Odman and co-workers pointed out how dental implants could be used as anchorage (Odman *et al.*, 1988; Thilander *et al.*, 2001). The limitation, however, is that the situation must be such that the dental implant is needed and can be placed before the orthodontic treatment is initiated.

The first case report introducing skeletal anchorage that did not originate from the dental implants described how a surgical wire inserted through a hole in the infrazygomatic crest could serve as anchorage for retraction of upper front teeth in patients with insufficient teeth for posterior anchorage (Melsen *et al.*, 1998). This method was used in 15 patients over the years, but soon the need for skeletal anchorage that could serve as a reactive unit for other types of tooth movements became obvious. Meanwhile, a case report published by Creekmore and Eklund (1983) demonstrated how a surgical screw could serve as anchorage for intrusion and proclination of the upper front teeth. When published, this paper attracted little interest; but many years later, when special orthodontic anchorage screws had been described by Kanomi (1997) and screws replacing the zygoma ligatures were used by Costa *et al.* (1998), Creekmore and Eklund's paper became a key reference.

Since the turn of the century, numerous skeletal anchorage systems have been introduced. The skeletal anchorage systems now referred to as temporary anchorage devices (TADs) came from two different sources. One

category originated from the dental implants, thus relying on osseointegration, with a specially treated surface comprising conventional implants. Onplants (Block and Hoffman, 1995) and specially produced small dental implants (Wehrbein and Merz, 1998) used as palatal anchorage or, as described above, as retromolar implants (Roberts *et al.*, 1990) are examples of this category. The other group comprised screws originating from the surgical world and included plates fixed with two or more screws (Umemori *et al.*, 1999; Sugawara, 2005). Some of the screws require predrilling correspond to the full length of the TAD, whereas others are self-drilling and can be inserted directly. The morphology of the head of the TAD varies and may accordingly allow for one-, two-, or three-dimensional control and does, as such, have a significant impact on the spectrum of usage of these units (Melsen, 2005).

The indication for the usage of skeletal anchorage has widened, and a multiplicity of different TADs have been introduced. The application of TADs has made it possible both to perform treatments otherwise considered impossible and to facilitate the outcome of conventional treatments, as the need for compliance could be often reduced. TADs make it feasible not only to avoid adverse effects to the reactive units, but also reduce treatment time, as it is possible to apply goal-oriented force systems displacing teeth more directly from the original to the planned position, thereby reaching the treatment goal in less time and without useless tooth displacement.

INCREASING THE RATE OF TOOTH MOVEMENT AND SHORTENING TREATMENT TIME

Increasing the rate of treatment had already been attempted by Yamasaki *et al.* (1984), who injected prostaglandin into the periodontal ligament, enhancing initial tooth displacement. The principle was abandoned as it appeared that the anabolic effect was not following the katabolic effect boosted by the prostaglandin. Electrical stimuli were suggested by Davidovitch *et al.* (1980). This attracted considerable interest for a period, but was later abandoned, possibly due to the complexity of the appliances. Lately, vibration has been introduced, and shockwaves generated are shown to speed up the rate of tooth movement (the brand name AcceleDent® reflects the goal of the appliance delivering the shockwave) (Nishimura *et al.*, 2008). Photobiomodulation (infrared light therapy) has also been suggested (Youssef *et al.*, 2008; Yoshida *et al.*, 2009; Yamaguchi *et al.*, 2010), but has not yet caught the general market. However, the first and foremost approach related to enhance the rate of tooth movement has been corticotomy, which was first presented in the German world by Byloff-Clar (1967a,1967b). However, the technique did not gain very much popularity, and almost 10 years passed before the first publication with the keyword corticotomy appeared in English (Lines, 1975). This paper described corticotomy as part of a rapid palatal expansion, and the subsequent papers focused on the combination of maxillofacial surgery and corticotomy. The influence on tooth movement was not brought to the attention of orthodontists until the principle was presented by the Wilcko brothers as "Wilckodontics" (Wilcko *et al.*, 2009). The corticotomy aims at the generation of a regional acceleratory phenomenon. When this occurs, the turnover is locally accelerated, which is then reflected in an increased rate of tooth movement (Iino *et al.*, 2007; Iglesias-Linares *et al.*, 2011). The "surgery first" approach recently introduced by Sugawara *et al.* (2010) is built on the same principle.

The corticotomy suggested by the Wilcko brothers included a full-thickness flap in addition to cutting and decortication. As a result, the bone goes through a phase of temporary osteopenia which facilitates the accelerated osteogenic osteotomy. However, recent studies performed on rats demonstrate that a similar acceleration of the molar movement can be obtained by performing three shallow holes 5 mm mesial to a rat molar prior to loading (Teixeira *et al.*, 2010).

Treatment time, on the other hand, is not only influenced by the rate of tooth movements, but also, as mentioned above, by the distance the teeth have to be displaced. When, as usually advocated, a treatment is started with a leveling with a round wire, a lot of adverse effects and undesirable displacements take place as the force system generated will be dictated not by the treatment goal, but by the inter-brackets configuration, as described by Burstone and Koenig (1974) (Figure 9.1). If the treatment is guided by goal-oriented tooth movement, minimizing the total displacement of the individual teeth, treatment time can be reduced. This implies that the treatment has to be divided into phases, each of which has a specific treatment goal. A database from the office of one of the authors (BM) demonstrates that, in that office, where the treatments are not dependent on growth (adult patients) the median treatment time was 15.6 months. This can be considered a short treatment time compared with the reported average treatment time of close to 2 years or more. A probable explanation may be that the individual tooth was displaced as closely as possible along a straight line to the treatment goal. The initial leveling was avoided, meaning not only less jiggling, but also reduced risk of root resorption (Chan and Darendeliler, 2004). When the treatment time in relation to treatment with Suresmile® was examined in a very large study and compared with the common treatment time, Sachdeva *et al.* (2012) found a reduction of 8 months from the 23 months reported by the control clinics to 15 months in the practices working with Suresmile® designed appliances. This difference can, as the previous survey, be well explained by the tooth movements being more goal oriented than with the plain straight-wire technique, where the displacements are determined by the geometries, the mutual relation of the

(a)

CLASS	I	II	III	IV	V	VI
$\dfrac{\theta_A}{\theta_B}$	1.0	0.5	0	−0.5	−0.75	−1.0
Lower left quadrant	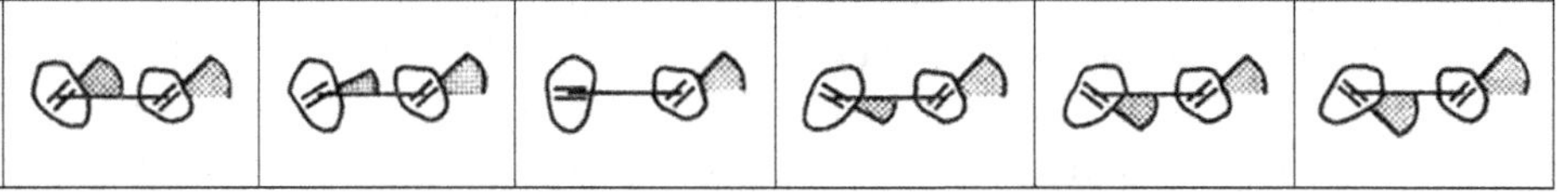					

(b)

OLAOO	I	II	III	IV	V	VI
$\dfrac{\theta_A}{\theta_B}$	1.0	0.5	0	−0.5	−0.75	−1.0
$\dfrac{M_A}{M_B}$	1.0	0.8	0.5	0	−0.4	−1.0
Force system on wire at yield L = 7mm	531.4 ⇅ 531.4 / 1860 1860	477.4 ⇅ 477.4 / 1488 1860	398.0 ⇅ 398.0 / 930 1860	265.4 ⇅ 265.7 / 1860	160.0 ⇅ 160.0 / 740 1860	1860 1860
Force system on wire at yield L = 21mm	177.0 ⇅ 177.0 / 1860 1860	160.0 ⇅ 160.0 / 1488 1860	133.0 ⇅ 133.0 / 930 1860	88.6 ⇅ 88.6 / 1860	53.3 ⇅ 53.3 / 740 1860	1860 1860

Figure 9.1 (a) Classification of the relationship between two teeth or units of teeth. The six basic geometries are based on the ratio between the angle of the bracket slots to a line connecting the midpoints of the brackets. The geometry is independent on the inter-bracket distance. *Source:* Burstone and Koenig (1974). Reproduced with permission of Elsevier and Dr Charles J. Burstone. (b) Force systems developed with respect to the bracket in the different geometries when a 0.016″ stainless steel wire is applied. Only the initial force is described; the effect within the bracket is disregarded. *Source:* Burstone and Koenig (1974). Reproduced with permission of Elsevier and Dr Charles J Burstone.

brackets, which in reality means that there is no way the displacement of the individual tooth can be predicted as the degree of freedom would be 6 (three directions and three moments) to the power of 12 when inserted into 12 brackets.

A different approach to the shortening of the treatment time would be to take advantage of the fact that trabecular bone has a higher turnover than the cortical bone. This fact was used by Ricketts when referring to "cortical anchorage" and recommending the orthodontist to move the roots against cortical bone and secondarily use these teeth as anchorage (Diedrich, 1993). Displacement of the roots first in relation to space closure is, on the other hand, based on the wish to move the roots forward within the trabecular bone, which is generally surrounding the apical part of the roots (Figure 9.2). Thereby,

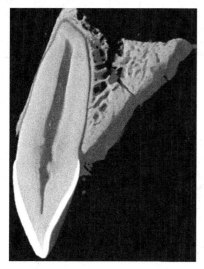

Figure 9.2 Sagittal cut through a micro-computed tomography reconstruction of a lateral incisor from a 30-year-old. Note the extremely thin cortex of the buccal alveolus with a fenestration at the mid-root level. Adapted from: Morten G Laursen, MSc thesis, Aarhus University, 2007, with permission from Dr Michel Dalstra.

a gradual modeling of the cortex is initiated, paving the way for the subsequent displacement of the tooth into even a narrowed or atrophic alveolar process or into an area with a maxillary sinus extension (Figure 9.3). This has sometimes been considered a limitation, but with a line of action of the force apical to the center of resistance of the tooth it can be done (Figure 9.4). With the control of the force system, even a significantly atrophied alveolar process or even a nonexisting alveolar process can be rebuilt (Figures 9.5 and 9.6). Moving the crowns first by means of tipping occurring during leveling will frequently lead to an adverse displacement of the apices in the opposite direction, leading to a need for an even larger movement of the root than at the start of treatment. This is especially relevant when vertical displacements are part of the leveling. The tooth to be extruded will simultaneously be subject to buccal root torque. On the contrary, the intrusion will lead to lingual root torque (Figure 9.7). The displacement of the roots through cortical bone can be facilitated by corticotomy, especially when space closure involves displacement of teeth through heavily atrophied alveolar processes. Corticotomy was introduced to surgeons in order to facilitate maxillary surgery and to orthodontists with the purpose of increasing the rate of tooth movement. However, new indications have emerged

(a)

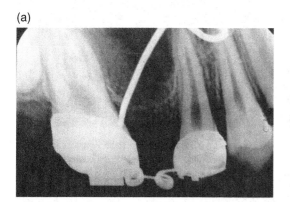

(b)

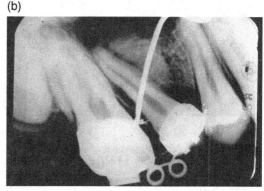

Figure 9.3 Periapical radiographs of a space closure bringing the premolar root distally against the maxillary sinus: (a) at the start of treatment; (b) 2 months later. As the uprighting of the premolar root took place it can be observed how the new bone is generated displacing the maxillary sinus.

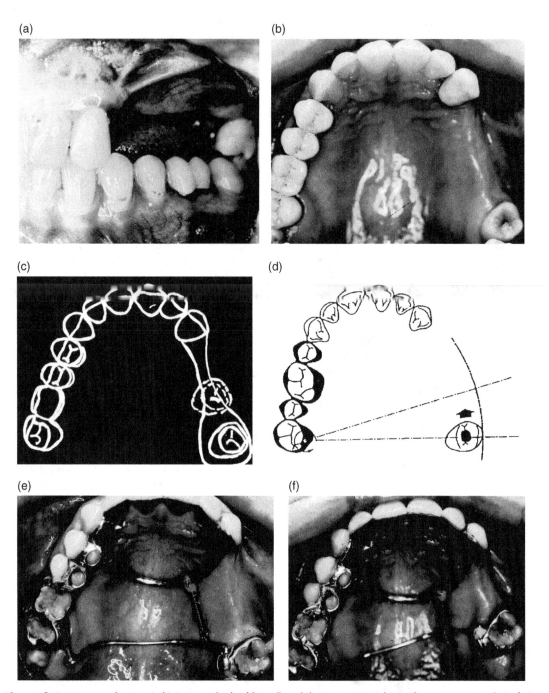

Figure 9.4 Hinge mechanics. (a,b) Patient who had lost all teeth between 23 and 28. The span was too long for a replacement with a bridge and the solution with more implants was not recommendable either, because of atrophy of alveolar bone and extension of the maxillary sinus leaving a paper-thin bone in the area. (c) Drawing illustrating the principle of hinge mechanics. (d) The anchorage unit was composed of all teeth apart from the third molar to be moved. These teeth were consolidated by a cast splint. The cast retention also comprised a transpalatal bar extending from nos. 14 to 24 and an extension palatally from no. 16. This extension was furnished with a vertical tube that served as the centre of rotation for the transpalatal arch serving as guiding mechanics for the mesialization of no. 28. The active unit was a coil spring at the level of the center of resistance from the anterior to the posterior transpalatal arch. The width of the arch is maintained by the guiding mechanics. (e,f) The situation at the end of treatment. (g–j) The tooth movement that has taken place through the maxillary sinus and widened the alveolar process. (Patient treated by Alain Fontenelle.)

(g)

(h)

(i)

(j)

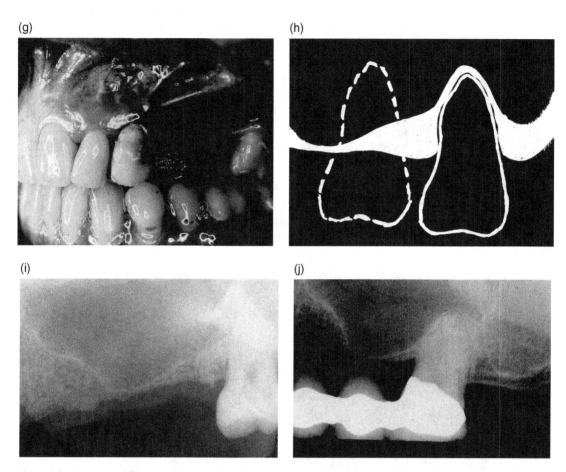

Figure 9.4 (*Continued*)

whereby the spectrum of orthodontics once more has been widened. The application of corticotomy combined with bone grafting has made it possible to move lower incisors buccally without iatrogenic damage to the cortical bone (De Clerck and Cornelis, 2006). The bone grafting combined with corticotomy has been recommended in patients with need for labial displacement of retroclined incisors, and the authors have demonstrated both increased rate of tooth movement and improved labial bone quality and quantity (Kim *et al.*, 2011; Shoreibah *et al.*, 2012). Especially the forward tipping of incisors has been warned against, but Allais and Melsen (2003; Melsen and Allais, 2005) demonstrated that by controlled tooth movement an overjet

could be reduced without iatrogenic damage, and a 20-year follow-up revealed that the results could be maintained (Figure 9.8) (Lindtoft, 2010). There is, however, no doubt that the combination of well-controlled force systems, corticotomy, and bone grafting will open the door to a different approach to the treatment of increased overjet, especially in adult individuals with lower alveolar retrusion. There are thus a number of factors that can contribute to the widening of the orthodontic possibilities, and this chapter is dedicated to the demonstration of how the application of skeletal anchorage can contribute to an improved service for our patients. It is not enough just to have access to absolute anchorage; the mechanics should

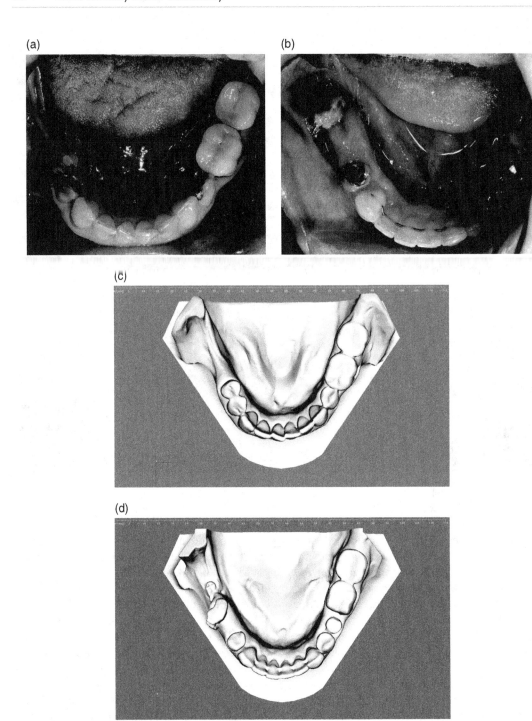

Figure 9.5 Images of a female patient who had lost all molars in the right side of the mandible due to caries. A prosthetic reconstruction of the bite was not possible owing the shortened dental arch. A tongue pressure had prevented the upper teeth from overeruption. (a) The alveolar process distal to the second lower premolar was totally atrophic. (b) Following treatment. (c,d) Digital models of the situation before and after treatment illustrating clearly the build up of bone. (Patient treated by Johan Knudsen, orthodontic department, School of Dentistry, Aarhus University.)

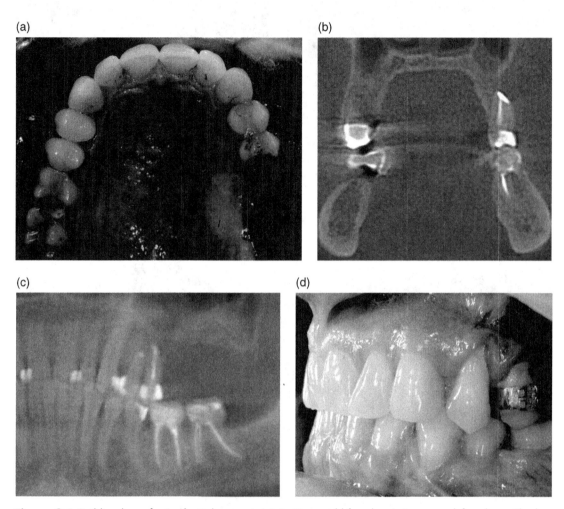

Figure 9.6 Building bone for implant placement. (a) A 40-year-old female missing upper left molars with alveolar bone as result of a severe infection. (b,c) Cone-beam computed tomography scanning demonstrated loss of all alveolar bone in the region of nos. 26, 27, and 28 and loss of apical and buccal bone in relation to no. 25. The apex of no. 25 fenestrated to the oral cavity due to absence of apical and facial bone. The prognosis of no. 25 was very poor and extraction of no. 25 would lead to extensive bone loss also in the second premolar region. An orthodontic treatment plan was established in order to build bone for an implant in the region of no. 25 by distal movement of the tooth. (d–f) Distal rotation of no. 25 was applied along with distal movement in order to build sufficient bone at the facial aspect of the alveolar process. The crown height of no. 25 was reduced to avoid occlusal interferences. Light forces were used in order to perform tooth movement with bone. The orthodontic displacement of no. 25 was anchored by a mini-implant placed in the palate and connected to no. 24. (g) At the end of orthodontic treatment sufficient bone was built for implant placement and the remaining attachment of no. 25 was minimal. (h) Before implant placement the site was carefully probed and demonstrated a complete bony support without fenestrations of the walls. (i) Dental implant in place in the region of no. 25. (Patient treated by Morten G. Laursen, Orthodontic Department, School of Dentistry, Aarhus University; implant inserted by Thomas Urban, Private Practice, Aarhus, Denmark.)

(e)

(f)

(g)

(h)

(i)

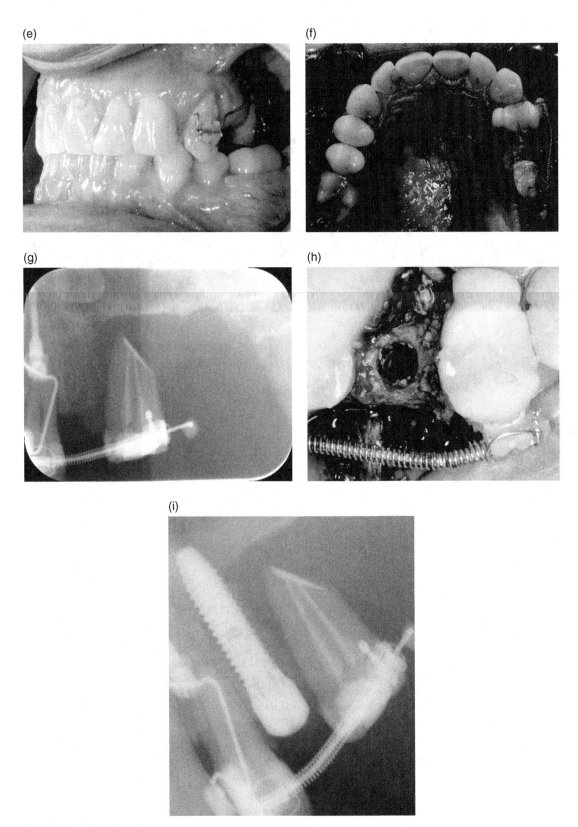

Figure 9.6 (*Continued*)

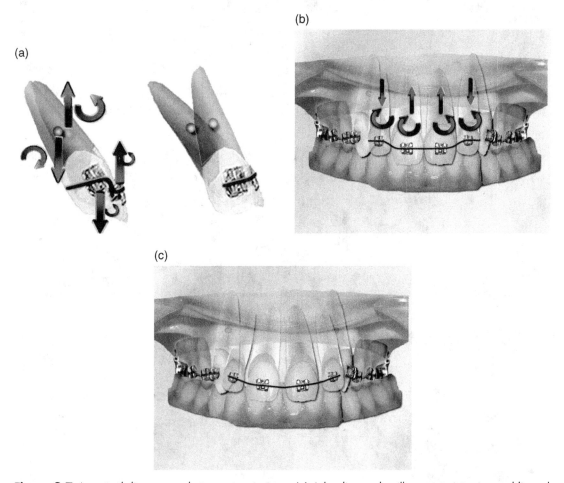

Figure 9.7 A vertical discrepancy between two incisors. (a) A leveling arch will generate intrusion and lingual root torque on the longer tooth, whereas extrusion and buccal root torque will be generated with respect to the short incisor. The situation is reflecting a geometry I according to Burstone and Koenig (1974). (b,c) When the situation is seen from the anterior aspect, a geometry is likewise present generating undesirable side effects with space opening. Courtesy of Dr G Fiorelli.

deliver a line of action of the force leading the tooth the shortest distance to the goal with a minimum variation in force direction and a low load–deflection rate. Well-controlled tooth movement can be used to build up bone, whether by displacing a molar through the maxillary sinus or an atrophic alveolar ridge. This was done by Fontenelle (1982) with a force system that allowed for the displacement of a molar mesially "with bone."

The following cases demonstrate further examples of how TADs and corticotomy can facilitate orthodontics.

CASE REPORTS

Case 1

Case 1 describes the treatment of a 34-year-old female patient with extensive, but inadequate,

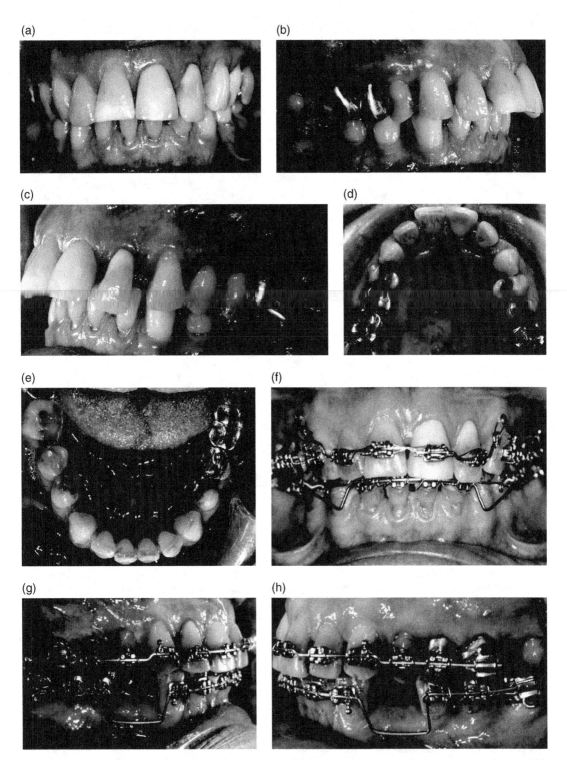

Figure 9.8 (a–m) Malocclusion presented by a 56-year-old woman. The increased overjet was partly caused by a retroclination of the lower front teeth following extraction of the lower first molars when she was still a child. Owing to her age, surgery was not an issue and it was considered unfortunate for the profile to extract upper premolars and retract the upper front teeth. It was therefore decided to protract the lower front teeth and generate space for an implant distal to the canines. (f–h) Sagittal expansion was done with a torque arch delivering buccal root torque to the lower incisors. This was combined with a bypass arch generating sagittal expansion.

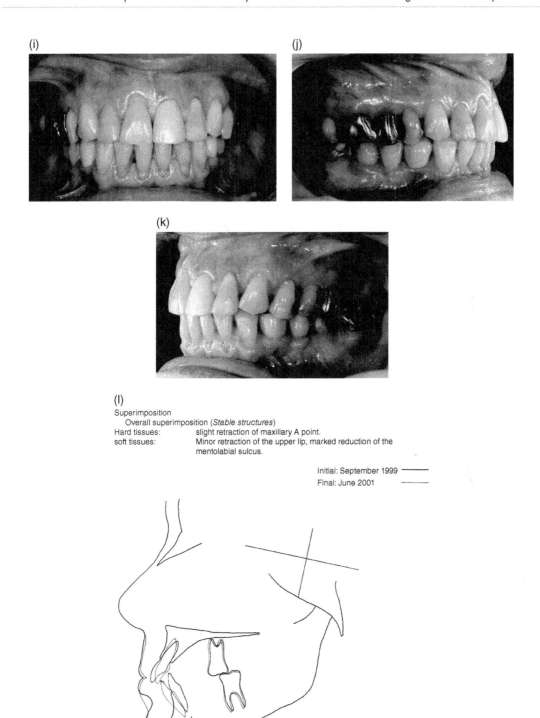

Figure 9.8 (*Continued*) (i–k) Status at the end of treatment. The treatment was finished by insertion of implants in the first premolar region. The patient then had "three lower premolars" in each side. The protrusion of the lower anterior segment was done as a controlled tipping generating bone on the anterior aspect of the lower alveolar

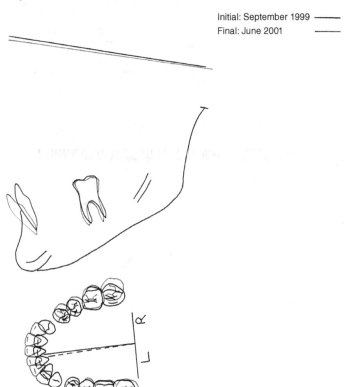

(m)
Mandibular superimposition (*Stable structures*)
Incisors: intrusion and protraction with a controlled tipping component.
Molars: mesial movement of the root
Mandibular rotation: slight anterior rotation
Occlusogram: advancement of the lower front of 5 mm.

Initial: September 1999 ——
Final: June 2001   ——

Figure 9.8 (*Continued*) process and without losing attachment or generating dehiscences. (l–m) Tracings demonstrating the tooth movements that took place during treatment.

prosthetic reconstruction in the upper arch. Several upper teeth and the lower left first molar were missing, and the upper left canine was impacted and palatally displaced (Figure 9.9). The patient's request to the prosthodontist was a new, functionally and esthetically pleasing prosthetic solution. The prosthodontist's wish was that the orthodontist would extrude the impacted tooth before he could perform a minimally invasive rehabilitation, reducing the present number of prosthetic elements.

The first part of treatment was forced eruption and distal tipping of the impacted canine. Access to the canine was obtained by an elevation of a palatal flap and a corticotomy to clear the canine crown onto which a gold-plated chain was bonded to the linguo-distal aspect (Figure 9.10). The flap was repositioned, leaving access to the crown. Furthermore, an Aarhus Mini-Implant® with 8.0 mm thread length, 2.5 mm neck length, and 1.5 mm diameter was inserted palatally in the area of the missing left first molar (Figure 9.11). One week after surgery, the sutures were removed and distal traction of the canine was performed with elastomeric chains extending from the

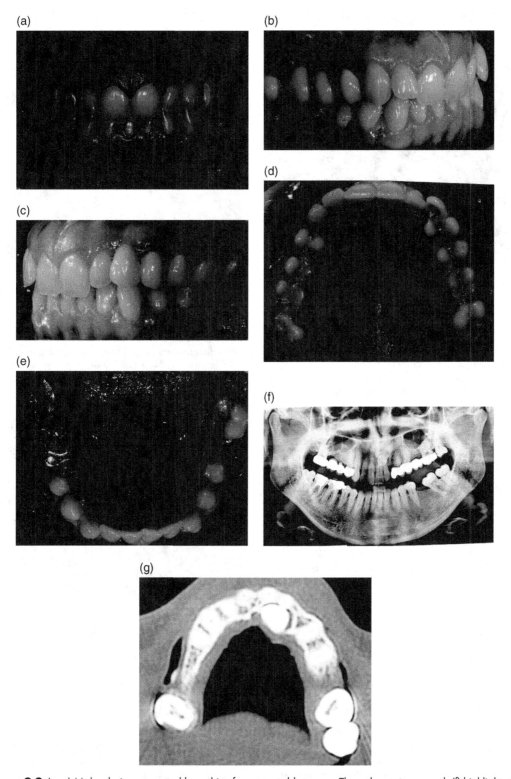

Figure 9.9 (a–g) Malocclusion presented by a thirty-four years old woman. The orthopantomograph (f) highlights the extensive inadequate prosthodontic rehabilitation of the upper arch, the impacted upper left canine and the missing lower left first molar. The detail of the computer tomography (g) highlights the palatal displacement of the impacted tooth.

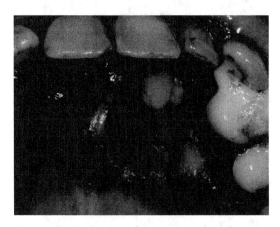

Figure 9.10 The day of surgery a palatal flap was elevated and the crown of the impacted canine was exposed. Cortical bone was removed by means of a piezoelectric instrument that was also used to perform cuts of the cortex bilaterally around the impacted tooth to facilitate and enhance tooth movement. Surgery performed by Dr Marco Sed.

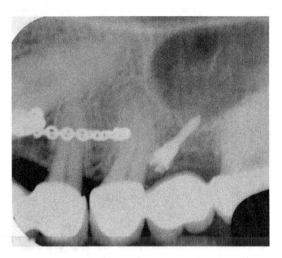

Figure 9.11 Radiographic control the day of surgery. A miniscrew was inserted in the edentulous area where tooth 26 was lost on the palatal side. Although the bidimensional X-ray shows proximity of the tip of the miniscrew to the maxillary sinus, no resistance indicating contact to the cortex on the sinus was encountered during insertion.

canine to the head of the inserted miniscrew (Figure 9.12). The elastomeric chains were changed every 2 weeks, and following 4 months of traction with nonvisible palatal mechanics the canine crown had erupted. The upper left prosthetic bridge was then removed and provisional single crowns were fabricated on the premolars and second molar. Brackets were bonded on both arches and leveling and alignment were progressively accomplished (Figure 9.13). At this stage the canine was simply ligated to the archwire, but no traction was performed as space in the arch had still to be gained. When alignment allowed for a rectangular 0.018″ × 0.025″ stainless steel archwire to be inserted in the upper arch, the mini-implant was used as direct anchorage for retraction of the two left premolars with sliding mechanics (Figure 9.14). Removal of the mini-implant was performed as soon as space closure was nearly finished, and the canine was finally brought into the arch (Figure 9.15) and de-rotated (Figure 9.16).

As a result of the previously extracted first molar in the left lower arch, the bucco-lingual ridge thickness was inappropriate for implant

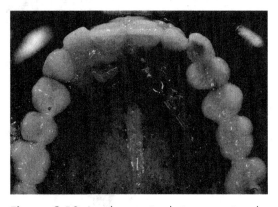

Figure 9.12 An elastomeric chain connecting the gold chain bonded to the canine crown and the head of the miniscrew, delivering approximately 50 cN of force, was inserted 1 week following surgery and renewed every 2 weeks until eruption of the cuspid.

placement without augmentation procedures, and mesio-distal space was insufficient for insertion of a molar crown. Therefore, space closure by mesial movement of teeth 37 and 38 was planned with the aim to substitute with the natural dentition the missing first molar. Orthodontic space closure was considered the

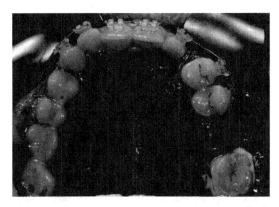

Figure 9.13 Four months following treatment start the cuspid crown erupted on the palate. Brackets were bonded on the upper teeth and a 0.014″ super-elastic leveling wire was inserted. At this stage the cuspid was simply ligated to the archwire.

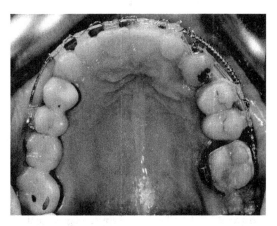

Figure 9.15 Once the canine was aligned, elastomeric thread was used on the two sides of the clinical crown, forming a couple, for de-rotation purposes.

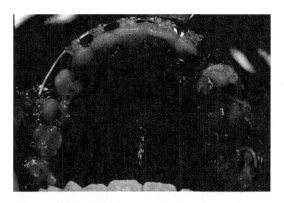

Figure 9.14 In order to generate space for the canine and to reduce the number of final prosthetic elements the premolars were retracted into the space of the missing first molar. A 0.018″ × 0.025″ stainless steel wire was used for sliding and an elastomeric chain, renewed every 2 weeks, was connected to the head of the miniscrew and was passed around the mesial aspect of the premolars and connected to the molar band on the buccal side. As soon as the cuspid had enough space for alignment, the miniscrew was removed and space closure was finalized with mesial molar displacement.

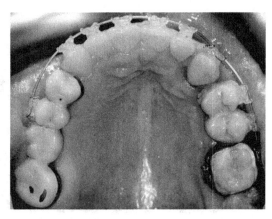

Figure 9.16 Following 2 months of de-rotation the cuspid reached the final position in the arch.

most biologic and minimally invasive procedure considering the good status of both the second and third molars. An Aarhus Mini-Implant with 8.0 mm thread length, 1.5 mm neck length, and 1.5 mm diameter was inserted

between the first and second premolar roots and used as direct anchorage for mesial traction of the molars (Figure 9.17). Although the edentulous ridge wad totally collapsed, tooth movement was accomplished "with bone" thanks to the use of a "V" bend, light forces, and bodily movement, allowing complete remodeling of the periodontium (Figure 9.18).

The case was finished after 28 months of active treatment (Figure 9.19); a fixed lower lingual anterior retainer was bonded and a removable plate was fabricated for night use. Orthodontic treatment made it possible for the

(a)

(b)

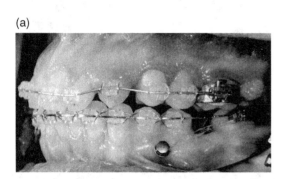
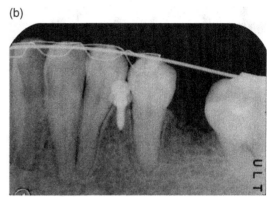

Figure 9.17 (a) Clinical and (b) radiographical views of the miniscrew inserted in the left mandible between first and second premolar. Elastomeric traction renewed every 2 weeks used for molar protraction sliding on a rectangular stainless steel 0.010" × 0.025" wire for space closure. Note the upper canine in the arch and under traction of a super-elastic rectangular wire finalizing the leveling phase.

(a)

(b)

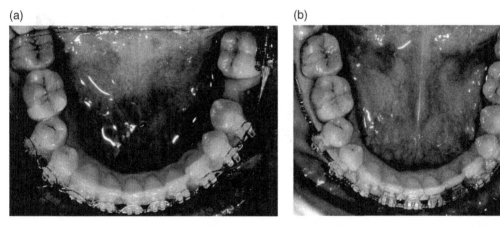

Figure 9.18 Lower arch (a) before and (b) after space closure. Note the extremely thin and collapsed alveolar ridge before space closure, inadequate for implant placement.

patient to avoid dental implants. The edentulous areas in the second and third quadrant were closed by means of orthodontic traction with the natural dentition, and only three final prosthetic ceramic crowns are planned for teeth 24, 25, and 27. The use of skeletal anchorage made this treatment possible by solving the problem of lack of teeth for anchorage in the left side of the upper arch during canine traction and posterior space closure, and in the lower left arch avoiding distal drift of the anterior teeth during mesial traction of the second and third molars. The use of

corticotomy around the impacted upper left canine enhanced the eruption, reducing the resistance of the periodontal structure during canine traction and increasing the local bone turnover.

Case 2

Case 2 describes the treatment of a 17-year-old female patient with severe dento-alveolar bi-protrusion and lip incompetence. The patient's request was to reduce the visibility of the

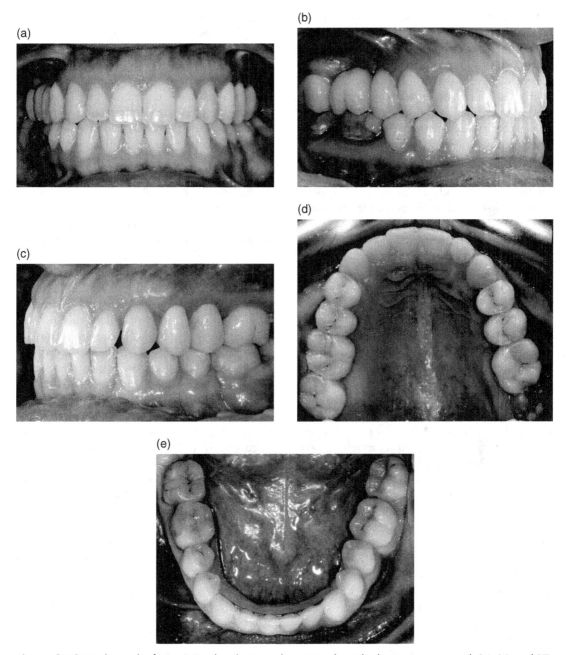

Figure 9.19 Final records of case 1. Final occlusion and provisional prosthodontic crowns on teeth 24, 25, and 27. Edentolous spaces have been closed, eliminating the need for dental implants. Prosthodontics: Dr Marco Sed.

dentition by "pulling it back." Class I skeletal and dental relationships were present with good arch forms and absence of crowding (Figure 9.20). The upper incisors were proclined relative to the palatal plane (U1/PNS–ANS = 130°) and the lower incisors to the mandibular plane (L1/Go–Me = 110°). These values confirmed the severe dento-alveolar biprotrusion and the need for extractions in order to achieve correct final inclinations with a reduced exposure of the dentition, improved lip competence, and enhanced facial appearance. The need of absolute posterior anchorage was evident.

Following bonding of full fixed appliances, leveling was accomplished in 3 months as no crowding was present. Extractions of four first premolars were performed when 0.019″ × 0.025″ stainless steel archwires had been inserted and two bracket-head Aarhus Mini-Implants with 8.0 mm thread length, 1.5 mm neck length, and 1.5 mm diameter were placed transcortically in the lower arch between the roots of the first and second molars, at the level of the muco-gingival line (Figure 9.21). No miniscrews were planned in the upper arch. Since the patient's request was to speed up treatment as much as possible, the decision was taken to perform flapless corticotomy. Surgery was planned and only vertical incisions of the soft tissues were made. Following incision, a piezoelectric hand-piece was used to achieve vertical cuts of the cortex. To enhance space closure, two vertical cuts were made bucally (Figure 9.22) in the lower extraction sites in order to reduce cortical resistance. The cuts were limited to the buccal cortex. Following sutures and radiographic periapical controls (Figure 9.23), orthodontic forces for space closure were were immediately applied. Corticotomy was not performed in the upper arch because maxillary cortical bone is thin and space

closure with regular tooth movement was thought to be less time consuming.

The sutures were removed 1 week following extractions and corticotomy. In order to take advantage of the lower skeletal anchorage for space closure in both arches, intra-arch elastomeric forces were planned in the lower jaw with elastic tie-backs, and inter-maxillary elastics were used for the upper jaw (Figure 9.24). The lower second premolars and first molars were tightly tied to the heads of the miniscrews with 0.012″ ligature wire in order to avoid any mesial displacement of the side segments during space closure. The positive patient compliance with the use of inter-maxillary elastic tractions resulted in rapid space closure. The finishing phase was performed with 0.018″ × 0.025″ stainless steel multistrand braided wires, and the patient was instructed to use vertical inter-maxillary elastics to improve intercuspation. Since second molars were not planned to be part of the anchorage during space closure, bonding of these teeth was only done during the last part of treatment when occlusal contacts were optimized with intermaxillary elastics. The case was finished after 18 months of active treatment (Figure 9.25), and a fixed lower lingual anterior retainer together with a removable plate fabricated for night use was used for retention. Class I molar and canine relationships were maintained, while the upper and lower incisor inclinations were successfully reduced, meeting posttreatment cephalometric norms. Lip competence improved, as well as facial esthetics. The final result and the posttreatment lateral cephalometry confirm the efficacy of the absolute posterior anchorage achieved by the use of TADs. Corticotomy in the lower arch enhanced the rate of space closure, especially in the first weeks of elastomeric traction. Overall, patient satisfaction was very high and treatment duration was relatively short.

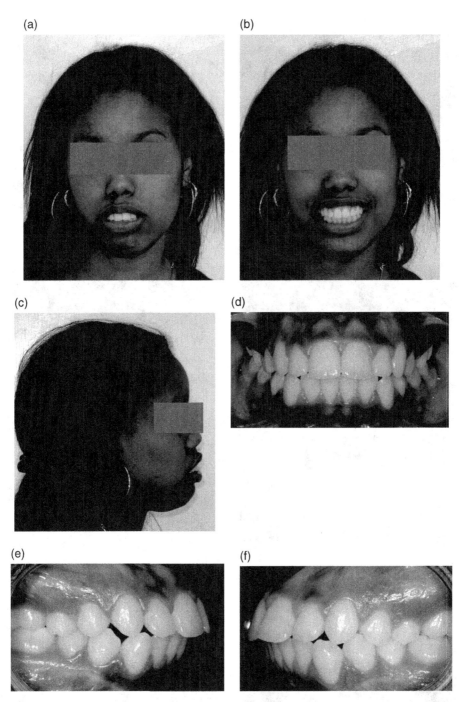

Figure 9.20 (a–l) Malocclusion presented by a 17-year-old woman. Severe dento-alveolar bi-protrusion with lip incompetence. The orthopantomogram (k) displays a complete dentition, and the lateral cephalogram (l) highlights the increased inclination of both the upper and lower incisors.

(g)

(h)

(i)

(j)

(k)

(l)

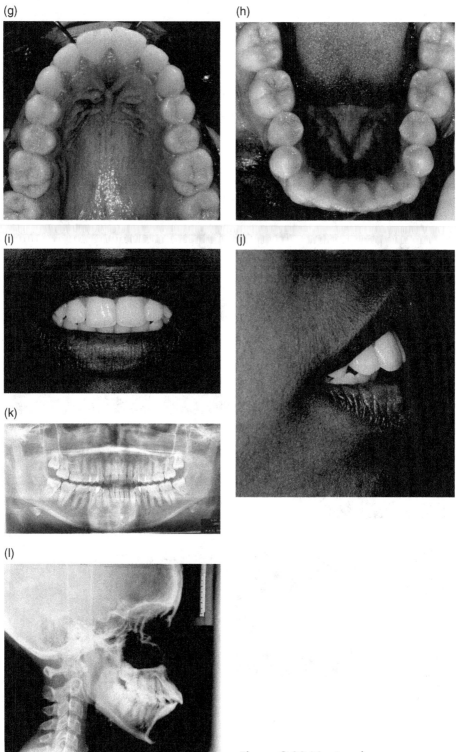

Figure 9.20 (*Continued*)

(a) (b)

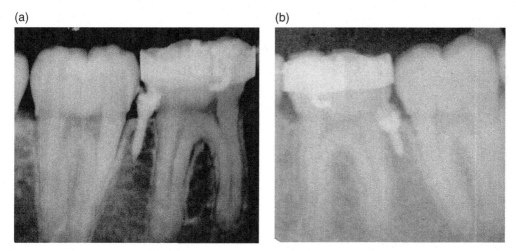

Figure 9.21 Periapical radiographs following insertion of two miniscrews bilaterally in the posterior mandible between first and second molars on the buccal alveolar process. Good clearance from the dental roots can be appreciated.

(a)

(b)

(c)

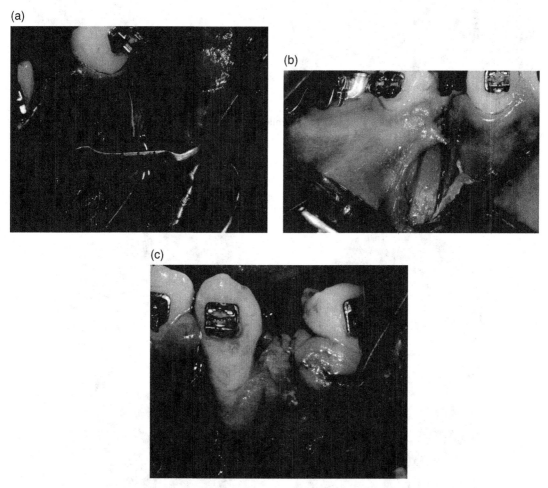

Figure 9.22 Flapless corticotomy with a "tunnel" technique. Following vertical incision of the soft tissues, a piezoelectric hand-piece was used (a) to perform two vertical cuts on each side of the mandible on the buccal aspect of the extraction sites (b,c) to reduce resistance of the bone and enhance tooth movement. Surgery was performed by Dr G Serino.

(a) (b)

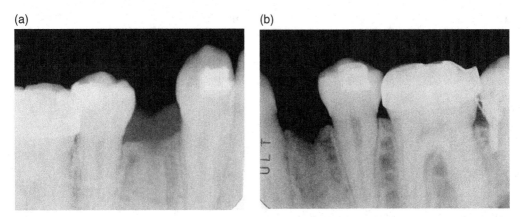

Figure 9.23 Periapical radiographs following corticotomy.

(a) (b)

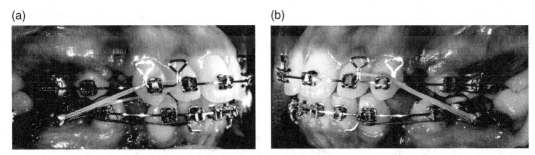

Figure 9.24 Clinical images during the space closure phase. The retraction of the upper front teeth is progressing with the use of inter-maxillary elastics, while the retraction of the lower front teeth is progressing with intra-arch elastic tie-backs. The lower first molars and second premolars are tied to the heads of the miniscrews, not allowing posterior anchorage loss.

(a) (b)

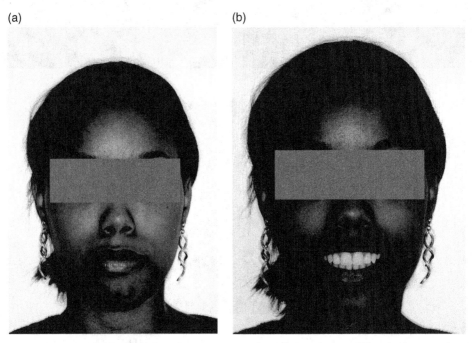

Figure 9.25 Final records of case 2 following 18 months of active treatment. The improvement of facial esthetics can be observed in the extraoral photographs. The intraoral pictures display a solid side occlusion and together with the lateral cephalogram demonstrate the pronounced change in the upper and lower incisor inclination.

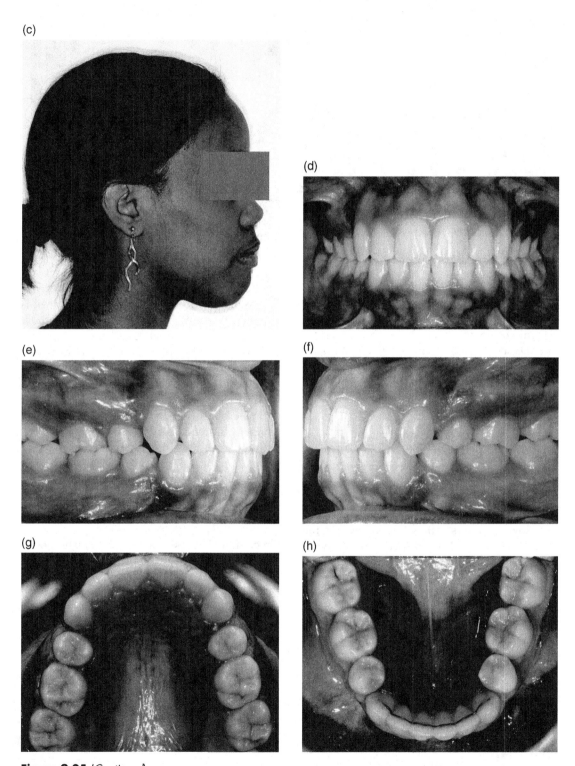

Figure 9.25 (*Continued*)

(j)

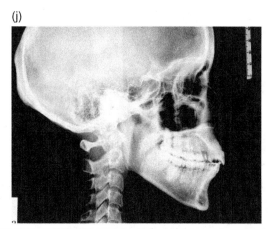

(i)

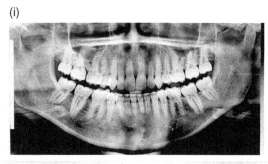

Figure 9.25 (Continued)

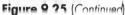

CONCLUSION

This chapter aimed at demonstrating how efficient mechanics with and without the application of TADs or/and corticotomy can modify the bony envelope claimed to limit orthodontic treatment.

References

Albrektsson T, Zarb G, Worthington P *et al.* (1986) The long-term efficacy of currently used dental implants: a review and proposed criteria of success. *International Journal of Oral and Maxillofacial Implants*, **1**, 11–25.

Allais D, Melsen B (2003) Does labial movement of lower incisors influence the level of the gingival margin? A case–control study of adult orthodontic patients. *European Journal of Orthodontics*, **25**, 343–352.

Bjork A, Skieller V (1972) Facial development and tooth eruption. An implant study at the age of puberty. *American Journal of Orthodontics*, **62**, 339–383.

Block MS, Hoffman DR (1995) A new device for absolute anchorage for orthodontics. *American Journal of Orthodontics and Dentofacial Orthopedics*, **107**, 251–258.

Burstone CJ, Koenig HA (1974) Forces from an ideal arch. *American Journal of Orthodontics*, **65** (3), 275–276.

Byloff-Clar H (1967a) Treatment of delayed (juvenile) cases using activators with and without corticotomy. Clinical and histologic study. *Stomatology (Heidelberg)*, **20**, 277–286 (in German).

Byloff-Clar H (1967b) Treatment with activator plates with and without corticotomy in late cases (juveniles). A clinical and histological study. *Stomatology (Heidelberg)*, **20**, 214–225 (in German).

Chan EK, Darendeliler MA (2004) Exploring the third dimension in root resorption. *Orthodontics and Craniofacial Research*, **7**, 64–70.

Costa A, Raffaini M, Melsen B (1998) Miniscrews as orthodontic anchorage: a preliminary report. *International Journal of Adult Orthodontics and Orthognathic Surgery*, **13** (3), 201–209.

Creekmore TD, Eklund MK (1983) The possibility of skeletal anchorage. *Journal of Clinical Orthodontics*, **17**, 266–269.

Davidovitch Z, Finkelson MD, Steigman S *et al.* (1980) Electric currents, bone remodeling, and orthodontic tooth movement. II. Increase in rate of tooth movement and periodontal cyclic nucleotide levels by combined force and electric current. *American Journal of Orthodontics*, **77**, 33–47.

De Clerck HJ, Cornelis MA (2006) Biomechanics of skeletal anchorage. Part 2: class II nonextraction treatment. *Journal of Clinical Orthodontics*, **40**, 290–298.

Diedrich P (1993) Different orthodontic anchorage systems. A critical examination. *Fortschritte der Kieferorthopädie*, **54**, 156–171.

Fontenelle A (1982) A periodontal concept of induced tooth movement: clinical evidence. *Revue Orthopedie Dento-Faciale*, **16**, 37–53 (in French).

Gainsforth BL, Higley LB (1945) A study of orthodontic anchorage possibilities in basal bone. *American Journal of Orthodontics and Oral Surgery*, **31**, 406–416.

Humphry GM (1878) On the growth of the jaws. *Journal of Anatomy and Physiology*, **12**, 288–293.

Iglesias-Linares A, Moreno-Fernandez AM, Yanez-Vico R *et al.* (2011) The use of gene therapy vs. corticotomy surgery in accelerating orthodontic tooth movement. *Orthodontics and Craniofacial Research*, **14**, 138–148.

Iino S, Sakoda S, Ito G *et al.* (2007) Acceleration of orthodontic tooth movement by alveolar corticotomy in the dog. *American Journal of Orthodontics and Dentofacial Orthopedics*, **131**, 448.e1–448.e8.

Kanomi R (1997) Mini-implant for orthodontic anchorage. *Journal of Clinical Orthodontics*, **31**, 763–767.

Kim SH, Kim I, Jeong DM *et al.* (2011) Corticotomy-assisted decompensation for augmentation of the mandibular anterior ridge. *American Journal of Orthodontics and Dentofacial Orthopedics*, **140**, 720–731.

Lindtoft H (2010) Post treatment changes in the clinical crown height and periodontal health occurring following an orthodontic treatment involving proclination of lower incisors. A prospective clinical study in adult orthodontic patients. Thesis, Aarhus University, Aarhus, Denmark.

Lines PA (1975) Adult rapid maxillary expansion with corticotomy. *American Journal of Orthodontics*, **67**, 44–56.

Linkow LI (1970) Endosseous blade-vent implants: a two-year report. *Journal of Prosthetic Dentistry*, **23**, 441–448.

Melsen B (2005) Mini-implants: where are we? *Journal of Clinical Orthodontics*, **39**, 539–547.

Melsen B, Allais D (2005) Factors of importance for the development of dehiscences during labial movement of mandibular incisors: a retrospective study of adult orthodontic patients. *American Journal of Orthodontics and Dentofacial Orthopedics*, **127**, 552–561.

Melsen B, Petersen JK, Costa A (1998) Zygoma ligatures: an alternative form of maxillary anchorage. *Journal of Clinical Orthodontics*, **32**, 154–158.

Nishimura M, Chiba M, Ohashi T *et al.* (2008) Periodontal tissue activation by vibration: intermittent stimulation by resonance vibration accelerates experimental tooth movement in rats. *American Journal of Orthodontics and Dentofacial Orthopedics*, **133**, 572–583.

Odman J, Lekholm U, Jemt T *et al.* (1988) Osseointegrated titanium implants – a new approach in orthodontic treatment. *European Journal of Orthodontics*, **10**, 98–105.

Roberts WE, Smith RK, Zilberman Y *et al.* (1984) Osseous adaptation to continuous loading of rigid endosseous implants. *American Journal of Orthodontics*, **86**, 95–111.

Roberts WE, Helm FR, Marshall KJ *et al.* (1989) Rigid endosseous implants for orthodontic and orthopedic anchorage. *Angle Orthodontist*, **59**, 247–256.

Roberts WE, Marshall KJ, Mozsary PG (1990) Rigid endosseous implant utilized as anchorage to protract molars and close an atrophic extraction site. *Angle Orthodontist*, **60**, 135–152.

Sachdeva RC, Aranha SL, Egan ME *et al.* (2012) Treatment time: SureSmile vs conventional. *Orthodontics (Chicago)*, **13**, 72–85.

Sherman AJ (1978) Bone reaction to orthodontic forces on vitreous carbon dental implants. *American Journal of Orthodontics*, **74**, 79–87.

Shoreibah EA, Ibrahim SA, Attia MS *et al.* (2012) Clinical and radiographic evaluation of bone grafting in corticotomy-facilitated orthodontics in adults. *Journal of the International Academy of Periodontology*, **14**, 105–113.

Steinberg B (1978) Tissue response to dental implants. *Journal of Oral Implantology*, **7**, 475–491.

Sugawara J (2005) Orthodontic reduction of lower facial height in open bite patients with skeletal anchorage system: beyond traditional orthodontics. *World Journal of Orthodontics*, **6** (Suppl), 24–26.

Sugawara J, Aymach Z, Nagasaka DH *et al.* (2010) "Surgery first" orthognathics to correct a skeletal class II malocclusion with an impinging bite. *Journal of Clinical Orthodontics*, **44**, 429–438.

Teixeira CC, Khoo E, Tran J *et al.* (2010) Cytokine expression and accelerated tooth movement. *Journal of Dental Research*, **89**, 1135–1141.

Thilander B, Odman J, Lekholm U (2001) Orthodontic aspects of the use of oral implants in adolescents: a 10-year follow-up study. *European Journal of Orthodontics*, **23**, 715–731.

Umemori M, Sugawara J, Mitani H *et al.* (1999) Skeletal anchorage system for open-bite correction. *American Journal of Orthodontics and Dentofacial Orthopedics*, **115**, 166–174.

Wehrbein H, Merz BR (1998) Aspects of the use of endosseous palatal implants in orthodontic therapy. *Journal of Esthetic Dentistry*, **10**, 315–324.

Wilcko MT, Wilcko WM, Pulver JJ *et al.* (2009) Accelerated osteogenic orthodontics technique: a 1-stage surgically facilitated rapid orthodontic technique with alveolar augmentation. *Journal of Oral and Maxillofacial Surgery*, **67**, 2149–2159.

Yamaguchi M, Hayashi M, Fujita S *et al.* (2010) Low-energy laser irradiation facilitates the velocity of tooth movement and the expressions of matrix metalloproteinase-9, cathepsin K, and alpha(v) beta(3) integrin in rats. *European Journal of Orthodontics*, **32**, 131–139.

Yamasaki K, Shibata Y, Imai S *et al.* (1984) Clinical application of prostaglandin E1 (PGE1) upon orthodontic tooth movement. *American Journal of Orthodontics*, **85**, 508–518.

Yoshida T, Yamaguchi M, Utsunomiya T *et al.* (2009) Low-energy laser irradiation accelerates the velocity of tooth movement via stimulation of the alveolar bone remodeling. *Orthodontics and Craniofacial Research*, **12**, 289–298.

Youssef M, Ashkar S, Hamade E *et al.* (2008) The effect of low-level laser therapy during orthodontic movement: a preliminary study. *Lasers in Medical Science*, **23**, 27–33.

Anterior open-bite treatment through orthodontically driven corticotomy

Nagwa Helmy El-Mangoury,[1] Helmy Y. Mostafa,[2,3] and Raweya Y. Mostafa[3,4]

[1]*Department of Orthodontics & Dentofacial Orthopedics, Cairo University Faculty of Dentistry, Cairo, Egypt*
[2]*Private Practice of Orthodontics, Binghamton & Endicott, New York, USA*
[3]*Mangoury & Mostafa Research Group*
[4]*Private Practice of Orthodontics, Cairo, Egypt*

INTRODUCTION

Astute orthodontists are always on a quest for implementing innovative techniques that enable them to serve their patients and deliver the expected services in an impeccable manner. During the last decade, new treatment modalities have been introduced into the orthodontic profession. Some of these modalities satisfied the efficiency parameters as far as speeding up the treatment; for example, via orthodontically driven corticotomy (ODC). In this chapter, our conceptual framework is tri-dimensional in nature: safe acceleration of tooth movements, efficient solving of clinical problems, and proficient expansion of orthodontic capabilities (Figure 10.1). Every effort was made to discuss anterior open-bite (AOB) treatment through evidence-based ODC. As shown in Figure 10.2, evidence-based orthodontics means to translate valid (El-Mangoury, 1981) research into judicious clinical orthodontics (Mostafa, 2005). In other words (Figure 10.2), decode the established reality into the practiced actuality (Mostafa, 2005).

Further, a firm biologic foundation (Figure 10.2) is necessary for any type of tooth movements. Mostafa *et al.* (1991) pointed out that: "Archimedes, the Greek mathematician and inventor, stated: 'Give me a firm place to stand, and I will move the earth.' To paraphrase Archimedes, the contemporary orthodontist would say, 'Give me a firm biologic basis, and I will move the teeth.'"

OPEN-BITE

If the overbite is negative, it is called open-bite (El-Mangoury *et al.*, 2014). Specifically, when the dentition is in centric occlusion, the

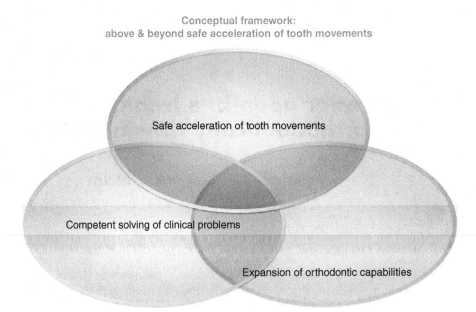

Figure 10.1 Conceptual framework: above and beyond safe acceleration of tooth movements.

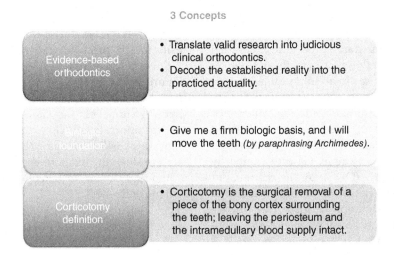

Figure 10.2 Three concepts: evidence-based orthodontics, biologic foundation, and corticotomy definition.

anterior open-bite manifests itself through a lack of vertical contacts between the maxillary and the mandibular incisors (Figure 10.3). According to Proffit *et al.* (2007), the open-bite prevalence in the USA is 3.3%. The open-bite could be moderate (0–2 mm), severe (3–4 mm), or extremely severe (more than 4 mm) as shown by Proffit *et al.* (2007). The open-bite could be either anterior or posterior, unilateral or bilateral, acquired or hereditary, as well as dental or skeletal (El-Mangoury *et al.*, 2014).

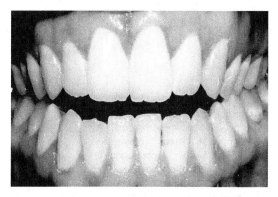

Figure 10.3 Anterior open-bite. When the dentition is in centric occlusion, the anterior open-bite manifests itself through a lack of vertical contacts between the maxillary and the mandibular incisors.

Dental open-bites are generally more responsive to treatment with orthodontics alone, whereas severe skeletal open-bites often require a combination of orthodontics and orthognathic surgery. Beane (1999) discussed the treatment principles for nonsurgical open-bites, and reviewed various treatment methods for skeletal open-bites.

Open-bites are challenging malocclusions; with a multifactorial etiology, varying clinical severity, and questionable stability (Mostafa *et al.*, 2009a). They should not be approached as a single disease entity; rather, they should be viewed as clinical manifestations of underlying dental and skeletal discrepancies.

Specific open-bite treatment plans should be based upon the underlying etiology. Early intervention might be necessary to resolve any developing open-bite skeletal deformity. Altering the mandibular plane may be recommended through either dentofacial orthopedic growth modifications or orthognathic surgery in cases of downward and backward mandibular rotations. The reverse curve of Spee and the proclination of the maxillary incisors must be corrected. Extraction mechanotherapies in the treatment of open-bite might be beneficial to level the curve of Spee together with normalizing the proclined maxillary incisors.

INTERVENTIONS FOR ACCELERATING ORTHODONTIC TOOTH MOVEMENT

In a systematic review about the interventions for accelerating tooth movement, Long *et al.* (2013) made the following four important conclusions:

- Corticotomy is effective and safe to accelerate orthodontic tooth movement.
- Low-level laser therapy was unable to accelerate orthodontic tooth movement.
- The current evidence does not reveal whether electrical current and pulsed electromagnetic fields are effective in accelerating orthodontic tooth movement.
- Dentoalveolar or periodontal distraction is promising in accelerating orthodontic tooth movement but lacks convincing evidence.

BRIEF DEFINITION OF CORTICOTOMY

As indicated in the introduction and previous chapters, osteotomy is often confused with corticotomy. By definition, corticotomy is the surgical removal of a piece of the bony cortex surrounding the teeth, leaving the periosteum and the intramedullary blood supply intact (Figure 10.2).

CORTICOTOMY BAKER'S DOZEN SYNONYMS

The baker's dozen phrase originated from the practice of medieval English bakers giving one or two extra loafs of bread when selling a dozen in order to avoid being penalized for selling short weight. Thus, 1 baker's dozen equals 13 or 14. There are at least 14 corticotomy synonyms.

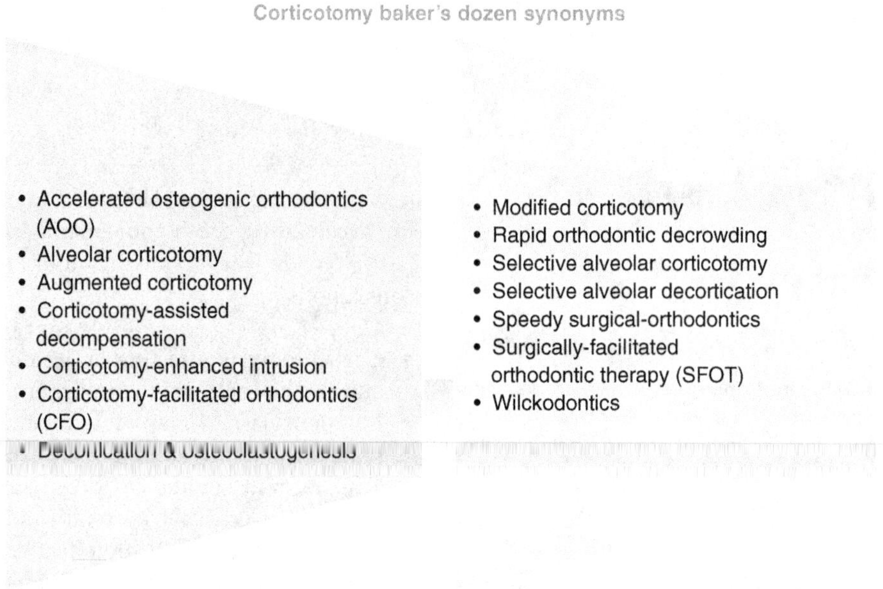

Corticotomy baker's dozen synonyms

- Accelerated osteogenic orthodontics (AOO)
- Alveolar corticotomy
- Augmented corticotomy
- Corticotomy-assisted decompensation
- Corticotomy-enhanced intrusion
- Corticotomy-facilitated orthodontics (CFO)
- Decortication & osteoclastogenesis

- Modified corticotomy
- Rapid orthodontic decrowding
- Selective alveolar corticotomy
- Selective alveolar decortication
- Speedy surgical-orthodontics
- Surgically-facilitated orthodontic therapy (SFOT)
- Wilckodontics

Figure 10.4 Corticotomy baker's dozen synonyms. One baker's dozen equals 13 or 14.

These synonyms are alphabetically organized in Figure 10.4. Chronologically arranged, these synonyms are: selective alveolar decortication (Mostafa *et al.*, 1985; Fischer, 2007; Baloul *et al.*, 2011; Hwang *et al.*, 2011), corticotomy-facilitated orthodontics (CFO) (Kerdvongbundit, 1990; Iino *et al.*, 2006; Fayed *et al.*, 2009; Mostafa *et al.*, 2009b; Aboul-Ela *et al.*, 2011; Shoreibah *et al.*, 2012a,b), rapid orthodontic decrowding (Wilcko *et al.*, 2003), modified corticotomy (Germeç *et al.*, 2006), alveolar corticotomy (Iino *et al.*, 2007; Sanjideh *et al.*, 2010), selective alveolar corticotomy (Oliveira *et al.*, 2008; Baloul *et al.*, 2011), speedy surgical-orthodontics (Chung *et al.* 2009a,b; Choo *et al.*, 2011), Accelerated Osteogenic Orthodontics® (AOO®) as indicated by (Wilcko *et al.*, 2009), decortication and osteoclastogenesis (Baloul *et al.*, 2011), Wilckodontics (Einy *et al.*, 2011), corticotomy-assisted decompensation (Kim *et al.*, 2011), augmented corticotomy (Ahn *et al.*, 2012), surgically facilitated orthodontic therapy (SFOT) as introduced by (Murphy *et al.*, 2012), and corticotomy-enhanced intrusion (Grenga and Bovi, 2013).

Most of these synonyms may directly be related to the concept of corticotomy (PAOO®) presented in detail throughout this book. The only technique that substantially differs from PAOO is speedy orthodontics (Chung *et al.*, 2009a,b; Choo *et al.*, 2011), because of the use orthopedic forces as opposed to the orthodontic ones. This is mainly due to the fact that the authors of speedy orthodontics espoused the bony-block movement, and therefore needed to use a stronger force to "bend" the medullary bone and move the bony block.

Chung *et al.* (2009a) described speedy orthodontics for treating severe protrusion in adults and concluded that this type of treatment mechanics can be an effective alternative to orthognathic surgery in adults. Later, Chung *et al.* (2009b) redescribed speedy orthodontics, which allows faster movements of the dental segments using skeletal anchorage. To minimize the risk of necrosis, two procedures were completed (Chung *et al.*, 2009b). During the initial surgery, bilateral and horizontal corticotomies were performed in the palatal area (Chung *et al.*, 2009b).

After 2–3 weeks, a second buccal corticotomy was done, and 500–900 g of force per side was immediately applied to the corticotomized segment (Chung *et al.*, 2009b). Successful alveolar bone bending could be obtained in cases of adult protrusion or open-bite (Chung *et al.*, 2009b). Speedy orthodontics allowed for more precise control of anterior segment retraction in adult protrusion patients and can be used for posterior segment intrusion (Chung *et al.*, 2009b). Additionally, Choo *et al.* (2011) pointed out that speedy surgical orthodontics can be an effective modality for adults with severe maxillary protrusion.

CORTICOTOMY AND TISSUE
ENGINEERING FOR
ORTHODONTISTS

About 30 years ago, Mostafa *et al.* (1985) were able to intrude overerupted maxillary molars through safe decortications and extremely simple biomechanics. Fischer (2007) was capable of reducing the orthodontic treatment duration for palatally impacted canines through selective alveolar decortication.

Iino *et al.* (2006) performed CFO on the lingual and buccal sides in the maxillary anterior as well as the mandibular anterior and posterior regions. Further, Mostafa *et al.* (2009b) studied six mongrel dogs, aged 6–9 months. Extraction of the maxillary second premolars and miniscrews placement were done bilaterally in the maxilla (Mostafa *et al.*, 2009b). The corticotomy was performed on the right side (Mostafa *et al.*, 2009b). The first premolars were distalized against the miniscrews with nickel–titanium coil springs on both sides (Mostafa *et al.*, 2009b).

The first premolar on the CFO side moved significantly more rapidly (Mostafa *et al.*, 2009b). Histologic findings showed more active

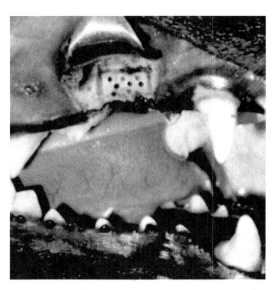

Figure 10.5 Corticotomy in a mongrel dog. Observe the horizontal and vertical cortical cuts, the cortical perforations, and the miniscrew. *Source:* Mostafa *et al.* (2009b). Reproduced with permission of Elsevier.

and extensive bone remodeling on both the compressive and tension sides in the CFO group (Mostafa *et al.*, 2009b). Actually, the CFO technique (Figure 10.5) doubled the rate of orthodontic tooth movement (Mostafa *et al.*, 2009b). Mostafa *et al.* (2009b) pointed out that the more active and extensive bone remodeling in the CFO group as well as the acceleration of tooth movement associated with corticotomy might be due to increased bone turnover based on regional acceleratory phenomena.

Moreover, Fayed *et al.* (2009) concluded that the CFO technique delayed the osseous bone formation around the miniscrews in comparison with the standard technique. During the first 2 months after corticotomy, Aboul-Ela *et al.* (2011) found that the average daily rate of canine retraction was significantly twice as high on the corticotomy side (Figure 10.6) than on the control side. This rate of tooth movement declined to only 1.6 times higher in the third month, and 1.06 times higher by the end of the fourth month (Aboul-Ela *et al.*, 2011). Thus, CFO can be a feasible

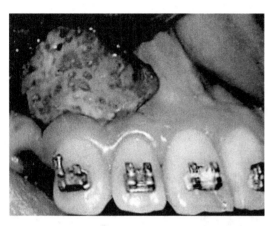

Figure 10.6 Corticotomy in the maxillary right canine region. Notice that the cortical perforations extend to the canine's apex. *Source:* Aboul-Ela *et al.* (2011). Reproduced with permission of Elsevier.

treatment modality for adults seeking orthodontic treatment with reduced treatment durations (Aboul-Ela *et al.*, 2011).

Further, the results of two additional studies suggest that CFO significantly reduced the total duration of treatment (Shoreibah *et al.*, 2012a,b). Moreover, the incidence of root resorption and adverse effect on teeth investing tissues associated with orthodontic tooth movement decreased (Shoreibah *et al.*, 2012a,b). The acceleration of tooth movement through the proposed technique improved patients' compliance (Shoreibah *et al.*, 2012a). Furthermore, the incorporation of bone graft material significantly increased the alveolar bone density in adult patients (Shoreibah *et al.*, 2012b).

Murphy *et al.* (2012) suggested that orthodontists should define themselves as dentoalveolar orthopedists, and restrict corticotomy procedures to "selective alveolar decortications," with or without grafting. Through a new vision or a "postmodern New Think" (orthodontic tooth movement, through a healing wound), orthodontists can modulate physiological internal strains (similar to those of distraction osteogenesis in long bones) to define novel

and more stable alveolus phenotypes; minimizing not only premolar extractions, but also orthognathic surgery morbidity (Murphy *et al.*, 2012).

ADVANTAGES OF ORTHODONTICALLY DRIVEN CORTICOTOMY

- In a systematic review, Long *et al.* (2013) found that corticotomy is effective and safe.
- Besides its effectiveness and safety, other advantages (Figure 10.7) are reduction of the active treatment duration, optimization of the treatment results, and avoidance (or at least minimization) of the adverse side effects.
- Specifically, accelerating the rate of tooth movement tends to reduce the active treatment duration, which is desirable not only to the patients, but also to the orthodontists, because prolonged treatment is linked to an increased risk of periodontal diseases, decalcifications, dental caries, root resorptions, and noncompliances.
- Notable significant improvements in smile esthetics (Mostafa *et al.*, 2009a).
- Rapid orthodontic decrowding and minimal apical root resorption resulting from increased regional bone turnover (the regional acceleratory phenomenon) and the associated osteopenia (i.e., calcium depletion and diminished bone density); precipitated by selective decortication (Wilcko *et al.*, 2003; Mostafa *et al.*, 2009b; Buschang *et al.*, 2012).
- Rapid orthodontic tooth movement, without any adverse effects on the periodontium and the vitality of the teeth (Germeç *et al.*, 2006); through rapid alveolar bone reaction in the bone marrow cavities, leading to less hyalinization of the periodontal ligament on the alveolar wall (Iino *et al.*, 2007).
- The experimental evidence indicates that corticotomies approximately double the amount of tooth movement produced with

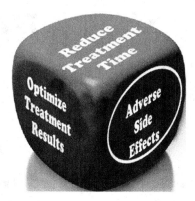

Figure 10.7 Main advantages of ODC: reduction of the active treatment duration, optimization of the treatment results, and avoidance (or at least minimization) of the adverse side effects.

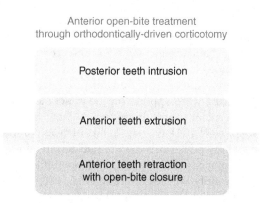

Figure 10.8 Anterior open-bite treatment through ODC: three suggested mechanotherapies.

orthodontic forces (Mostafa *et al.*, 2009b; Aboul-Ela *et al.*, 2011; Buschang *et al.*, 2012). However, the experimental effects are limited to a maximum of 1–2 months in the canine model, suggesting that the effects of corticotomies in humans may be limited to 2–3 months, during which 4–6 mm of tooth movement might be expected to occur (Buschang *et al.*, 2012).

ANTERIOR OPEN-BITE TREATMENT THROUGH ORTHODONTICALLY-DRIVEN CORTICOTOMY

Simply stated, the anterior open-bite is treated by increasing the overbite. The observed increase in overbite is attributable to small but clinically significant changes in relative mandibular vertical growth, bodily incisor movement toward the occlusal plane, and lingual tipping of the lower incisors (Bazzucchi *et al.*, 1999). Based on a thorough orthodontic diagnosis, the clinician should be able to elucidate the underlying open-bite causative factors. The treatment plan is to be tailored, targeting these etiologic fea-

tures. For the sake of clarity, the following topics will be discussed (Figure 10.8):

- posterior teeth intrusion;
- anterior teeth extrusion;
- anterior teeth retraction with open-bite closure.

Posterior teeth intrusion

Kanno *et al.* (2007) introduced a new efficient technique composed of corticotomy and compression osteogenesis in the posterior maxilla for treating severe anterior open-bite. In a similar vein, a severe anterior open-bite was treated by intrusion of the maxillary posterior teeth through one-stage osteotomy (Tuncer *et al.*, 2008). A segmental osteotomy was done, and the miniplates were fixed to the zygomatic buttress area (Tuncer *et al.*, 2008). The intrusive force was accomplished with nickel–titanium closed coil springs (using a force of 250 g between the miniplates and the maxillary first and second molar buccal tubes) as indicated by Tuncer *et al.* (2008). The intrusion was completed 2.5 months after osteotomy (Tuncer *et al.*, 2008). The maxillary molars were impacted 4 mm, and the mandibular plane showed a counterclockwise autorotation of 3° (Tuncer *et al.*, 2008).

Akay *et al.* (2009) determined the effects of combined treatment with corticotomy and skeletal anchorage in open-bite correction. Combined subapical corticotomy, skeletal anchorage procedure, and intrusion forces of 200–300 g were applied on the attachments of each molar and both premolars during 12–15 weeks (Akay *et al.*, 2009). Intrusion of the maxillary posterior teeth granted counterclockwise mandibular rotation, and open-bite was successfully corrected (Akay *et al.*, 2009). The Sella–Nasion–B point angle increased and the A point–Nasion–B point angle decreased (Akay *et al.*, 2009). Significant decreases were noticed for vertical skeletal characteristics, and overbite increased accordingly (Akay *et al.*, 2009). The results indicated that the use of combined treatment with corticotomy and skeletal anchorage provided safe and noncompliance intrusion of posterior teeth in a short period, and may be regarded as an alternative method for skeletal open-bite correction in adults who reject orthognathic surgery (Akay *et al.*, 2009).

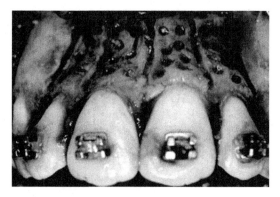

Figure 10.9 Corticotomy in the maxillary anterior region. Note the interradicular cortical cuts and the cortical perforations for treating an anterior open bite. Source: Mostafa *et al.* (2009a). Reproduced with permission of Quintessence Publishing Co. Inc.

Anterior teeth extrusion

The following anterior teeth extrusion topics will be briefly presented:

- Maximizing tissue response;
- Case selection criteria;
- Mechanotherapy.

Maximizing tissue response for anterior teeth extrusion

Mostafa *et al.* (2009a) described a method for maximizing tissue response in the treatment of selected subjects with anterior open-bites. Twelve subjects with anterior open bites and insufficient incisor displays underwent a limited corticotomy (Figures 10.9–10.11) to augment the alveolar bone response by creating an anteroposterior intra-arch anchorage differential (Mostafa *et al.*, 2009a). Pre-treatment and post-treatment cephalometric radiographs were recorded (Mostafa *et al.*, 2009a).

The changes in perceived smile esthetics were assessed by a visual analog scale (Mostafa *et al.*, 2009a). All open-bites were closed after a mean of 6 weeks (Mostafa *et al.*, 2009a). Radiographic evaluation showed significant maxillary incisor extrusion and retrusion (Mostafa *et al.*, 2009a). Moreover, there was a notable improvement in smile esthetics after treatment (Mostafa *et al.*, 2009a). Mostafa *et al.* (2009a) concluded that it is possible to close anterior open-bites rapidly, with significant improvement in smile esthetics.

Case selection criteria for anterior teeth extrusion

See Figure 10.12.

- Anterior dental open-bite.
- Insufficient amount of maxillary incisors display at rest and/or smiling.
- No signs of excessive vertical facial development.
- Exaggerated curve of Spee in the maxillary arch.
- Healthy periodontium.

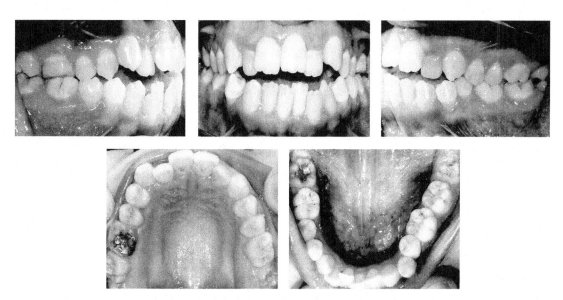

Figure 10.10 Pre-treatment anterior open-bite, intraoral views. Top: right profile, frontal, and left profile views. Bottom: maxillary occlusal and mandibular occlusal views. *Source: Mostafa et al.* (2009a). Reproduced with permission of Quintessence Publishing Co. Inc.

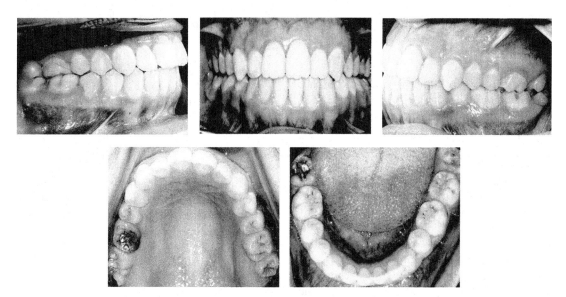

Figure 10.11 Post-treatment anterior open-bite, intra-oral views. Top: right profile, frontal, and left profile views. Bottom: maxillary occlusal and mandibular occlusal views. *Source: Mostafa et al.* (2009a). Reproduced with permission of Quintessence Publishing Co. Inc.

Case selection criteria
for anterior teeth extrusion

Anterior dental open-bite

Insufficient maxillary incisors display at rest &/ or smiling

No signs of excessive vertical facial development

Exaggerated curve of spee in the maxillary arch

Healthy periodontium

Complete permanent dentition (excluding third molars)

Absence of systemic disorders

Figure 10.12 Case selection criteria for anterior teeth extrusion: seven criteria.

- Complete permanent dentition (excluding third molars).
- Absence of systemic disorders (e.g., Down's syndrome).

Mechanotherapy for anterior teeth extrusion

In their effective mechanotherapeutic approach for safe anterior teeth extrusion, Mostafa *et al.* (2009a) recommended the following simple 12-step reliable clinical routine:

- Start with bonding/banding and sequential leveling wires.
- After placing maxillary archwire 0.016″ nickel-titanium and mandibular archwire 0.016″ × 0.022″ stainless steel, instruct the patient to use vertical intermaxillary elastics, and schedule for corticotomy.
- Perform the corticotomy under conscious sedation or bromazepam premedication and local anesthesia.
- Reflect a mucoperiosteal flap extending one tooth distal to the open-bite area bilaterally.
- Using a number 2 round bur in a high-speed hand-piece under copious irrigation, make

interradicular vertical corticotomy cuts; starting 2–3 mm apical to the alveolar crest and extending beyond the root apices.
- Make horizontal cuts to connect the vertical ones.
- Whenever possible, perforate the cortex over the roots' prominences.
- Assess the depth of the cuts by observing the bleeding from the cortical bone.
- After the corticotomy, carefully reposition the flap and close it with interrupted loop sutures.
- Instruct the patient to resume wearing the elastics on the day following the surgery.
- Schedule the patients every 2 weeks.
- In cases of denuded roots after the surgery, cover the roots with a mixture of equal parts of demineralized freeze-dried saline and clindamycin phosphate.

Anterior teeth retraction with open-bite closure

Through speedy surgical-orthodontics, Chung *et al.* (2009b) found that successful alveolar bone bending could be obtained in cases of adult protrusion or open-bite.

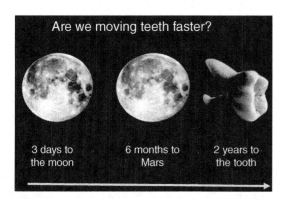

Figure 10.13 Are we moving teeth faster? Not yet: 3 days to the moon, 6 months to Mars, and 2 years to move teeth.

STABILITY OF ORTHODONTICALLY DRIVEN CORTICOTOMY

The teeth are more stable because of less disruption of the periodontal ligament through osteoclastic activity, and/or callus formation through bone healing (Kerdvongbundit, 1990). Further, there is a stable skeletal position of the maxilla at 14 months follow-up with satisfactory results and no complications after orthodontic treatment (Kanno *et al.*, 2007).

In a meta-analysis, Greenlee *et al.* (2011) studied the long-term stability of surgical and nonsurgical therapies for anterior open-bites. The pretreatment adjusted means were −2.8 mm for the surgical group and −2.5 mm for the nonsurgical group (Greenlee *et al.*, 2011). Closures up to +1.6 mm (surgical) and +1.4 mm (nonsurgical) groups were achieved (Greenlee *et al.*, 2011). Pooled results indicated reasonable stability of both the surgical (82%) and nonsurgical (75%) groups at a minimum of 12 months posttreatment (Greenlee *et al.*, 2011). Treatment success for both groups was greater than 75%; however, because the groups were examined in different studies and applied to different clinical samples, no direct assessment of comparative

To do the right thing right

We need to have

Control

Figure 10.14 Doing the right thing right. We need to have control.

effectiveness was possible (Greenlee *et al.*, 2011). Greenlee *et al.* (2011) stated that the pooled results should be viewed with caution because of the lack of within-study control groups and the variability among studies.

THREE CONCLUDING REMARKS

- The conceptual framework of ODC is one whose time has come. Remember that, about 30 years ago, Mostafa *et al.* (1985) were able to intrude overerupted maxillary molars through harmless decortications and very simple biomechanics.
- It takes 3 days to arrive on the moon, 6 months to get to Mars, and 2 years to move the teeth (Figure 10.13). El-Mangoury *et al.* (1987) pointed out that: "By definition, philosophy is a good think (with a 'k' rather than a 'g' at the end – not a typographic error)." The philosophy of the present authors is that orthodontists should move teeth faster, and with more control (Figure 10.14), through meticulous diagnosis and treatment planning, sound biomechanics, and the effective and safe ODC.
- In this chapter, our conceptual framework is above and beyond safe acceleration of tooth movement (Figure 10.1). This

framework is tri-dimensional in nature: safe acceleration of tooth movements, competent solving of clinical problems, and proficient expansion of orthodontic capabilities.

ACKNOWLEDGMENTS

We express our genuine appreciations to Dr Yehya A. Mostafa, Dr Larry W. White, Dr Ahmed M. Heider, Dr Fouâd A. El-Sharaby, and, above all, to the memory of Professor Mohammed-Helmy El-Mangoury.

References

Aboul-Ela SM, El-Beialy AR, El-Sayed KM et al. (2011) Miniscrew implant-supported maxillary canine retraction with and without corticotomy-facilitated orthodontics. *American Journal of Orthodontics and Dentofacial Orthopedics*, **139**, 252–259.

Ahn HW, Lee DY, Park YG et al. (2012) Accelerated decompensation of mandibular incisors in surgical skeletal class III patients by using augmented corticotomy: a preliminary study. *American Journal of Orthodontics and Dentofacial Orthopedics*, **142**, 199–206.

Akay MC, Aras A, Günbay T et al. (2009) Enhanced effect of combined treatment with corticotomy and skeletal anchorage in open bite correction. *Journal of Oral and Maxillofacial Surgery*, **67**, 563–569.

Baloul SS, Gerstenfeld LC, Morgan EF et al. (2011) Mechanism of action and morphologic changes in the alveolar bone in response to selective alveolar decortication-facilitated tooth movement. *American Journal of Orthodontics and Dentofacial Orthopedics*, **139**, S83–S101.

Bazzucchi A, Hans MG, Nelson S et al. (1999) Evidence of correction of open bite malocclusion using active vertical corrector treatment. *Seminars in Orthodontics*, **5**, 110–120.

Beane RA Jr (1999) Nonsurgical management of the anterior open bite: a review of the options. *Seminars in Orthodontics*, **5**, 275–283.

Buschang PH, Campbell PM, Ruso S (2012) Accelerating tooth movement with corticotomies: is it possible and desirable? *Seminars in Orthodontics*, **18**, 286–294.

Choo H, Heo HA, Yoon HJ et al. (2011) Treatment outcome analysis of speedy surgical orthodontics for adults with maxillary protrusion. *American Journal of Orthodontics and Dentofacial Orthopedics*, **140**, e251–e262.

Chung KR, Kim SH, Lee BS (2009a) Speedy surgical-orthodontic treatment with temporary anchorage devices as an alternative to orthognathic surgery. *American Journal of Orthodontics and Dentofacial Orthopedics*, **135**, 787–798.

Chung KR, Mitsugi M, Lee BS et al. (2009b) Speedy surgical orthodontic treatment with skeletal anchorage in adults – sagittal correction and open bite correction. *Journal of Oral and Maxillofacial Surgery*, **67**, 2130–2148.

Einy S, Horwitz J, Aizenbud D (2011) Wilckodontics – an alternative adult orthodontic treatment method: rational and application. *Alpha Omegan*, **104**, 102–111.

El-Mangoury NH (1981) Orthodontic cooperation. *American Journal of Orthodontics*, **80**, 604–622.

El-Mangoury NH, Shaheen SI, Mostafa YA (1987) Landmark identification in computerized posteroanterior cephalometrics. *American Journal of Orthodontics and Dentofacial Orthopedics*, **91**, 57–61.

El-Mangoury NH, Mostafa HY, Mostafa RY et al. (2014) *Illustrated Orthodontic Series*, Avicenna, Cairo.

Fayed MM, Mehanni S, Elbokle NN et al. (2009) Immediately loaded mini screws: histological study of the effect of two different orthodontic tooth movement techniques. *Progress in Orthodontics*, **10**, 38–46.

Fischer TJ (2007) Orthodontic treatment acceleration with corticotomy-assisted exposure of palatally impacted canines. *Angle Orthodontist*, **77**, 417–420.

Germeç D, Giray B, Kocadereli I et al. (2006) Lower incisor retraction with a modified corticotomy. *Angle Orthodontist*, **76**, 882–890.

Greenlee GM, Huang GJ, Chen SS *et al.* (2011) Stability of treatment for anterior open-bite malocclusion: a meta-analysis. *American Journal of Orthodontics and Dentofacial Orthopedics*, **139**, 154–169.

Grenga V, Bovi M (2013) Corticotomy-enhanced intrusion of an overerupted molar using skeletal anchorage and ultrasonic surgery. *Journal of Clinical Orthodontics*, **47**, 50–55.

Hwang DH, Park KH, Kwon YD *et al.* (2011) Treatment of class II open bite complicated by an ankylosed maxillary central incisor. *Angle Orthodontist*, **81**, 726–735.

Iino S, Sakoda S, Miyawaki S (2006) An adult bimaxillary protrusion treated with corticotomy-facilitated orthodontics and titanium miniplates. *Angle Orthodontist*, **76**, 1074–1082.

Iino S, Sakoda S, Ito G *et al.* (2007) Acceleration of orthodontic tooth movement by alveolar corticotomy in the dog. *American Journal of Orthodontics and Dentofacial Orthopedics*, **131**, 448.e1–448.e8.

Kanno T, Mitsugi M, Furuki Y *et al.* (2007) Corticotomy and compression osteogenesis in the posterior maxilla for treating severe anterior open bite. *International Journal of Oral & Maxillofacial Surgery*, **36**, 354–357.

Kerdvongbundit V (1990) Corticotomy-facilitated orthodontics. *Journal of the Dental Association of Thailand*, **40**, 284–291.

Kim SH, Kim I, Jeong DM *et al.* (2011) Corticotomy-assisted decompensation for augmentation of the mandibular anterior ridge. *American Journal of Orthodontics and Dentofacial Orthopedics*, **140**, 720–731.

Long H, Pyakurel U, Wang Y *et al.* (2013) Interventions for accelerating orthodontic tooth movement: a systematic review. *Angle Orthodontist*, **83**, 164–171.

Mostafa YA (2005) Before we continue: une pause. *World Journal of Orthodontics*, **6** (Suppl), 27–30.

Mostafa YA, Tawfik KM, El-Mangoury NH (1985) Surgical–orthodontics treatment for overerupted maxillary molars. *Journal of Clinical Orthodontics*, **19**, 350–351.

Mostafa YA, Iskander KG, El-Mangoury NH (1991) Iatrogenic pulpal reactions to orthodontic extrusion. *American Journal of Orthodontics and Dentofacial Orthopedics*, **99**, 30–34.

Mostafa YA, El-Mangoury NH, Abou-El-Ezz AM *et al.* (2009a) Maximizing tissue response in selected subjects with anterior open bites. *World Journal of Orthodontics*, **10**, 187–195.

Mostafa YA, Fayed MMS, Mehanni S *et al.* (2009b) Comparison of corticotomy-facilitated vs standard tooth-movement techniques in dogs with miniscrews as anchor units. *American Journal of Orthodontics and Dentofacial Orthopedics*, **136**, 570–577.

Murphy NC, Bissada NF, Davidovitch Z *et al.* (2012) Corticotomy and tissue engineering for orthodontists: a critical history and commentary. *Seminars in Orthodontics*, **18**, 295–307.

Oliveira DD, de Oliveira BF, de Araújo Brito HH *et al.* (2008) Selective alveolar corticotomy to intrude overerupted molars. *American Journal of Orthodontics and Dentofacial Orthopedics*, **133**, 902–908.

Proffit WR, Fields HW, Sarver DM (2007) *Contemporary Orthodontics*, 4th edition, Mosby, St Louis, MO.

Sanjideh PA, Rossouw PE, Campbell PM *et al.* (2010) Tooth movements in foxhounds after one or two alveolar corticotomies. *European Journal of Orthodontics*, **32**, 106–113.

Shoreibah EA, Salama AE, Attia MS *et al.* (2012a) Corticotomy-facilitated orthodontics in adults using a further modified technique. *Journal of the International Academy of Periodontology*, **14**, 97–104.

Shoreibah EA, Ibrahim SA, Attia MS *et al.* (2012b) Clinical and radiographic evaluation of bone grafting in corticotomy-facilitated orthodontics in adults. *Journal of the International Academy of Periodontology*, **14**, 105–113.

Tuncer C, Ataç MS, Tuncer BB *et al.* (2008) Osteotomy assisted maxillary posterior impaction with miniplate anchorage. *Angle Orthodontist*, **78**, 737–744.

Wilcko MT, Wilcko WM, Pulver JJ *et al.* (2009) Accelerated osteogenic orthodontics technique: a 1-stage surgically facilitated rapid orthodontic technique with alveolar augmentation. *Journal of Oral and Maxillofacial Surgery*, **67**, 2149–2159.

Wilcko WM, Ferguson DJ, Bouquot JE *et al.* (2003) Rapid orthodontic decrowding with alveolar augmentation: case report. *World Journal of Orthodontics*, **4**, 197–205.

Orthodontically Driven Corticotomy: Tissue Engineering to Enhance Orthodontic and Multidisciplinary Treatment,
First Edition. Edited by Federico Brugnami and Alfonso Caiazzo.
© 2015 John Wiley & Sons, Inc. Published 2015 by John Wiley & Sons, Inc.
Companion Website: www.wiley.com/go/Brugnami/Corticotomy

Printed in the United States
By Bookmasters